Diagnostic Breast Imaging

Diagnostic Breast Imaging

Mammography, Sonography, Magnetic Resonance Imaging, and Interventional Procedures

Sylvia H. Heywang-Köbrunner, M.D.
Associate Professor and Substitute Director
Diagnostic Radiology
Martin Luther University Halle-Wittenberg
Halle, Germany

Ingrid Schreer, M.D.
Assistant Professor
University Hospital
Hamburg, Germany

D. David Dershaw, M.D.
Director, Breast Imaging Section
Department of Radiology
Memorial Sloan-Kettering Cancer Center
New York, NY USA

In collaboration with Professor Roland Bässler, M.D.

Translated by Peter F. Winter, M.D.

674 illustrations

Thieme
Stuttgart · New York 1997

Roland Bässler, M.D.
Professor, Institute of Pathology
Municipal Clinics
Pacelliallee 4
36043 Fulda, Germany

D. David Dershaw, M.D.
Director, Breast Imaging Section
Department of Radiology
Memorial Sloan-Kettering Cancer Center
1275 York Avenue
New York, NY 10021 USA

Sylvia H. Heywang-Köbrunner, M.D.
Associate Professor and Substitute Director
Diagnostic Radiology
Martin Luther University Halle-Wittenberg
Magdeburger Strasse 16
06097 Halle, Germany

Ingrid Schreer, M.D.
Assistant Professor
University Hospital
Martinistrasse 52
20246 Hamburg, Germany

Translated by:
Peter F. Winter, M.D.
Clinical Assistant Professor
University of Illinois
College of Medicine at Peoria
530 N.E. Glen Oak Avenue
Peoria, IL 61637 USA

Rüdigerstrasse 14, 70469 Stuttgart, Germany
Thieme Medical Publishers, Inc.
381 Park Avenue South
New York, NY 10016 USA

Typesetting by primustype Robert Hurler GmbH
73274 Notzingen, Germany

Illustrations by Barbara Gay and Uwe Neumann

Printed in Germany by Grammlich, Pliezhausen

ISBN 3-13-102891-2 (GTV, Stuttgart)
ISBN 0-86577-636-9 (TMP, New York)

1 2 3 4 5

Library of Congress Cataloging-in-Publication Data

Heywang-Köbrunner, Sylvia H.,1956 –
[Bildgebende Mammadiagnostik, English]
Diagnostic breast imaging / Sylvia H. Heywang-Köbrunner, Ingrid Schreer, D. David Dershaw : in collaboration with Roland Bässler ; translated by Peter F. Winter.
p. cm.
Includes bibliographical references and index.
ISBN 3-13-102891-2 (GTV). – ISBN 0-86577-636-9 (TMP)
1. Breast–Imaging, 2. Breast–Diseases–Diagnosis. I. Heywang-Köbrunner, Sylvia H., 1956– II. Schreer, Ingrid, II. Dershaw, D. David. IV. Title
[DNLM : 1. Breast Diseases-diagnosis. 2. Breast Neoplasms–diagnosis, 3. Diagnostic Imaging-methods. WP 815 H622b 1997a]
RG493.5.D52H913 1987
618.1' 90754–dc21
DNLM/DLC 96–44581
for Library of Congress CIP

This book is an authorized, updated, and adapted translation of the German edition published and copyrighted 1996 by Georg Thieme Verlag, Stuttgart, Germany. Title of the German edition: Bildgebende Mammadiagnostik: Untersuchungstechnik, Befundmuster und Differentialdiagnostik in Mammographie, Sonographie und Kernspintomographie

Preface

Breast carcinoma is one of the most feared diseases among women. As the most frequent cancer and the leading cause of death in woman between the ages of 40 and 60 years, it is a source of great personal and familial suffering.

During the past decades, breast cancer screening has decisively improved early detection as well as the potential of breast preservation and longer survival. Complementary imaging modalities and new biopsy techniques can eliminate uncertainties and reduce the large number of surgical biopsies performed for benign conditions. Making the right decision in critical cases requires knowledge of all methods and cognizance of their potential, limitations, appropriate application, and respective roles. To turn the potential of breast imaging into a reality requires thorough training as well as constant attention to quality.

This book reviews the basic knowledge and current status of breast imaging techniques comprehensively and systematically while putting both into perspective. Based on current understanding and in accordance with the experience of the authors, it presents basic clinical and histopathologic information, the status of current technology and standards, diagnostic image presentation of benign and malignant diseases of the breast, the application of diagnostic modalities for screening and further evaluation, and the approach to the differential diagnosis. Its primary audience is radiologists in practice and training as well as gynecologists or surgeons interested in mammography.

This text addresses the fundamentals of diagnosis, including taking the patient's history, talking with the patient, and performing the physical examination. A large segment of the text covers the physical and technical aspects pertaining to imaging and diagnostic intervention, including quality control, since quality results can only be achieved by maintaining the highest standards.

The image presentation of benign and malignant conditions and their variations is systematically correlated with the underlying histopathology. The role and indications of various imaging technologies and interventions for the evaluation of the individual presentations are discussed.

The text concludes with practical applications of breast imaging for screening and with strategies for establishing a diagnosis on the basis of imaging findings.

Throughout this text, we have tried to incorporate the most up-to-date information. We trust that the reader will understand that the influence of personal experience cannot be avoided. We hope that this book will improve the skills of the reader experienced in breast imaging and provide the novice with a systematic approach to breast imaging diagnosis.

Acknowledgements

This book encompasses much of the knowledge the authors have gathered over the last 15 to 20 years. We, the authors, wish to thank the teachers and sponsors who have been instrumental in guiding and assisting us:

First, we wish to express our gratitude to Professor Dr. Frischbier for encouraging, supporting, and stimulating critical analysis and for sharing his profound knowledge with us and many other colleagues over many decades.

Furthermore, I (S.H.K.) wish to thank M.A. Thomas, R.L. Egan and M.B. McSweeney for relating their immense knowledge and constructive appraisal. I thank Professor Dr. J. Lissner for supporting my continuing education in the United States and at the Klinikum Grosshadern of the University of Munich and for promoting my scientific work.

My training, as well as numerous research projects conducted over many years, would have been impossible without the support of the Deutsche Krebshilfe (German Cancer Foundation), and I will always be grateful for their patronage.

We were fortunate to have had the excellent collaboration of physicians and other coworkers in the Department of Radiology at the University of Halle and the Department of Gynecologic Radiology at the Women's Hospital of the University of Hamburg as well as the support of the University of Munich and the University of Leipzig.

Our special thanks go to members of our "mammographic team," in particular to Dr. Hilbertz, Dr. Beck, and Dr. Viehweg, as well as to Ms. Andersen, Ms. Schäper and Ms. Dickhaut, who always supported our scientific work and extensive collection of cases.

We thank our gynecological and surgical colleagues and our contact persons at the Pathologic Institutes of the University of Munich, University of Leipzig, University of Halle, and University of Hamburg.

We would like to extend our special appreciation to Mr. Hoberg for providing us with relevant information and active support for the chapter on mammographic technique and quality control. We also thank Dr. Aichinger, Dr. Neitzel, Dr. Schätzl, Ms. Samorra, and Ms. Sonnenberger for their constructive contributions and valuable advice. We also wish to acknowledge Ms. Fulbrecht for her fast and reliable typing of the manuscript.

We are grateful to Dr. Winter for his excellent translation and editorial assistance and, at Georg Thieme Verlag, to Dr. Bergman, Mr. Krüger, and Ms. Schmidt Ryan for their outstanding editorial and production work.

Dr. Dershaw would like to express his appreciation to his colleagues in the Breast Imaging Section of the Department of Radiology at Memorial Sloan-Kettering Cancer Center in New York: Dr. Laura Liberman, Dr. Andrea F. Abramson, Dr. Elizabeth A. Morris, and Dr. Lucy Hann. Without their support, projects such as this would not be possible. He also wishes to thank the other members of the radiology faculty and their chairman, Dr. Ronald Castellino, for making it possible to work on this text.

Sylvia H. Heywang-Köbrunner, M.D.
Ingrid Schreer, M.D.
D. David Dershaw, M.D.

Contents

I. Methods

1. Patient History and Communication with the Patient 2

Scheduling 2
Patient Information 2
Patient History 3
References 6

2. Clinical Findings 7

Visual Inspection 7
Palpation 8
References 10

3. Mammography 11

Purpose, Accuracy, Possibilities, and Limitations 11
Indications 11
Accuracy 11
Screening 12
Problem Solving 13
Mammographic Technique 13
Components of the Mammographic Imaging Technique 14
Specific Requirements and Solutions 23
Image Sharpness 23
Contrast 26
Noise 33
Radiation Dose 34
Positioning and Compression 37
Compression 37
Positioning for Standard Views 39
Positioning for Additional Views 43
Film Labelling 44
Spot Compression and Magnification Technique 49
Positioning of Breasts with Implants 53
Specimen Radiography 56
Quality Factors 57
Hardware Factors that Influence Image Quality 57
Influence of the Screen–Film System and Film Processing on Image Quality 58
Quality Assurance in Mammography 59
Reporting and Documentation Findings 62
Clinical Findings 62
Mammography Report 62
Digital Mammography 67
Galactography 69
Appendix: Sonographic Imaging of Lactiferous Ducts 73
Pneumocystography 76
References 78

4. Sonography 81

Purpose, Accuracy, Possibilities, and Limitations 81
Diagnosing Cysts 81
Differentiating Solid Lesions 81
Diagnosing Carcinomas 81
Equipment Requirements 83
Selecting the Transducer 83
Image Quality 83
Examination Technique 86
Time-gain Compensation 86
Stand-off 87
Focusing 87
Examination Technique 88
Interpreting Sonographic Findings 88
Normal Sonographic Findings 88
Focal Ultrasound Lesions 90
References 91

5. Magnetic Resonance Imaging (MRI) 92

Purpose, Accuracy, Possibilities, and Limitations 92
Accuracy 92
Indications 93
Technical Requirements 93
Examination Procedure 95
Planning the Examination 95
Examination Procedure 96
Interpretation Criteria and Documentation of Findings 96
Documenting Findings 96
Interpretation Criteria 97
References 99

6. Percutaneous Biopsy Methods 101

Purpose, Definition, Accuracy, Indications, Contraindications, and Side Effects 101
Purpose 101
Definitions 101
Accuracy 101
Indications 102
Contraindications 102
Side Effects 103
Informing and Preparing the Patient .. 103
Biopsy Materials 103
Localization and Biopsy Techniques 104
Stereotaxic Biopsy 104
Ultrasound-guided Needle Biopsy . 108
MR-guided Needle Biopsy 110
Percutaneous Biopsy of Palpable Lesions 110
References 111

7. Preoperative Localization 112

Purpose, Definition, Indications, and Side Effects 112
Methods and Technique 113
Mammographically Guided Localization Techniques 113
Ultrasound-guided Localization ... 117
MR-guided Localization 118
Galactographically Guided Localization 118
Localization Materials 118
Problems and Their Solutions 119
References 120

II. Appearance

8. The Normal Breast 122

Anatomy ... 122
The Adolescent Female Breast ... 122
Histology ... 122
Clinical Examination ... 122
Mammography ... 122
Sonography ... 122
The Mature Female Breast ... 125
Histology ... 125
Clinical Examination ... 125
Mammography ... 125
Sonography ... 126
Magnetic Resonance Imaging ... 128
Involution ... 130
Histology ... 130
Clinical Examination ... 130
Mammography ... 130
Sonography ... 130
Magnetic Resonance Imaging ... 131
Abnormalities ... 131
Asymmetry ... 132
Clinical Examination ... 132
Mammography ... 132
Macromastia ... 133
Clinical Examination ... 133
Mammography ... 133
Sonography ... 133
Accessory Breast Tissue (Polymastia) ... 134
Clinical Examination ... 134
Mammography ... 134
Sonography and Magnetic Resonance Imaging ... 134
Inverted Nipple ... 134
Clinical Examination ... 134
Mammography ... 134
Sonography ... 134
Mammography ... 135
Sonography ... 134
Magnetic Resonance Imaging ... 135
Pregnancy and Lactation ... 136
Histology ... 136
Clinical Examination ... 136
Mammography ... 136
Sonography ... 138
Magnetic Resonance Imaging ... 138
Breast Response with Hormone Replacement Therapy ... 138
Mammography ... 138
Sonography ... 138
Magnetic Resonance Imaging ... 139
Percutaneous Biopsy ... 139
References ... 140

9. Benign Breast Disorders 141

Pathogenesis ... 141
Incidence ... 141
Histopathology ... 141
Clinical Findings ... 143
Diagnostic Strategy and Objectives ... 143
Mammography ... 144
Sonography ... 149
Magnetic Resonance Imaging ... 151
Percutaneous Biopsy ... 154
References ... 155

10. Cysts 156

Histology ... 156
Medical History and Clinical Findings ... 156
Breast Examination ... 157
Objectives of Diagnostic Studies ... 157
Diagnostic Strategy ... 157
Sonography ... 157
Aspiration of the Cyst ... 160
Pneumocystography ... 161
Mammography ... 161
Magnetic Resonance Imaging ... 162
Appendix: Galactoceles ... 164
References ... 164

I Methods

1. Patient History and Communication with the Patient

Providing the patient with some essential information concerning breast imaging may help gain her understanding and cooperation. Furthermore obtaining a limited history is very helpful both for separating screening patients from those who need a diagnostic breast study and to support image interpretation in diagnostic breast studies.

Both information about the patient and her history can be obtained orally or by use of an information sheet, a checklist, or a questionnaire.

■ Scheduling

The issue of whether mammography should be scheduled according to the menstrual cycle is controversial. In many institutions the patient's menstrual cycle is disregarded. At the University of Halle, it is routine to perform mammographic imaging during the first part of the menstrual cycle. During this time, the breast is more compressible, and compression is less painful, which is appreciated by the patients. In some patients, due to the better compression the glandular tissue may even appear less dense on the mammogram, which facilitates diagnosis.

In contrast-enhanced (c.e.) magnetic resonance imaging (MRI), nonspecific enhancement in benign tissue may be encountered at the end of the menstrual cycle and during menses, while it is less frequent between days 6 to about 17 of the cycle. Therefore c.e. MRI should—if possible—be scheduled between days 6–17 of the cycle.

■ Patient Information

If the patient asks specific questions, they should, of course, be discussed or answered by the technologist or physician. Furthermore, the following essentials concerning the imaging techniques involved may be helpful to gain the patient's understanding and cooperation.

■ Mammography

- The patient should understand the importance and necessity of compression. Adequate compression helps visualize small carcinomas since normal tissue usually can be spread out while carcinomas persist. Compression also helps to reduce the radiation dose (see Chapter 3, p. 29).
- Any fears that compression might cause cancer should be allayed.
- Possible fear of radiation exposure from mammography should be addressed by putting the risk into proper perspective. For example, the theoretical risk (so small that it can only be extrapolated) of dying from cancer caused by a mammogram is comparable to the risk of dying of lung cancer from smoking three cigarettes (see Chapter 3, p. 34).

As in any other radiologic examination, question appropriate women about pregnancy.

■ Sonography

Ultrasound examinations are generally very well accepted by patients. It should, however, be explained that, in general, ultrasonography cannot replace mammography for excluding the presence of cancer.

■ Magnetic Resonance Imaging with Contrast Medium

Contrast-enhanced MRI—like the other methods that do not use ionizing radiation—is well accepted by the patients except for those who suffer from claustrophobia. Contrast-enhanced MRI is used as an additional imaging modality for specific indications. Before performing c.e. MRI, ask for any contraindications and document their absence. These include cardiac pacemakers, intracerebral vascular clips, clips from surgery performed within the last 2 months, implantable drug infusion pumps, and certain types of cardiac valve prostheses.[1]

Finally, the patient should be informed of the necessity of injecting contrast medium. The few contraindications concern rare cases of allergy against paramagnetic contrast medium, and severe hepatic or renal insufficiency. Extensive tolerance data are available for the paramagnetic contrast medium Gd-DTPA (studies in over 5 million patients).[2, 3] Tolerance of this contrast medium is excellent. Side effects occur significantly less frequently than with radiographic contrast media.

Paramagnetic MRI contrast media may even be used in the presence of an allergy against radiographic contrast medium since there are no allergic cross reaction.[2]

■ Interventions

When a puncture is planned (aspiration of a cyst, aspiration cytology, or needle biopsy), the patient should be informed about possible hematoma formation and about the very low risk of infection. The patient should be questioned about any coagulatory disorders, aspirin intake, or anticoagulation treatment. Provided the direction of puncture is strictly parallel to the chest wall, injury to the chest wall can be excluded, and the very rare complication of iatrogenic pneumothorax need not be mentioned. If a silicone implant is present and might be damaged, the patient must also be informed. At some centers, it is routine to obtain informed consent before any of these procedures.

■ Patient History

To save time, many centers have the patient fill out a questionnaire (Fig. 1.**1**). The questions may concentrate on data that are significant for assessing risk and interpreting the images.

■ Risk Factors

The most important risk factors involve:

- Family history. A history of breast cancer in immediate relatives such as the mother or sister, the number of family members affected, and the time at which the cancer appeared (premenopausal or postmenopausal) are significant.[4–7]
- The patient's personal history. The history of an invasive or in situ breast carcinoma is significant, as is a history of proliferative breast disease (confirmed in earlier biopsies), particularly when atypias were present.[4, 5, 8, 9]
- Immunodeficiency disorders can result in an increased risk of malignancy. They include ataxia telangiectasia,[10], Li-Fraumeni syndrome,[11] BRCA-1 alterations,[12], HRAS-1 alterations,[13] and other gene alterations.[7, 14]. These effects constitute a predisposition for various tumor disorders frequently occurring before age 40, yet on the whole they are rare.[7]
- Early menarche or late menopause and the frequency and duration of breast feeding have a slight impact on overall risk. In combination with other risk factors, first childbirth after the age of 30 or the absence of breast feeding unfavorably influence the prognosis.[4, 5]
- Other factors include the patient's history and family history of ovarian, endometrial, or colonic cancer.[4–7]

Table 1.**1** provides an overview of the significance of individual risk factors or combinations of these factors.

Absence of risk factors, however, does not exclude the possible occurrence of breast cancer. In fact, 70% of breast cancers occur in patients without any risk factors.[4]

Table 1.**1** Relative risk of breast cancer related to one or more risk factors (according to Maass[4] and Stoll,[5] used with permission)

Risk doubles
Menopause after age 50
Menarche before age 12
Nulliparity
Obesity in postmenopausal women
Epithelial hyperplasia
Risk increases by a factor of 2 to 4
First childbirth after age 30
Breast cancer in mother or sister
Comination of nulliparity and epithelial hyperplasia
Previous ovarian, endometrial, or colon cancer
Risk increases by factor of more than 4
Prior breast cancer
Breast cancer in mother and sister
Premenopausal bilateral breast cancer in the mother or sister
Atypical hyperplasia
Family history combined with late first pregnancy or nulliparity

■ Medical History Data Helpful for Image Interpretation

The following data may be helpful in image interpretation:

Recent pregnancy or breast feeding. This can be the cause of extensive proliferation of glandular tissue, which may be misinterpreted if the physician is unaware of the patient's history.

- Administration of female hormones. In some postmenopausal patients, hormone replacement therapy may involve extensive proliferation of glandular tissue. Newly occurring or increasing densities can be mistaken for suggestive findings if the physician is unaware of the patient's history.
- Thyroid hormone. Published studies have described that administration of thyroid hormone can promote fibrocystic changes in the breast.
- Surgery or radiation therapy. Changes after surgery or radiation therapy can produce masses, distortions or microcalcifications that can simulate or obscure a carcinoma (see Chapter 16). Here, careful documentation of scars and their location in the breast is important. Architectural distortion outside the scar area may be a sign of malignancy. The period of time that has elapsed since surgery or irradiation may also be valuable for correct image interpretation.

Furthermore the following symptoms may be a hint to malignancy:

- Any—even slight—changes of the nipple, such as a recent deviation or inversion of the nipple, are important. Even though deviation or inversion of the nipple can be congenital or can occur following inflammation, new development may be an important and early hint of malignancy.
- Spontaneous discharge. Significant factors here include color, occurrence over time (association with pregnancy), number of involved ducts (single versus multiple), and the results of cytologic smears where available.

Significant aspects of any clinical findings (skin dimpling, skin changes, palpable findings) include:

- Time when the condition was first noticed,
- Changes since the condition was first noticed (decrease, increase, time span)
- Results of previous examinations (such as surgical biopsy, core biopsy or cytology)

If *previous imaging studies* exist, ask for the name and, if known, the address of the physician who performed them. It may be useful to obtain these films for comparison. Whenever available, *compare findings with earlier imaging studies*, since this might improve diagnostic accuracy.

■ References

1 Barentsz JO, Debruyne FMJ, Ruijs SHJ. M.R.I. of carcinoma of the urinary bladder. Dordrecht: Kluwer Academic; 1990;27

2 Niendorf HP, Alhassan A, Geens VR, Clauss W. Safety review of gadopentetate dimglumine: extended clinical experience after more than 5 million applications. Invest Radiol. 1995;29:179–82

3 Niendorf HP. Gadolinium-DTPA: a well-tolerated and safe contrast medium. Insert Eur Radiol. 1994;4:1–2

4 Maass H. Mammakarzinom: Epidemiologie. Gynakologe. 1994;27:3

5 Stoll BA. Defining breast cancer prevention. In: Stoll BA, ed. Approaches to breast cancer prevention. London: Kluwer; 1991

6 Easton D, Peto J. The contribution of inherited predisposition to cancer incidence. Cancer Surv. 1990;9:395

7 Friedrichs K. Genetische Aspekte des Mammakarzinoms. Gynakologe. 1994;27:7

8 Prechtel K, Gehm O, Geiger G, Prechtel P. Die Histologie der Mastopathie und die kumulative ipsilaterale Mammakarzinomsequenz. Pathologe. 1994;15:158

9 Dupont WD, Page DL. Risk factors for breast cancer in women with proliferative disease. N Engl J Med. 1985;312:146

10 Swift ML, Sholman L, Perry M, Chase C. Malignant neoplasms in the families of patients with ataxia – teleangiectasia. Cancer Res. 1976;36:209

11 Malkin D, Li FP, Strong LC et al. Germline p 53 mutations in a familial syndrome of breast cancers, sarcomas and other neoplasms. Science. 1990;250:1233

12 Hall J, Ming KL, Newmann B et al. Linkage of early-onset familial breast cancer to chromosome 17q 21. Science. 1990;250:1990

13 Krontiris TG, Devlin B, Karp D et al. An association between the risk of cancer and mutations in the HRAS 1 minisatelite locus. N Engl J Med. 1993;329:517

14 Zuppan P, Hall JM, Lee MK et al. Possible linkage of the estrogen receptor gene to breast cancer in family with late onset disease. Am J Hum Genet. 1991;48:1065

2. Clinical Findings

A complete breast examination includes the physical examination as well as a mammogram. In a screening setting, about 10% of breast cancers will only be detectable by physical examination.

Additionally, it is important at the time of diagnostic mammography to correlate mammographic findings with physical findings and vice versa. Competence in physical examination of the breast is therefore a desirable skill for the mammographer.

■ Purpose

Initial examination of the breast involves visual inspection and palpation. When the physical examination is abnormal, subsequent diagnostic imaging studies should always be interpreted together with clinical findings. The physician must also ensure that the examination includes the marginal areas of the breast, namely the area close to the sternum, the inframammary fold, the lateral border of the glandular body, and the axilla, which may be poorly imaged at mammography.

Visual Inspection

■ Technique

Observe the breast with the patient's arm raised as well as with her hand placed on her hip. Alternatively, the patient may be seated with her arms extended, next to her body pressing on the edge of the table. Observe and document any findings with respect to:

- Breast size and symmetry
- Contour
- Skin changes
- Nipples

■ Findings

The *size* of the breast can vary considerably among individual patients. Small breasts are generally easy to examine clinically, while macromastia will limit the amount of information provided by palpation. It is important to determine whether asymmetry in breast size (anisomastia) is an indication of:

- Individual variation
- A postoperative condition
- Retraction in the presence of disseminated tumor (reduction in breast size combined with palpable thickening)

Normal *breast contour* is convex. Flattening or dimpling can result from surgery or from retraction due to a subjacent tumor.

Skin changes may be generalized or circumscribed. Examples of such changes include:

- Erythema (mastitis, inflammatory breast carcinoma, or acute radiation reaction)
- Skin thickening
- Peau d'orange (skin thickening with inversion of the pores indicative of lymphedema)
- Prominent veins (supraclavicular, infraclavicular, or mediastinal mass producing venous compression)
- Hyperpigmentation or teleangiectasia (sequela of radiation therapy)

Circumscribed skin changes include:

- Verrucae
- Nevi
- Atheromas
- Fibroepitheliomas
- Sebaceous cysts
- Scars
- Long area of retraction associated with thrombophlebitis (Mondor disease)

Inversion of the nipple can be:

- Congenital
- Acquired as a result of surgery
- The result of breast inflammation or a malignant tumor
- Associated with retraction

Deviation of the nipple or lack of symmetry when compared to the opposite side can be an indication of beginning retraction. Asymmetric depigmentation of the nipple can occur as a result of radiation therapy.

Crusty deposits on the nipple can be a sign of pathologic discharge. Eczematous changes in the nipple can be a sign of Paget disease.

Any abnormalities in breast size or contour and any skin or nipple changes should be noted along with the probable causes suggested by the clinical examination or the patient's history. The radiologist should be aware of any benign skin lesions that might simulate a focal lesion at mammography. Cutaneous lesions may calcify, which should be considered in the mammographic differential diagnosis.

Precisely document any scars since they may explain mammographically detectable structural changes (Fig. 2.**1**).

Palpation

Technique

Palpation should be performed gently, allowing for the patient's individual sensitivity to pain.

- Using the fingertips of both hands, separate the glandular tissue from the underlying and surrounding tissue and palpate it
- Examine the breasts individually and systematically
- Assess the individual consistency of the gland, looking for circumscribed areas of altered (i. e., firmer) consistency
- Always palpate both breasts for comparison
- Assess the mobility of the nipple
- Also assess the mobility of the breast tissue with respect to the skin and chest wall

Move your fingers toward each other and grasp the glandular tissue to assess whether a plateau appears as a sign of a desmoplastic reaction in the subjacent tissue (the Jackson sign).

Palpation is initially performed with the patient standing, after which the examination is continued with the patient supine. The final procedure is the examination of the lymph drainage routes. These include the axillary tail of the breast, the axilla, the infraclavicular region, and the supraclavicular region. Palpate axillary lymph nodes by examining the patient with her arms hanging down. Move your fingertips as far superiorly into the axilla as possible. Applying moderate pressure against the lateral chest wall, move slowly down the lateral chest wall. Lymph nodes will typically slide away under the fingertips. Palpate the axillary tail, the infraclavicular region, and the supraclavicular region using the same technique as for glandular tissue.

Findings

Palpation provides information about:

- The structure of glandular tissue
- Possible asymmetry
- Lumps and their consistency and relation to the surrounding tissue, skin (the Jackson sign), pectoralis muscle, and painful sensation
- Nipple and the subareolar tissue
- Lymph drainage routes

The structure of the glandular tissue can be soft or, in the presence of breast disorders, firm or granular. Granular texture may be finely, medium, or coarsely nodular. Documenting these palpatory findings is very valuable for interpreting subsequent findings. Asymmetry can be an

Physician´s Work Sheet

Clinical findings:

Palpable Findings:
(please check applicable finding)

Generally **soft** breast: ____________ **Firm** glandular tissue: ____________

Finely nodular glandular tissue: ____________ **Coarseley nodular** glandular tissue: ____________

Additional findings:
(please number if more than one)

- Mobile lumps: ○
- inverted **nipple**: △
- **Retraction** (skin, nipple): □
- Cutaneous **verruca** or similar finding: ●
- Immobile **lumps**: 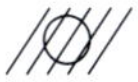
- **Thickening:** 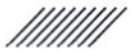
- **Scar:** 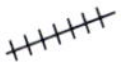

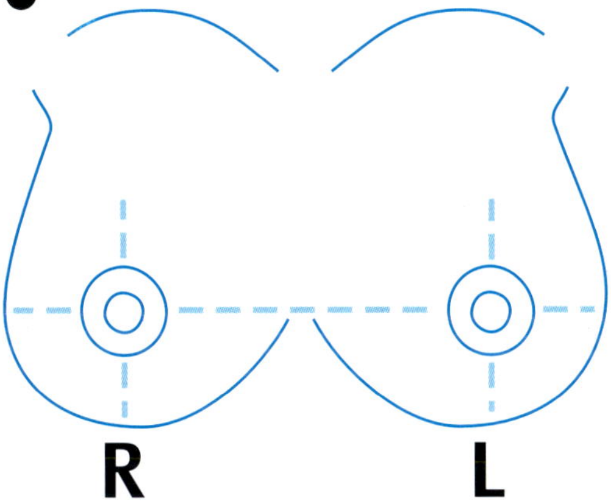

Finding number:	Approximate size:	First noticed when:	Change in size: ↑ ↓ =
1.	____________	____________	____________
2.	____________	____________	____________
3.	____________	____________	____________
4.	____________	____________	____________

Status of lymph nodes:

____

____

____

____

____

Fig. 2.**1** Physician's Work Sheet

initial sign of a disseminated or focal carcinoma, but it can also be congenital.

For every circumscribed palpable finding, assess the following parameters:

- Consistency
- Contour
- Mobility and the relation to surrounding tissue (skin and pectoralis muscle). A malignant tumor can cause a desmoplastic reaction, and/or tumor infiltration may form a plateau accompanied by peau d'orange. This sign can be detected even before a tumor can be reliably palpated.

Circumscribed lumps can be soft (lipomas, fibroadenolipomas, partially filled cysts, or medullary and mucinous carcinomas) or of firmer consistency (cysts, fibroadenomas, or carcinomas).

Involuted fibroadenomas, oil cysts, and circumscribed scarring can have the same hard consistency as a carcinoma.

Fibrocystic masses, distended or chronically inflamed cysts, and hematomas are painful, whereas malignant tumors are less often so. Some women with good body perception will feel localized pain or sense a change at the site of a tumor that may not even be palpable. This may be due to the disturbed parenchymal structure and consistency caused by the tumor.

When the nipples are examined, mobility should be assessed. Mobility can be compromised by a tumor in the subjacent tissue or by subacute or chronic mastitis or scarring.

Small (i. e., ≤ 10 mm), smooth, mobile, generally firm lymph nodes can be normal findings in the axilla but are pathologic in the supraclavicular or infraclavicular regions. Enlarged lymph nodes and/or lymph nodes with poor mobility should be regarded as pathologic until proven otherwise.

Ectopic glandular tissue may be present in the axilla, above or below the breast. This will be apparent as relatively soft circumscribed palpable findings. The patient may report changes in size or painfulness related to the menstrual cycle.

Problems

Palpation can reveal small carcinomas in superficial sites or in small breasts. However, tumors exceeding 2 cm in diameter may go undetected in the deeper tissue of large or lumpy breasts. In fact, less than 50% of the tumors smaller than 1.5 cm and even less than 50% of the tumors between 1 and 1.5 cm in size are palpable.[1, 2]

Palpating disseminated carcinomas such as disseminated invasive lobular carcinomas is particularly difficult. More than 90% of intraductal carcinomas are nonpalpable. Extensive nodular breast disorders can greatly limit the diagnostic accuracy of palpation.

Any atypical palpable findings and any findings suggestive of carcinoma should be further assessed by mammography or other diagnostic studies. A clinical examination conducted by a physician familiar with the mammographic findings will permit improved diagnostic interpretation of asymmetries or circumscribed areas of increased density.

Summary

Careful palpation is essential even with regular mammographic screening. The reasons for this are:

1. Mammography has limited sensitivity, especially in radiodense tissue. Approximately 10% of malignancies are only discovered because they are palpable. This means that palpable findings, even with negative mammography, may require further workup or biopsy.
2. Palpation can detect malignant processes along the periphery of the glandular body or in the axillary tail which may escape detection at mammography.

Mammography does not replace careful physical examination. However, whenever a questionable or suggestive clinical findings exists, further workup (by mammography, possibly ultrasound and/or percutaneous biopsy) should follow to avoid missing nonpalpable additional lesions or unnecessary biopsy (of lipomas, definite fibroadenomas, hamartomas, oil cysts or simple cysts).

References

1 Ciatto S, Roselli-del-Turco M, Cantarzi et al. Causes of breast cancer misdiagnosis at physical examination. Neoplasma. 1991;38(5):523–31

2 Reintgen D, Berman C, Cox C et al. The anatomy of missed breast cancers. Surg Oncol. 1993;2(1):65–75

3. Mammography

Purpose, Accuracy, Possibilities, and Limitations

Indications

Mammography is the single most important imaging method in diagnosing breast disease. Its areas of application include:

- Screening. Mammography is the only imaging method to date that is suitable for screening.
- Problem solving. Aside from a few exceptions (such as unequivocal sonographic diagnosis of a cyst, unequivocal clinical diagnosis of an abscess, and very young patients), mammography is always indicated as a diagnostic method in symptomatic patients. In applicable cases, it may be used with other methods.

A basic knowledge of the accuracy of mammography is an important prerequisite to properly judge its value in screening and clinical use.

Accuracy

General Aspects

The sensitivity and specificity of the method cannot be precisely quantified. While high image quality and experienced examiners are essential prerequisites, accuracy also depends on the following factors:

- Patient selection: Screening versus diagnostic problem solving, type of screening (number of views, use of clinical data, and screening interval), distribution of findings in the study group, and the extent to which other methods of preoperative diagnosis are used.
- The threshold of the individual examiner. Experience being equal, a low threshold will lead to a high sensitivity at the expense of specificity, whereas a high threshold increases specificity and the positive predictive value at the expense of sensitivity.[1, 2]

The individual threshold represents a compromise arrived at by assessing the tradeoff between the false negative rate and the false positive rate. It is also influenced by other factors such as limited funds of a screening program, restrictions concerning the accepted rate of excisional diagnostic biopsies, or the accepted number of additional examinations).

Sensitivity

Realistically, mammography has a sensitivity of about 90%, i. e., about 10% of all carcinomas are not detected initially by mammography. When mammographic screening is performed, about 25–35% of the carcinomas become apparent between screening examinations, usually by manifesting clinical symptoms. They are called interval carcinomas. Finally it is important to know that numerous carcinomas detected at screening are retrospectively visible on the previous examination, mostly as some uncharacteristic change.[3, 4, 5]

Thus mammography does not provide a 100% sensitivity. There exists a threshold for mammographic detection of malignancy, which depends on tumor size, tumor type, and surrounding tissue. These limitations must be kept in mind, particularly for diagnostic mammography.

For screening, however, mammography is the only method that allows reproducible and reliable detection of a prognostically relevant number of nonpalpable carcinomas, at an acceptable rate of false positive calls and at acceptable expense.

Overall sensitivity of mammography in fatty tissue is excellent. It decreases as radiodensity increases. This means that mammography has a lower sensitivity in radiodense tissue and, therefore, a negative mammogram does not eliminate the need for further workup of otherwise indeterminate or suggestive palpable findings in dense tissue.[6, 7]

Mammography is highly sensitive in detecting carcinomas containing microcalcifications, and this sensitivity is largely uninfluenced by the radiodensity of the surrounding tissue. These carcinomas account for about 50% of all cancers, including approximately 30–40% of all invasive carcinomas and about 90% of carcinomas in situ currently detected. Since these are generally not palpable but have excellent cure rates, mammography plays a decisive role in early detection.

Specificity

Mammography is specific in only a few cases:

- Absence of malignancy can be diagnosed reliably in fatty breasts (provided the area in question is included on the mammogram).
- A definitive diagnosis of a benign lesion is possible for a typical oil cyst, a hamartoma, a lipoma, a typically calcified fibroadenoma or lymph nodes with typical mammographic features.
- A quite reliable diagnosis of a benign tumor or cyst (> 98% correct) is possible in the case of a typical well-circumscribed mass.

In the majority of clinically or mammographically detected changes, mammography, however, is nonspecific and only permits likelihood statements.[8, 9]

- The specificity of the diagnosis of a carcinoma is quite high for spiculated masses, as well as for pleomorphic and cast-like microcalcifications with ductal distribution. However, a spiculated mass can also be caused by an area of fat necrosis or a radial scar. (Rarely, even suspicious microcalcifications are associated with papillomatosis, papilloma, fibroadenoma, plasma cell mastitis or fat necrosis).

In addition to the factors already mentioned (threshold and selection of patients), the size of the findings decisively influences the expected specificity of the mammographic study. In fact, most nonpalpable carcinomas, in particular small carcinomas, appear as nonspecific changes.[10, 1, 11, 12, 13] Unless the examiner is only looking for large, obvious findings, one has to be aware that only 1 of every 5 to 10 mammographically suspicious changes will correspond to malignancy.[8, 1]

Further diagnostic studies, including additional views, sonography, and percutaneous biopsy, can improve this rate so that more than half of the excisional biopsies of nonpalpable abnormalities will be performed for a malignancy.[14]

Screening

Due to the high sensitivity of mammography in fatty tissue and its ability to reveal microcalcifications, mammography can detect small carcinomas at an early and prognostically favorable stage.

Mammographic screening has resulted in a 30–70% reduction in mortality (see Chapter 19). To date, neither physical examination nor chemotherapy or hormonal therapy has been able to achieve comparable results.

Mammography is the only imaging modality suitable for screening. In addition to good sensitivity and acceptable specificity, it offers the following important advantages:

- It is the most cost-effective noninvasive examination method.
- Mammographic studies are reproducible and easily documented.
- It requires relatively little physician time (in contrast to breast ultrasound).
- It is the only technique that reliably visualizes microcalcifications—which are associated with about 30–40% of the invasive breast cancers and almost all presently detected intraductal cancers.

Yet despite the many advantages, one should bear these points in mind:

- Negative screening results do not exclude a carcinoma. Supplementary studies are always indicated in the presence of new or existing problems.
- In screening as in diagnostic use, best results are achieved by evaluating the mammographic studies in conjunction with clinical data and the patient's medical history. Clinical examination and patient history should not be neglected. About 10% of breast cancers are detected only by physical examination.
- The results are highly dependent on image quality and the examiner's level of experience.

■ Problem Solving

Problem solving begins when clinical data, the patient's medical history, or imaging studies (usually mammography) reveal an abnormality. The most important objective is to verify or exclude the presence of a carcinoma with the highest possible degree of certainty. Considering the general intraoperative and perioperative risk (embolism) of surgery, the physiological and psychological stress on the patient, patient compliance and costs, biopsies of benign lesions should be avoided whenever possible. Furthermore, severe or multiple scars may impair later diagnosis. However, a high degree of certainty is necessary to exclude a suspected malignancy.

The following should be remembered for problem solving:

1. The sensitivity of mammography is excellent (approaching 100%) in fatty breasts or in all fatty areas of the breast. This means that in the absence of mammographic findings, malignancy can be excluded with a high degree of certainty even in the presence of palpable abnormality in this area.[15] This applies only if the palpable findings in question
   - have been included mammographically (note that the axillary tail and areas close to the chest wall can be a problem)
   - lie entirely within fatty tissue

   For this reason it is useful to place a radiopaque marker over palpable lesions to localize them on the mammogram.
2. It is particularly important to remember that the sensitivity of mammography is significantly reduced in areas containing a high proportion of glandular or connective tissue.[6, 7] Carcinomas without microcalcification can be overlooked in such areas. Thus, in tissue that is not mammographically equivalent to fat, any suggestive palpable findings require further workup.
3. Only a few entities have such a distinct mammographic appearance that no further diagnostic studies are necessary. These include:
   - lipomas
   - typical hamartomas
   - characteristically calcified fibroadenomas
   - oil cysts and some galactoceles
   - intramammary lymph nodes
4. Whenever a mammographically, clinically or otherwise detected abnormality does not exhibit a pathognomonic appearance, further workup is necessary.

Another important task of mammography concerns detection of secondary lesions. For this reason, even with palpable lesions undergoing surgical biopsy, mammography is always indicated preoperatively to be certain when a second nonpalpable lesion that requires biopsy is not present.

Mammographic Technique

Compared to radiographic studies of other parts of the body, mammography places particularly stringent demands on equipment and image quality. The stringent demands of technique and positioning make mammography one of the most diffcult examinations in conventional radiology.

The specific requirements can be **summarized as follows:**

- Extremely fine microcalcifications and fibrotic strands (tiny structures with a size of about 100 µm with only slight differences in density to the surrounding tissue) must be imaged sharply, with high contrast and with a low level of image noise.
- Despite the highest possible contrast, mammography must permit adequate assessment of areas of greatly varying density. These include fatty areas behind the nipple or close to the skin in small breasts, areas of radiodense fibrocystic tissue in large breasts and the tissue overlying the pectoralis muscle. This requires an imaging system with a wide object range.
- In view of the sensitivity of mammary tissue to radiation (especially in younger women), the examination should involve the minimum dose of radiation sufficient to produce an image of acceptable quality.
- Imaging the complete body of the gland is imperative for an accurate assessment in both screening examinations and diagnostic problem solving. This is possible only with a consistent effort to achieve optimum standard positioning. Knowledge and application of additional views, whenever indicated, is necessary.

These stringent requirements apply to the choice of equipment and film as well as to the level of training and experience of physicians and technical staff. Radiologists and radiologic technologists must ensure a standard of image quality that permits detection of early malignancy.

It is therefore *essential that radiologists and radiologic technologists* be thoroughly familiar with mammographic technique and constantly monitor quality. Studies have shown that only optimal imaging technique ensures early detection of breast cancer.[16] Where this is not the case, early stage carcinomas with excellent cure rates will not be detected with sufficient certainty. This has serious negative repercussions because the mammographic examination will give the patient and her referring physician a false sense of security, and both may underestimate the significance of early clinical signs of malignancy.

Components of the Mammographic Imaging Technique

(Fig. 3.**1**)

■ The X-ray Tube

Mammography requires *special tubes* that produce particularly *low-energy radiation* in comparison to other diagnostic X-ray tubes. This is achieved by use of special targets and filters. Mammography requires low-energy radiation to achieve the required high tissue contrast.

Since the radiation needed originates in a small focal spot and the exposure time should be as short as possible (to avoid motion blurring), the tubes used for mammography must be powerful.

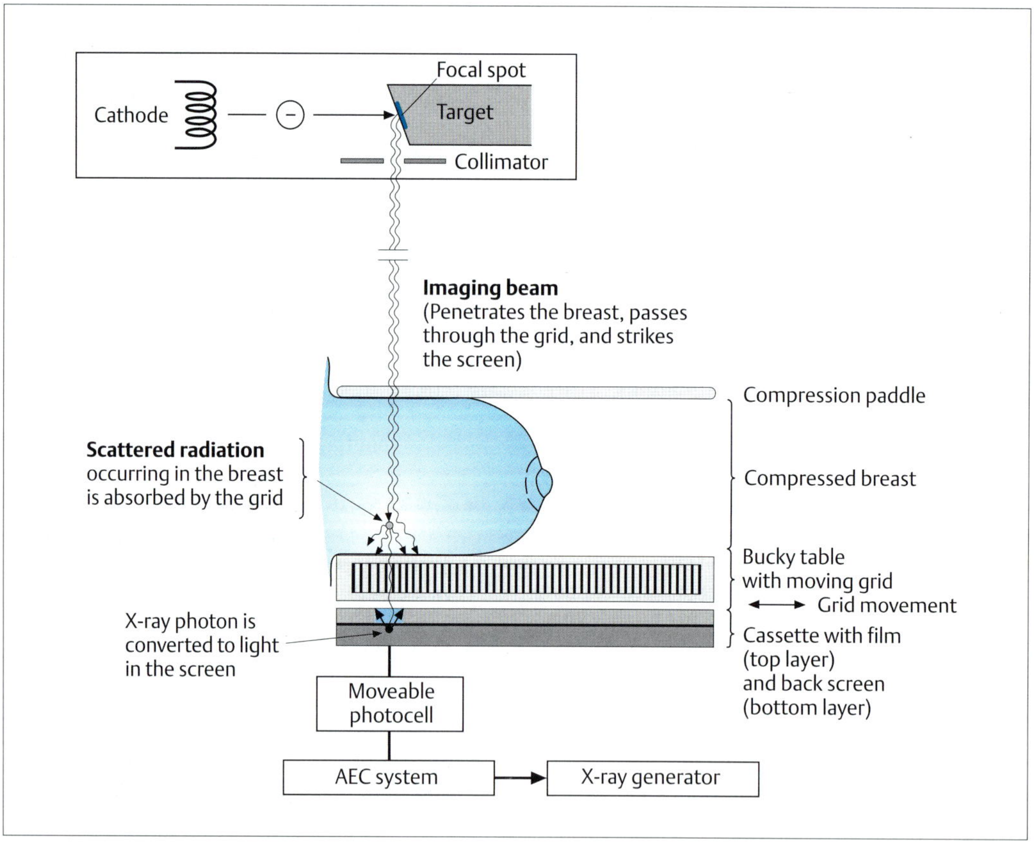

Fig. 3.**1** Mammographic imaging technique. Overview of components

Sharpness: Focal Spot Size and Geometry (Source to Image–Receptor Distance = SID)

To achieve the required sharpness (spatial resolution), mammography tubes must have an extremely small focal spot. A *nominal focal spot size smaller than 0.4* is required today.

Note: A nominal focal spot size of 0.4 means that the (diameter) in each direction will be between 0.4 mm and 0.6 mm. The local projection of the width of the focal spot will vary according to:

- its distance from the chest wall
- the angulation of the tube

In addition to minimal focal spot size, the proper geometric configuration of the focal spot, object, and image receptor is important in achieving the necessary sharpness. Use of a *small focal spot*, the *shortest possible distance between the object and the film and the longest possible distance between the focus and the film* will minimize the penumbra (geometric blurring) (Fig. 3.**2**).

Radiation Spectrum: Penetration and Contrast

The radiation produced in X-ray tubes is not monoenergetic but consists of a spectrum of radiation energies. This spectrum comprises X-ray bremsstrahlung and the characteristic radiation determined by the target material.

Since the spectrum of imaging radiation greatly influences contrast and radiation dose, the following physical aspects should be considered:

- With *low-energy radiation*, slight differences in the radiodensity of soft tissue of the breast that would otherwise remain undetected can be visualized with *high contrast.*
- *Increasing energy* of the radiation *decreases soft-tissue contrast.*

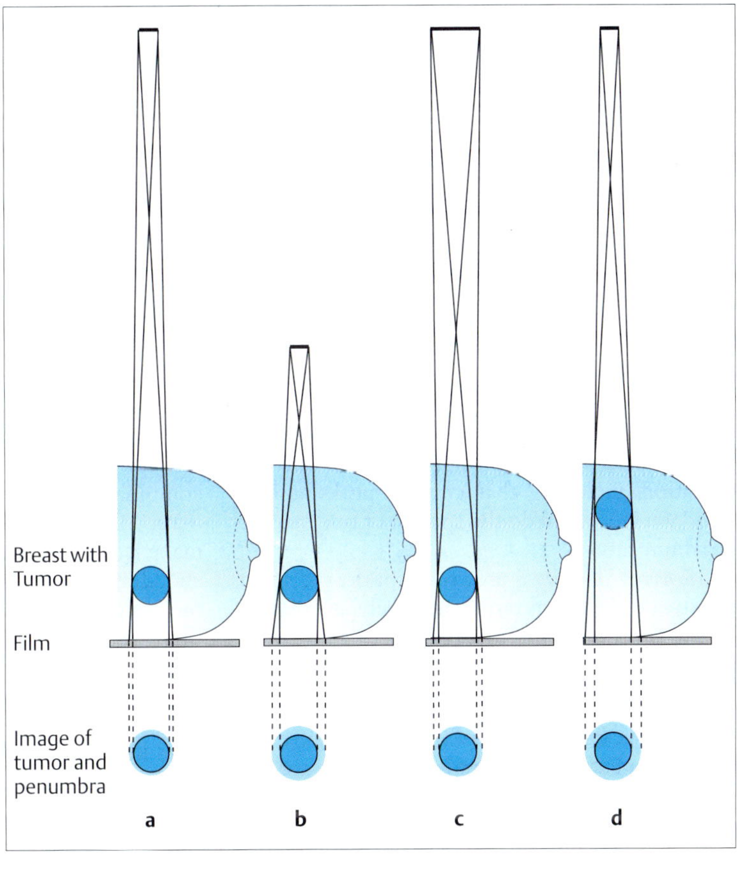

Fig. 3.**2** A long SID (source-to-image receptor distance), small focal spot, and short distance between the object and the film minimize penumbra and optimize image definition (**a**). The penumbra increases with a short SID (**b**), large focal spot (**c**), and a long distance between object and film (**d**)

- But, the radiation spectrum *must* have *sufficiently high energy for adequate penetration* of thick breasts and breasts with abundant fibrotic or glandular tissue.
- Radiation with insufficient energy will not penetrate the breast even with long exposure time. Such radiation is not suitable for imaging at all. It will unnecessarily increase the radiation dose and, since dense tissue cannot be penetrated, it will produce an inadequate image.

Thus, *higher-energy* radiation is required in *dense breasts* (in the presence of abundant fibrotic tissue, glandular tissue, or mastopathy) and in thick *breasts.*

With the optimum radiation energy selected, the *absorption is higher in radiodense tissue (fibrotic tissue, glandular tissue, and malignant tissue) than in radiolucent tissue (fat or loose connective tissue).* These *differences in absorption* produce the image pattern.

Since too large a component of high energy reduces the contrast and too high a component of low energy results in excessive radiation exposure, it is advisable to adapt the radiation spectrum as closely as possible to the thickness and density of the breast.

The radiation spectrum is determined by the following factors:

1. The *target/filter combination* of the X-ray tube
2. The *peak kilovoltage (kVp)* setting on the X-ray unit

Target/Filter Combination

The radiation spectrum created at the target depends on the *kVp setting* and on the *target material.*

The radiation spectrum of molybdenum targets contains a higher proportion of low-energy radiation (including characteristic peaks at 17.5 and 19.6 keV) than do the spectra of tungsten or rhodium tubes.

Selective filtering is used to adapt the radiation spectrum of a given target as closely as possible to the specific requirements.

Selective filtering:

- Suppresses the low-energy components of the spectrum that would represent unnecessary radiation exposure because they are absorbed in the breast (like the standard aluminum filter)
- Reduces the energy components above the K absorption edge characteristic of the selected filter material, essentially permitting a narrow spectral range directly below the K absorption edge to pass. Any filter is particularly efficient at absorbing that part of the radiation whose energy exceeds a limit, referred to as the K absorption edge, specific to the filter material.

The effective spectral range can thus be defined by selecting the target and filter material and the thickness of the filter (Fig. 3.3).[17, 18]

Commercially available *target/filter combinations* include molybdenum/molybdenum, molybdenum/rhodium, rhodium/rhodium or tungsten/molybdenum, and tungsten/rhodium.

- The radiation quality from a molybdenum/molybdenum or tungsten/molybdenum target/filter combination is suitable for most breasts.
- The combinations tungsten/molybdenum, molybdenum/rhodium, tungsten/rhodium, and rhodium/rhodium provide, in this order, increasingly high-energy radiation spectra. They permit better penetration of large and mastopathic breasts with abundant glandular, fibrotic, and connective tissue, resulting in higher image quality and a reduction and unnecessary radiation exposure.

Peak Kilovoltage (kVp)

A higher kVp setting increases the relative proportion of high-energy radiation in the respective spectrum, whereas a lower kVp setting increases the relative proportion of low-energy radiation.

Selecting the proper kVp setting, target material, and filter material according to breast thickness and density: Since the optimum kVp for a target/filter combination is not applicable to others, automatic exposure control systems are provided to make it easier to match kVp to breast thickness and density. Depending on the manufacturer, the system can select or suggest the proper settings (see p. 21).

Penetration: Heel Effect

The heel effect of the X-ray tube is also exploited to compensate for varying penetration in the chest wall and nipple.

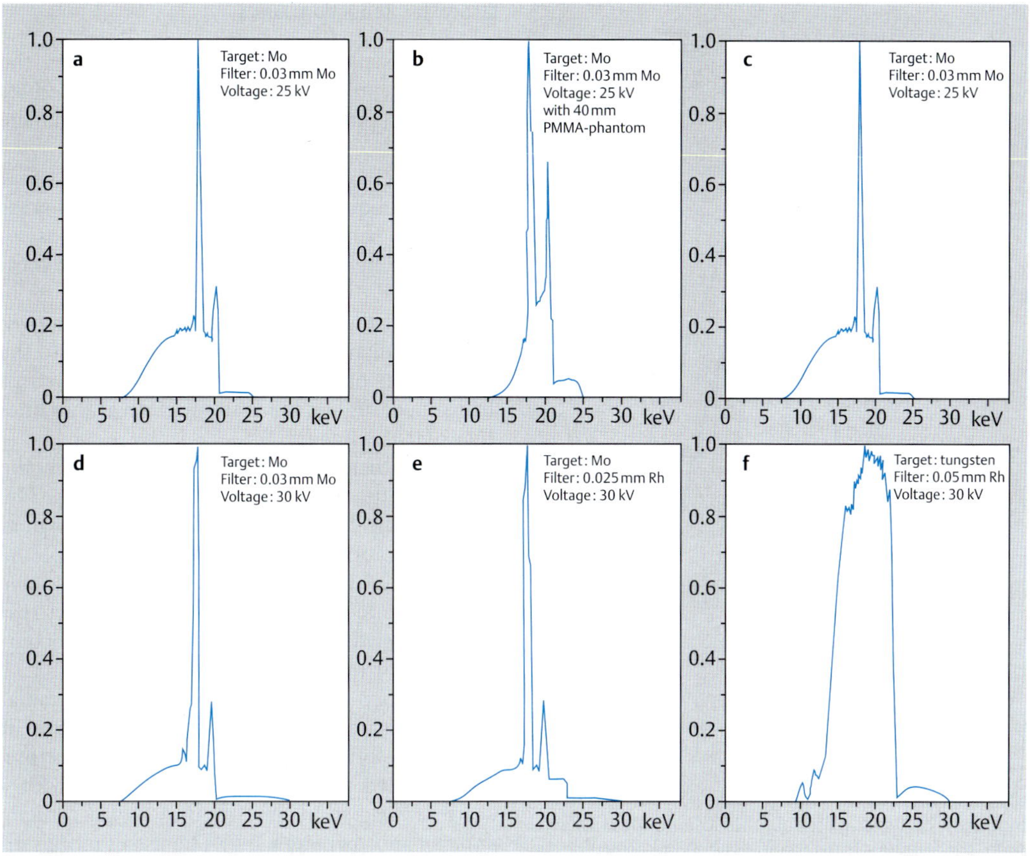

Fig. 3.**3 a–f** Radiation spectra of various target/filter combinations
a and **b** The illustration shows the photon spectrum of a molybdenum/0.030-mm molybdenum filter combination at 25 kV peak kilovoltage as it is emitted from the X-ray tube (**a**), and as it is measured at the image receptor after penetrating a 4-cm breast phantom (**b**). The respective spectra of radiation in the right and left pictures are normalized according to the maximum energy (= 100%) present in the respective spectrum.
Comparing the left and right illustration reveals that the low energies are absorbed in the breast. Thus, they cannot contribute to visualization but only increase the dose. The more breast thickness increases, the more low-energy components of the spectrum are absorbed in the glandular tissue.
Increasing the average energy of the spectrum in proportion to breast thickness and density is recommended to achieve sufficient penetration and avoid an excessive dose due to absorption of the low-energy radiation
c–f One way of increasing the high-energy components in the spectrum is to increase the kVp setting. Changing the filter material and/or filter thickness or choosing another target material make it possible to adapt the radiation spectrum even more closely to the thickness and density of the breast. (This increases the high-energy components in the spectrum and better filters out the low-energy components, which increase the dose, particularly in dense breasts.) This may be illustrated in the spectra of various target/filter combinations

The heel effect (Fig. 3.**4**) means that the intensity of rays emitted by the target is not uniform throughout the beam.[19]

More of the rays that leave the target at obtuse angle will be absorbed by the target than those leaving the target at acute angle, due to the longer path they have to travel in the target.

Since the thickness of the breast is greater close to the chest wall than near the nipple, it is best when the area of maximum radiation inten-

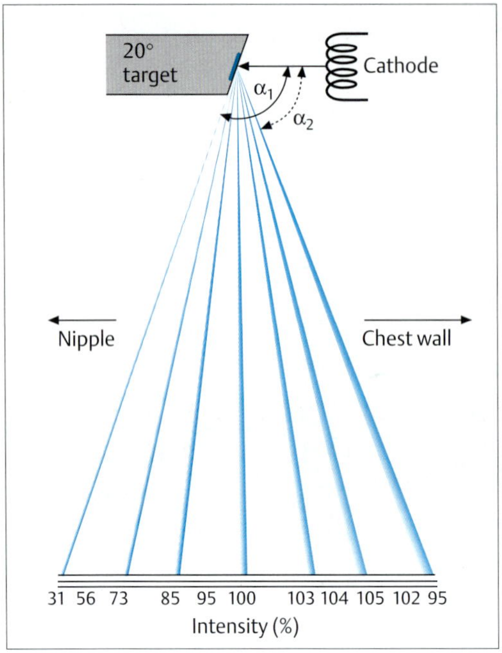

Fig. 3.**4** Heel effect
The beam created at the target focus is weaker on the target side than on the cathode aside. The illustration shows the radiation intensity referred to the central ray (100%). The intensity varies depending on the angle of egress of the radiation from the target. This effect is used in mammography by locating the cathode closer to the chest wall than the anode. Thus the radiation intensity will be greater close to the chest wall and less near the nipple, where the breast is thinner

sity lies near the chest wall. This is achieved by positioning the target opposite the cathode, which is closer to the chest wall. The intensity distribution of the radiation can be influenced by slightly angling (i. e., tipping) the X-ray tube. However, this alters the projection of the focal spot.

Scattered Radiation

In every radiograph of the breast, *scattered radiation* is produced in the tissue. In denser and thicker glandular tissue, more scattered radiation occurs than in the thinner, fatty, transparent tissue. Increasing amounts of scattered radiation result in progressive loss of contrast.

Scatter Reduction: Grids

The grid is placed between the breast and the image receptor (screen–film system) to reduce undesired scattered radiation that impairs image quality.

Grids (Fig. 3.**1**) consist of strips of lead that absorb obliquely oriented radiation, whereas radiation parallel to the lead strips passes through. The lead strips are focused on the focal spot.

During the exposure, the grid rapidly moves perpendicular to the path of the beam and to the orientation of the strips to prevent the strips from appearing on the mammogram as thin lines that mar the image.

The efficiency of the grid depends on the height of the strips and the strip spacing. The ratio of strip height to strip spacing is known as the grid ratio. The larger the grid ratio, the greater the efficiency of the grid but also the greater the required radiation dose. For this reason, only grid ratios of 4:27 or 5:30 are recommended for mammography.[19, 20]

Since the grid absorbs both scattered radiation and a small proportion of useful radiation, it requires a longer exposure time and, therefore, an increased radiation dose. Exposures with a scattered radiation grid require a *grid exposure factor* of approximately 2.5. The use of more sensitive screen–film systems has compensated for this increased dose, compared with earlier gridless mammographic techniques.

The *significant increase in image quality* fully justifies the increased radiation dose required by the grid, and *grid mammography* has superseded gridless mammography.

Gridless mammography can only be performed without significant loss of quality in very small, compressed, and fatty breasts in the interest of reducing radiation exposure.

Scatter Reduction: Compression

The second important method of *reducing scattered radiation* consists of sufficient *compression of the breast.* By reducing breast thickness, compression reduces the proportion of scattered radiation, thus reducing the dose and improving the image contrast (see p. 24).[21, 20]

Other options for reducing scattered radiation include air-gap technique. The air gap, which is effective only in conjunction with good collimation, is used for scatter reduction in magnification mammography.[20, 22] Slot mammography represents another effective method of scatter reduction (see p. 68).

■ Image Receptor System

After passing through the breast and the grid, the imaging radiation reaches the *image receptor system*. In modern screen–film mammography, this system consists of *a single intensifying screen* with luminescent coating and *a special single-emulsion film* (Fig. 3.**5 a**).

The film emulsion and the coated side of the screen face each other. To obtain a sharp focus, the two must be in direct contact. Insufficient screen–film contact will cause significant local blurring.

Screen–film systems with dual-emulsion mammography films should not be used because the light photons, which are emitted from the film emulsion facing away from the screen, cause additional blurring (crossover effect). For reasons dictated by radiation geometry, the screen lies behind the film (back screen), maximizing image definition (Figs. 3.**5 b** and **c**).

Every quantum of radiation absorbed in the luminescent layer of the screen excites the phosphorus, causing it to emit several quanta of light. The resulting intensifying effect of the screen depends on the intensifying substance, the density of the luminescent layer, the distribution of the coating, and the screen dye. All the currently available intensifying screens contain gadolinium oxysulfide as an intensifying substance.[19]

While greater screen thickness and coarse crystal structures increase the intensifying effect of the screen, they also decrease the resolution. In addition to this, high intensification is accompanied by a significant increase in image noise (due to the lower number of X-ray photons that are needed). Thus to achieve the resolution required in mammography, only very high-definition intensifying screens (speed class 12) that

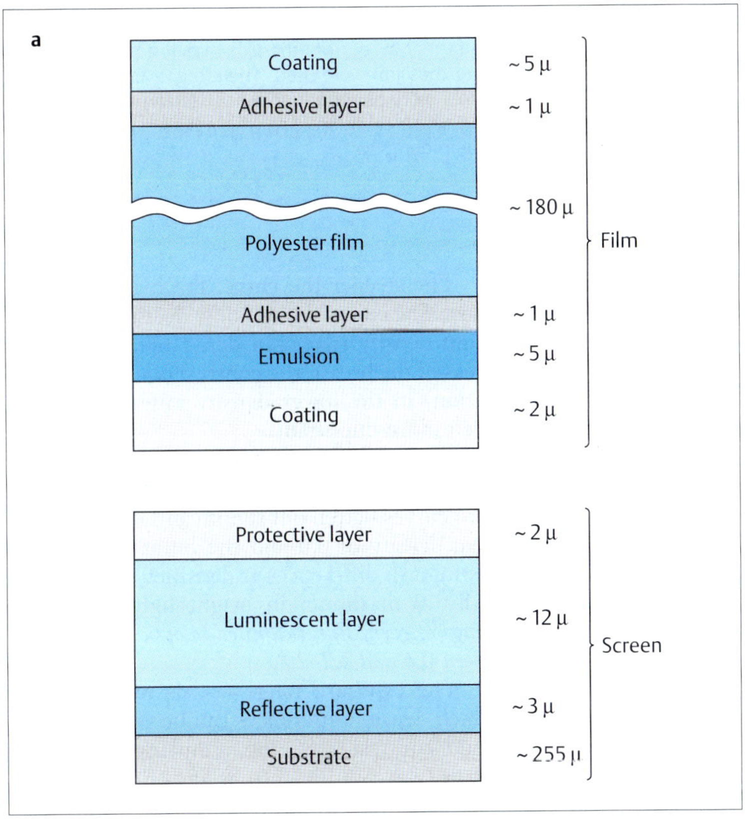

Fig. 3.**5 a–c** Influence of the arrangement of film and intensifying screen on image sharpness
a Mammography film and screen

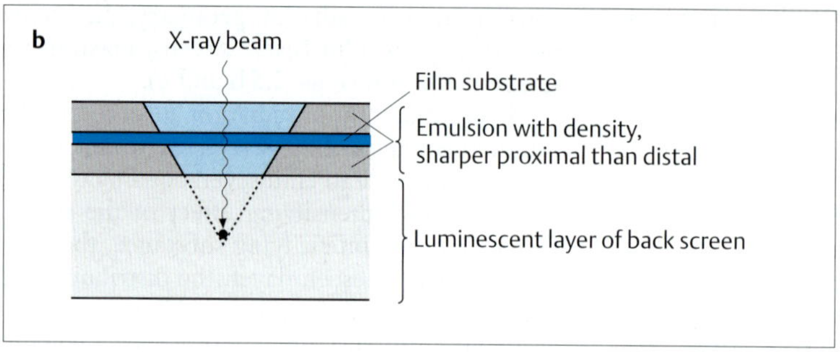

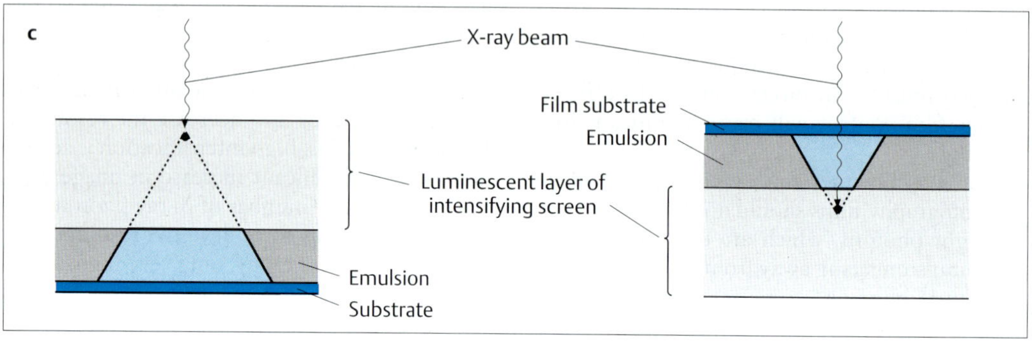

Fig. 3.**5b** The photons released from the luminescence centers of the intensifying screen are nondirectional in contrast to X-ray beams. For this reason, the diameter of the dense spot will increase with the distance between the film emulsion and the screen. This is illustrated by the diagram of a dual-emulsion film with a screen behind the film. Because of this phenomenon, only single-emulsion films are used in mammography
c Due to absorption of the X-ray beam within the intensifying screen, the majority of luminescence centers contributing to the image will be on that side of the screen, where the X-ray beam enters the screen. If a front screen were used, the majority of luminescence centers would be farther away from the film than if a back screen (behind the film) were used. Therefore, a front screen produces more blurring than a back screen. For this reason, only single-emulsion films with a back screen are used in mammography

achieve resolutions of 14–18 lines per millimeter should be used (see p. 24) for the importance of the screen–film system in optimizing resolution).[20, 23]

While the *sharpness* of a screen–film system is determined primarily *by the screen*, the *contrast* of the system is determined *by the film* and by the processing. Since the differences between the currently available high-resolution screens of the same class are slight, the sensitivity of a screen–film system and thus the required dose are then influenced by the choice of film.[23]

The contrast behavior of a mammographic film is shown in its respective *characteristic curve*. The characteristic curve shows the relationship between film density and the dose of radiation incident on the film. Optical density (blackening) is plotted against the logarithm of the radiation dose (Fig. 3.**6**).

The steeper the curve, the higher the contrast. The contrast is not only decisive in the medium density range. In dense breasts or dense areas of the breast, the contrast (and thus visualization) in the lower density range (0.5–1.5) is even more important.

For diagnostic purposes, uniformly high contrast in every density range would be desirable. Since the film curves flatten out significantly below an optical density of 0.6 and the human eye cannot distinguish differences at densities exceeding 2.2 (2.8–3.0 maximum in bright light), *the useful range of every film is limited to optical densities between 0.6 and 2.2–2.8.*

The exposure range (x-axis of Fig. 3.**6**) in which density differences can be visualized with good contrast, i. e., the useful optical density range (y-axis in Fig. 3.**6**), is known as the *imageable object range or latitude.*

If the film contrast is too high, the latitude will be too narrow. This means that the imageable object range will not include areas of very high or of very low density in the breast, and these areas can no longer be visualized in the useful density range. Density differences in these relatively *overexposed or underexposed areas* will no longer be adequately visualized (despite or because of the particularly high contrast in areas of medium density). Such overexposed or underexposed areas can appear particularly in large or dense breasts since their differences in absorption are especially high. To minimize these problems, the resulting contrast must be carefully optimized but should not be too high.[24]

The contrast is essentially determined by the choice of film, the quality of radiation (exposure voltage, target and filter), and the film processing.[20, 23]

■ Exposure

After selecting the proper film–screen system (FSS) and after adapting the radiation quality to the thickness and density of the breast, the film must be exposed in such a manner that all details relevant to the diagnosis are visualized in the optimum density range. This means that the mean optical density should lie approximately in the middle of the useful optical density range, i. e., between 1.2 and 1.6. (Recent studies have shown a mean density of 1.2–1.6 preferable to the mean density of 1.0–1.4 mentioned in medical guidelines.)

Film density ranges below 0.6 and above 2.2 (or 3.0 in bright light) permit only limited visualization at best.

The *exposure* is the *product of tube current (mA) and exposure time (second)*, expressed as the milliampere–second product, or mAs product. One method of adjusting the exposure is by *selecting the settings manually*, i. e., all exposure parameters can be freely selected. However, this requires a fair amount of experience because the exposure varies with both breast thickness and breast density.

Even experienced radiologists and radiologic technologists will use *automatic exposure control systems* to minimize the chance of incorrect exposure. The purpose of an automatic exposure control system (a required feature on every mammography unit) is to ensure a reproducible mean optical density of 1.2–1.6 on the film regardless of breast thickness and density.

The automatic exposure control system (see Figs. 3.**1** and 3.**7**) utilizes a *photocell* placed beneath the cassette containing the film and screen. The chamber measures the dose behind the image receptor in a representative area. When the *cutoff dose* for the selected mean optical film density is reached (this depends on the screen–film system used), the *system switches off the exposure.*

Since the sensitivity of the photocell varies with different radiation energies (that result from beam hardening behind breasts of different thickness or density and behind the image receptor), the automatic exposure control system must compensate for the variable breast thickness and density when determining the optimum cutoff dose.

The quality of the automatic exposure control system determines how well it can achieve a constant film density independent of breast thickness and density. (see pp. 32)[17, 25, 24, 20]

The position of the photocell has to be adjusted. To ensure that the automatic exposure control system will function optimally, position the *photocell* so that it lies *under a representative part of the glandular tissue (which is in the anterior third of the breast).* The correct position of the photocell will depend on the size of the breast. Improper positioning of the photocell will result in incorrect exposure. Problems may occur with very small breasts that cannot cover the photocell or with silicon implants (see pp. 31 and 32).

■ Film Processing

Since deviations in chemical composition or developing time and temperature can cause problems with image contrast, noise, sensitivity, and fog, *it is essential to process the film strictly according to the manufacturer's recommendations and regularly monitor processing* (see pp. 33 and 37). Carefully controlled film processing becomes all the more important when it is understood that most acute changes in image quality are caused by deviations in film processing.[26, 27]

Prolonging the developing time (for example from 90 to 180 seconds, i. e., extended processing) while keeping temperature constant can increase image quality with certain film types by increasing contrast and sensitivity. However, since many factors influence quality (including film type, the existing steepness of the gradation curve, film throughput, and so forth), no generalized recommendations can be made.[28]

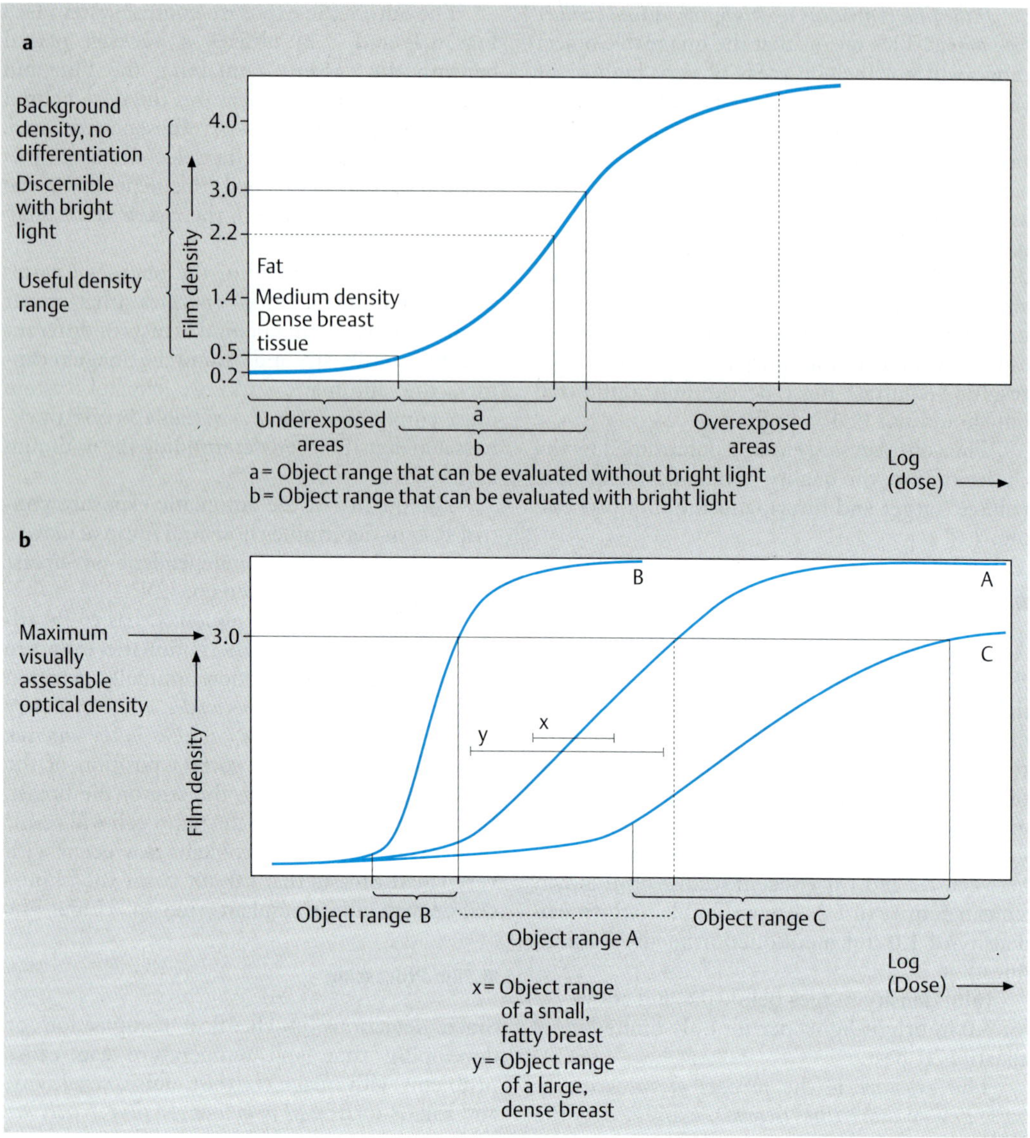

Fig. 3.**6 a** and **b**

■ Viewing the Image

Proper evaluation of the complete density range of a well exposed mammogram requires a viewbox that provides *homogeneous illumination at the required intensity*. Viewboxes must provide adjustable luminance in the range of 2000–3000 cd/m² at a color temperature of 4500–6500 K. An additional *bright spotlight* must be available for illuminating areas of high exposure. This light should provide luminance up to 20000 cd/m². Focused illumination of images that cover a wide density range with bright light will make details in highly dense areas appear more readily visible. However, this is only possible up to an optical density of 2.8–3.0. Focused illumination provides important additional information, although this is always limited and is usually not able to compensate for incorrect exposure, an excessively high-contrast film, or excessively high contrast due to errors in processing the film.

◁ Fig. 3.**6 a** and **b** The significance of characteristic curves
a Principle curve
b Exaggerated gradation curves of different films:
Film A shows a wide object range within which details are visualized with good contrast and can be easily discerned.
Film B is more sensitive (left shifted) and images the details in the center section of the curve with greater contrast. However, its object range is narrower so that details beyond this range are visualized with poor contrast (underexposed or overexposed).
Film C requires a high dose yet images a narrower density range. In spite of this, it visualizes a wide object range with uniform albeit relatively low contrast.
Imaging a small breast requires a narrower object range than imaging a large, dense breast.
The mean exposure (center of the object range of the breast to be imaged) is adapted to the sensitivity of the screen–film system by selecting a higher or lower mAs product (right or left shift in the object range of the breast to be imaged). Changing the mAs product will not influence the width of the object range. This means that a small breast can be imaged with all three films. At optimum exposure settings, film B will produce the highest-contrast image. This image will be perceived as the sharpest, although there is no objective difference in the definition of films A, B, or C.
Film B cannot adequately image a dense breast. The object range of this film is narrower than that required for imaging dense breasts, and overexposed and underexposed areas will result. For this reason, film B should not be used although it produces better images of small breasts. Film A is the optimal film since it can image both large, dense breasts and small breasts with good contrast. Here, precise exposure settings are essential to avoid overexposed or underexposed areas since its object range is only slightly larger than a large, dense breast requires. Film C can image both small and large dense breasts in an acceptable range, albeit with slightly less contrast. This film should be considered if achieving precise exposure is a problem (as can occur with older automatic exposure control system with insufficient density compensation). Experience has shown that both microcalcifications and structures relevant to the diagnosis can be discerned, although they are less obvious.

All viewing areas for mammography, including the work area for technologists, should be furnished with identical illumination. All light bulbs should be changed routinely throughout these viewing areas and the viewboxes cleaned weekly. The films are to be read in a darkened room with matting of the viewbox to the size of the film, when possible. These latter techniques minimize ambient light and thereby increase contrast when viewing the films. A *magnifying lens* with magnification by at least a factor of 2 should be available for evaluating the mammogram.

Specific Requirements and Solutions

The ability to recognize structures on the mammogram is determined by:

- *Resolution*
- *Image noise*
- *Contrast*

These variables must be optimized using the lowest possible radiation dose.

The following sections will explain factors that influence these variables.

■ Image Sharpness

Image sharpness is determined by motion blur, geometric blurring, and the blurring of the image receptor system.[29, 20, 23] (Table 3.**1**)

Motion blurring is caused by patient motion and, less pronounced, by arterial pulsation. It can be minimized by:

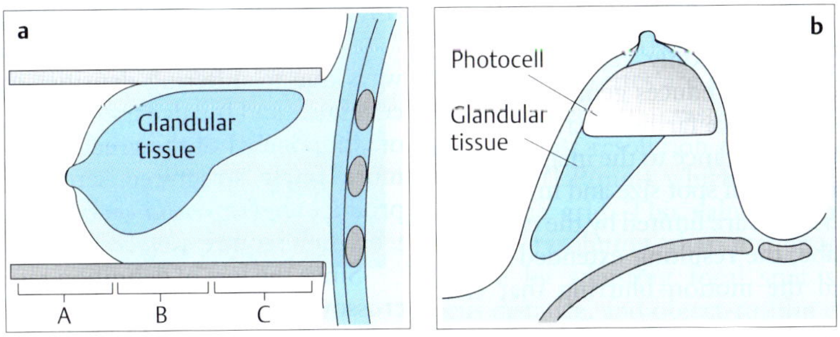

Fig. 3.**7 a** and **b** Positioning the photocell
a Lateral view of the compressed breast
Position A is poor (beam must pass through too much air).
Position B is optimal.
Position C is poor (beam must pass through too much fat).
b View of breast from above showing optimal photocell position

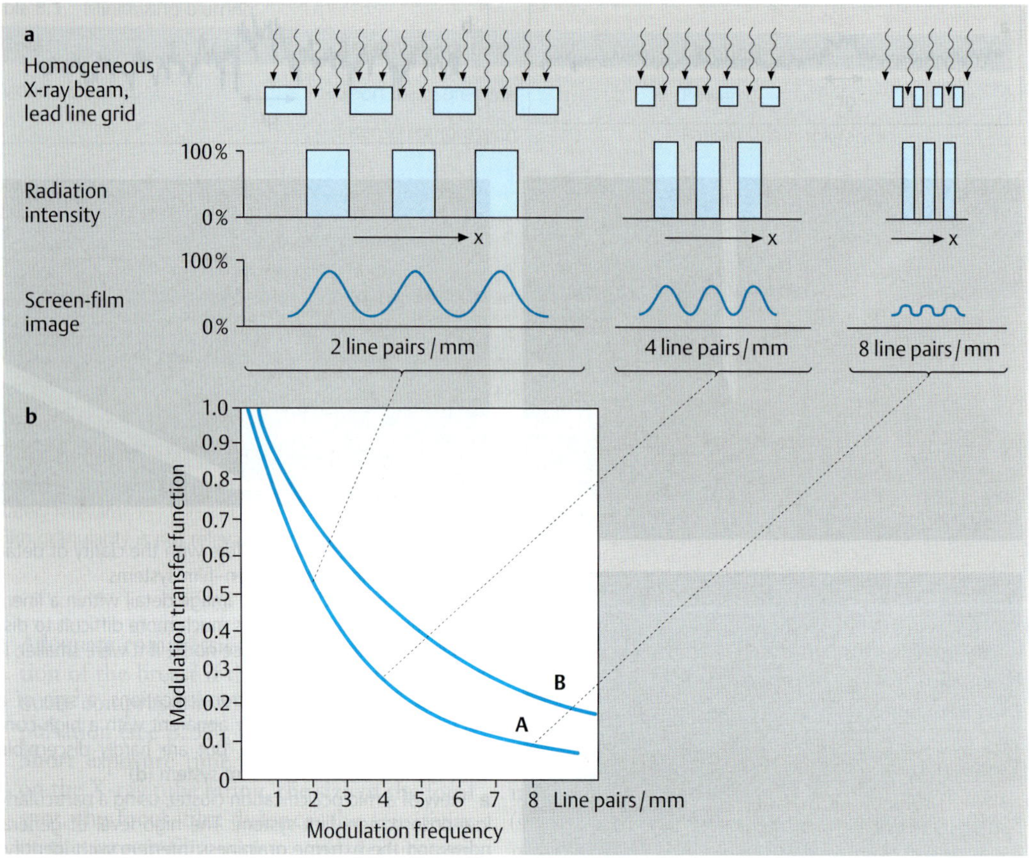

Fig. 3.**9 a** and **b** Modulation transfer function (MTF) and structural resolution
a A lead line grid imaged with a homogeneous beam. The radiation density in the image of the line grid is alternately 0 and 100%. Light scattering in the screen–film system in particular causes the sharp edges of the grid to appear fuzzy. The finer the grid, the more the differences in intensity will be equalized in the image
b The resulting relationship that renders structures less detectable as they become finer (local modulation frequency of intensity) is described by the modulation transfer function of a component (in this case, the screen–film system). As the fineness of the lines increase, the MTF decreases from an initial value of 1 (no loss of information), thus limiting the resolving power of the components.
Curve B shows a better modulation transfer function than curve A

very slight differences in density. Therefore, whether they can be detected is highly dependent on contrast and image noise. The clarity of details as a function of their size is expressed by the modulation transfer function, MTF (see Fig. 3.**9**).[19] This means that for a given image receptor system, large objects will appear with high contrast, whereas fine objects will be imaged with low contrast and will thus have poor resolution. Thus, despite its capability for a high-contrast resolution of 14–18 line pairs, an optimum technical system will be limited to detecting microcalcifications measuring *0.1–0.2 mm* or larger (corresponding to 10 or 5 LP/mm).

Contrast

Contrast can be defined as the relative difference in density between an object and its surroundings referred to the surrounding density:[19]

$$\text{Contrast} = \frac{\text{Density}_{\text{obj.}} - \text{Density}_{\text{surroundings}}}{\text{Density}_{\text{surroundings}}} \times 100$$

Fig. 3.**23 b** and **c**

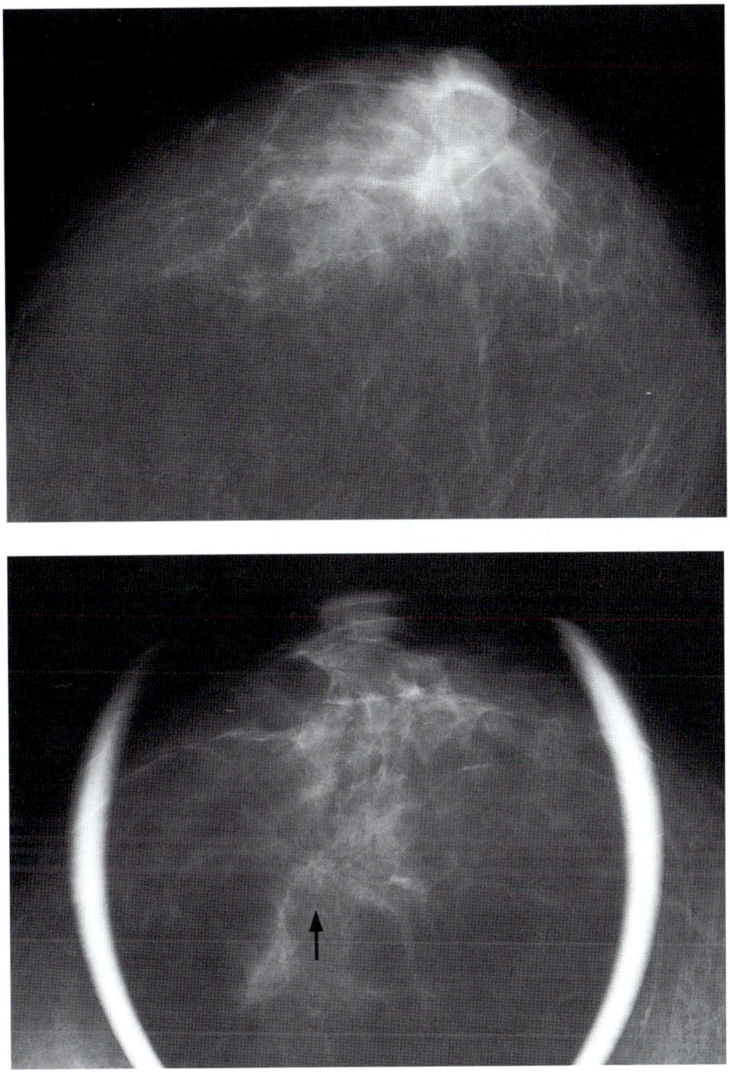

Fundamental Considerations in Magnification Mammography

The total resolution (definition) in an unmagnified image is limited by geometric blurring, resolution of the screen–film system, and, in applicable cases, motion blurring.

Total resolution is also influenced by the contrast of the detail being imaged and by image noise.

Magnification mammography has the following effects:[20, 65, 22]

1. Magnifying details by the factor *f* and projecting them on the screen–film system improves that proportion of the resolution (definition) determined by the screen–film system by precisely this factor *f*.
2. Increasing the magnification while keeping the size of the focus constant would significantly increase the geometric blurring due to the larger penumbra (geometric blurring). The geometric threshold resolution has definitely been reached when the size of the penumbra equals or exceeds that of an imaged detail. For this reason, magnification mammography requires a *microfocus with a nominal maximum value of 0.1–0.15* (depending on the magnification factor). The size of the

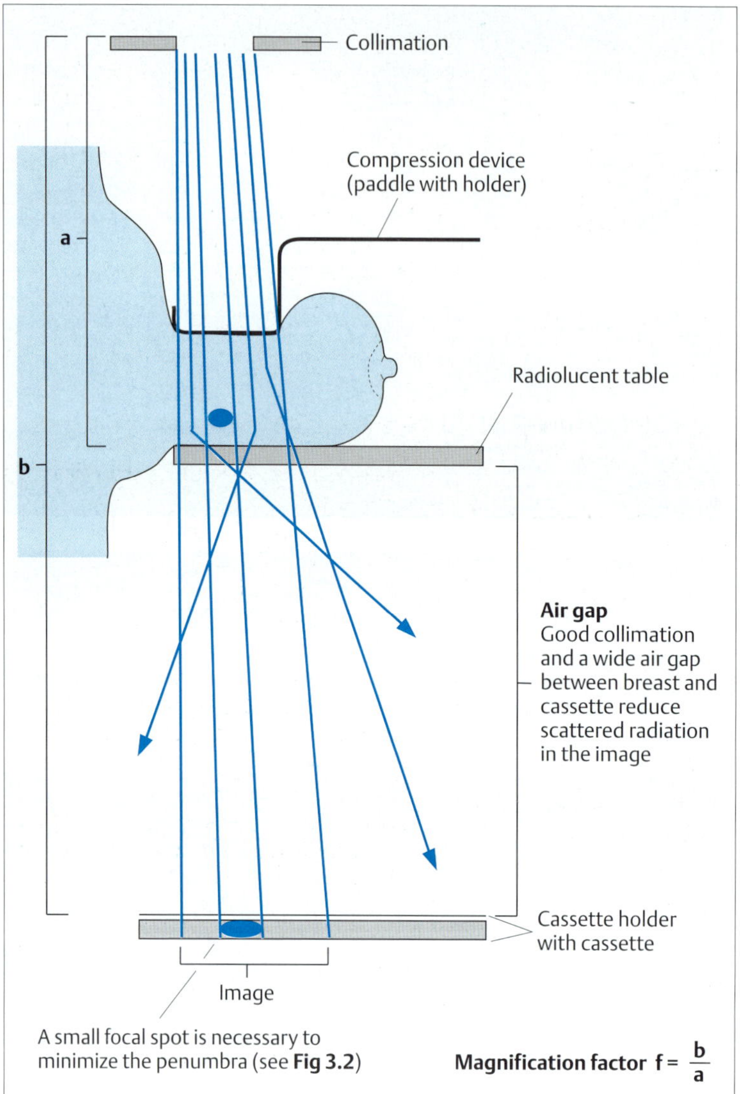

Fig. 3.**24** Magnification mammography

focus in turn limits the maximum feasible *magnification factor to 1.4–2.0* on standard units.

3. The minimal size of the focal spot is currently limited by the load rating of the microfocus.
4. Bearing in mind the limited power of the microfocus, we recommend the following measures to minimize exposure time (in the interest of reducing motion blurring and dose, and avoiding reciprocity law failure of the film):
   - Use a faster low-dose screen–film system (e. g., sensitivity class 25. At the given magnification factor, the screen–film system no longer influences maximum resolution).
   - Increase kVp by approximately 2 kV compared with the corresponding nonmagnified exposure. This allows a decrease in the exposure time (mAs) while the density remains comparable to the nonmagnified view. Otherwise, the small focal spot would require a long exposure, and patient motion may be a problem.

5. To maintain an adequate signal-to-noise ratio, the dose required to produce the image increases as the square of magnification factor. If all other parameters are kept constant, magnifying the image by a factor of 1.4 will double the dose, and magnifying the image by a factor of 2 will quadruple the dose. Minimizing the dose is necessary in the interest of minimizing the patient's exposure to radiation and to avoid exceeding the load rating of the microfocus. This is achieved by increasing the voltage by approximately 2 kV and eliminating the grid.
6. For magnification mammography, the grid is removed. This is necessary to limit the radiation dose to the breast and to reduce the exposure time, which otherwise might become very long (due to the increased dose required for magnification and due to the limited load rating of the small focus). To avoid motion blurring and the reciprocity law failure, the exposure time should not be too long. Removing the grid results in decreased radiation and shorter exposure time with less patient motion.
7. Scatter reduction, which improves contrast in magnification mammography, is achieved by the "air gap" combined with good collimation. The air gap itself allows reduction of scatter since part of the scattered radiation will pass beyond the film. Even though magnification without collimation is possible, good collimation significantly enhances the effect of the air gap. Only with good collimation (≤5 cm) can the lack of the grid be compensated by the air gap.

Advantages

- Improved resolution of fine details by overcoming blurring due to the screen–film system.
- Magnified details are easier to observe, i. e., there is more information on the film of the area imaged.
- When spot compression is used along with magnification, structures are less obscured by displacing the superimposed tissue.
- Dense areas representing summation of superimposed tissue can be differentiated from real findings (see also spot compression).

Disadvantages

- Magnification mammography increases the dose required, but this is largely compensated for by using a low-dose screen–film system, increasing the kVp, and eliminating the grid.
- Contrast could be decreased due to the lack of a grid and the higher kVp setting. This can largely be compensated for with good compression of the area of interest (pushing superimposed tissue aside) and good collimation (air gap reduces scattered radiation).

Indications

- Determining whether microcalcifications are present.
- Analyzing the geometry and distribution and of microcalcifications (Fig. 3.**25**).
- Detecting additional fine calcifications for improving the differential diagnosis of microcalcifications.
- Excluding or verifying the presence of multiple foci and assessing the extent of carcinomas with microcalcifications (Fig. 3.**26**).
- Analyzing the contours of masses, i. e., smooth, lobulated, spiculated (Fig. 3.**27**).
- Differentiating dense areas resulting from summation of superimposed structures from real masses (see also spot compression; Fig. 3.**22**).

Positioning of Breasts with Implants

Surgical technique and type and location of the implant determine the available mammographic imaging options. Following subcutaneous mastectomy and implant placement, usually only a small amount of tissue will remain around the implant. The distribution and architecture of the breast parenchyma can vary considerably. After augmentation mammoplasty, all of the breast tissue that was originally present will usually be superficial to the implant. Achieving good results in mammography depends upon the type of previous surgery and the type and position of implant material.

Standard mammography of these women usually requires manual exposure settings for those views that include the implants since the implant usually overlies the phototimer, attenuating the X-ray beam and causing the image to be overexposed.

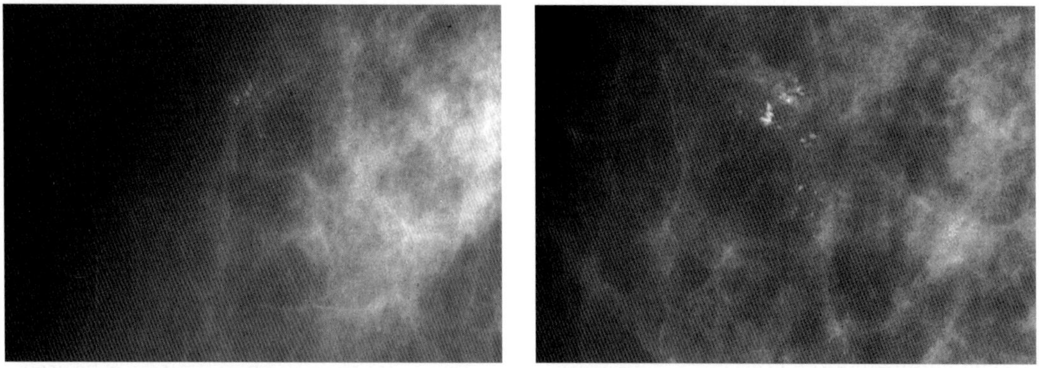

a b

Fig. 3.**25 a** and **b** The craniocaudal view shows a group of pleomorphic microcalcifications at the margin of the parenchyma (**a**). An additional magnification view (**b**) clearly reveals them to be suggestive of malignancy

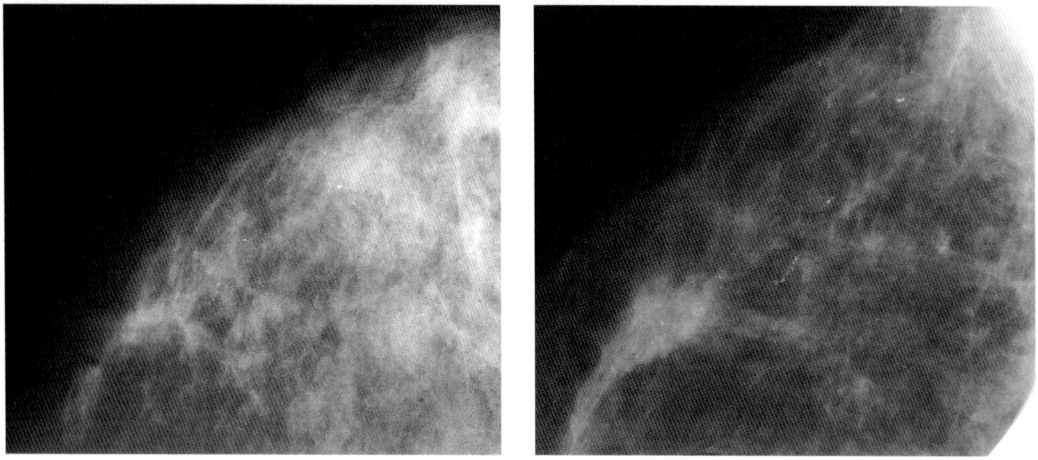

a b

Fig. 3.**26 a** and **b** The craniocaudal view reveals a focal density with ill-defined contour with central and marginal microcalcification (**a**). The magnification mammogram (**b**) with spot compression clearly demonstrates highly suspicious spiculations. In addition to the above mentioned suspicious microcalcifications, more pleomorphic microcalcifications are shown on this magnification view extending toward the nipple

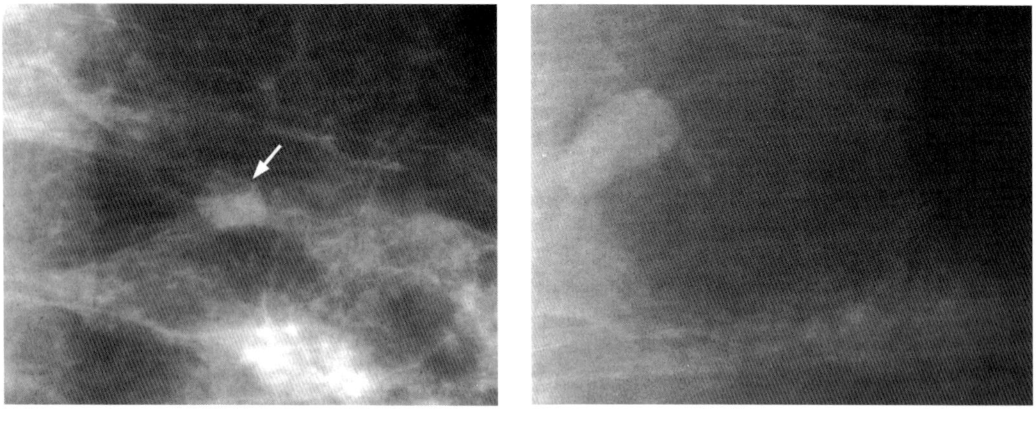

a b

The augmented breast should not be imaged as a screening study but always as a diagnostic mammogram. Full imaging of the augmented breast requires four views, not just the routine two views. MLO and CC views of the breasts, including the implant, are done to see tissue back to the chest wall and to image the implant. Compression used should be adequate to stabilize the breast so there is no motion on the image. Compression beyond this should not be used for fear of rupturing the implant. An additional two views should be performed according to the procedure described by Eklund:[66] pull the glandular tissue anteriorly away from the implant, push the implant posteriorly, and gradually slide the compression paddle over the breast tissue anterior to the implant. This pushes the implant posteriorly, allowing better compression of the glandular tissue itself (Fig. 3.**28**). Imaging should be done in the CC and the MLO or 90° lateral projections. It should be possible to obtain these displacement views in about 80% of women with implants. In those women who have hard, noncompressable implants (capsular contracture) or for whom the displacement maneuver is painful, it will not be possible to obtain these additional two views. Since these views are done with the implant out of the way, phototiming can be used.

Mammography as described by Eklund is generally no longer possible after subcutaneous

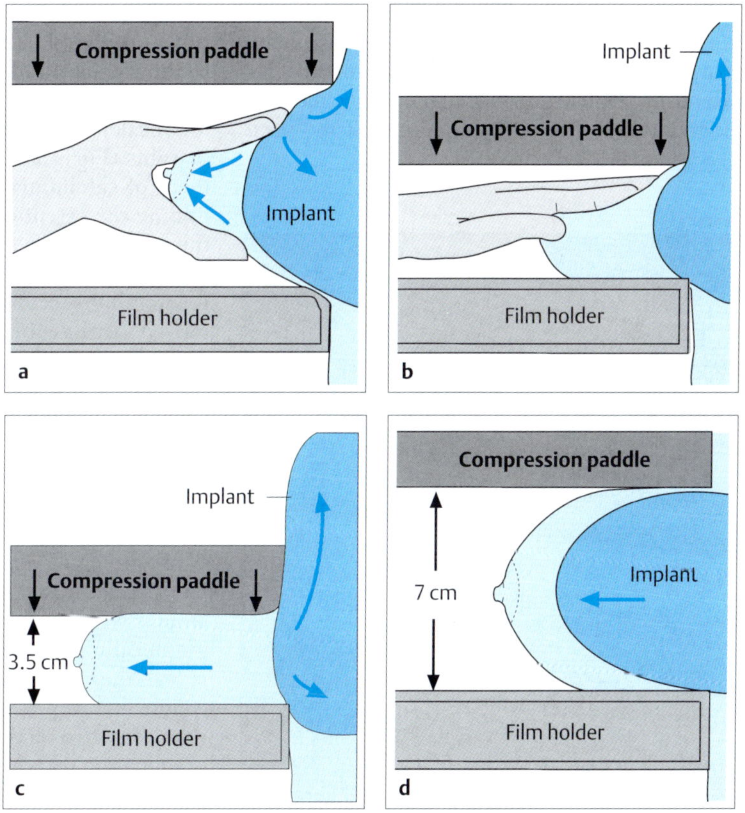

Fig. 3.**28 a–d** Eklund's method of imaging a breast with an implant following augmentation mammoplasty. The glandular tissue is pulled forward away from the implant, which is displaced posteriorly, as the technologist lowers the compression paddle over the breast tissue, and compresses it. This displaces the implant posteriorly so that it no longer covers the glandular tissue (as decribed by Eklund et al.[66])

Fig. 3.**27 a** and **b** The mediolateral oblique view shows an indeterminate mass measuring 7 mm located at the superior margin of the parenchyma (**a**). Spot compression reveals this to be a smooth-contoured lesion, compatible with a lymph node mastectomy and breast reconstruction. Mammography can still be performed to clarify clinical findings, but the radiologist should be aware that only the tissue layers tangential to the beam not obscured by the implant can be assessed. For this reason, mammography is usually performed in several planes, though it will not be possible to image all of the tissue surrounding the implant in these patients.

■ Specimen Radiography

Nonpalpable, mammographically confirmed lesions requiring excision must be localized preoperatively (see Chapter 7). After excision, specimen radiographs, i. e., radiographs of the surgical specimen, are obtained to verify whether it contains the mammographic findings leading to the excision, and to identify the location of the lesion in the specimen for histologic analysis. If the biopsied lesion is malignant and it extends to the margin of specimen, specimen radiography can also be used to suggest the need for further surgical excision. Specimen radiography can be performed using a mammography unit or a Faxitron, a tabletop X-ray unit designed for specimen radiography. If a mammography unit is used, manual settings instead of automatic exposure settings should be employed.

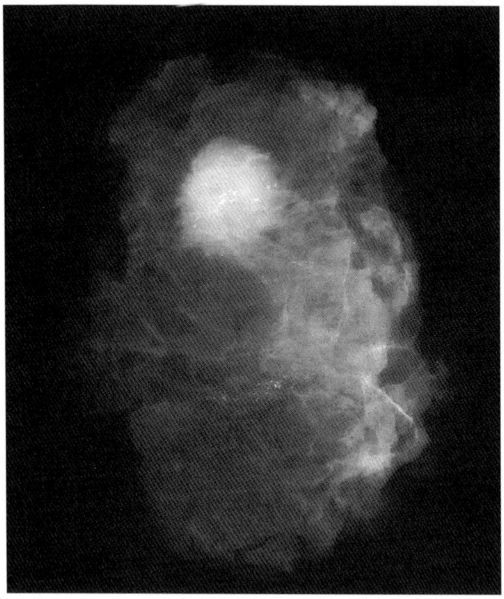

Fig. 3.**29** A magnification radiograph of a specimen clearly reveals not only the calcifications within the center of the tumor but two additional remote foci of microcalcifications

Histology: Highly fibrotic invasive ductal breast cancer measuring 17 mm; intraductal tumor is shown adjacent to the mass. Furthermore, another focal ductal carcinoma in situ was verified 15 mm distant from the invasive tumor

Compression of the specimen may improve the image, especially when the biopsy has been performed for an uncalcified mass. Compression equalizes differences in thickness, reduces scattered radiation and spreads out the overlying tissue.

A radiograph in a second plane may be necessary to localize small foci of disease or to determine if the lesion has been transsected during surgery. Areas in the specimen that require histologic analysis should be indicated for the pathologist so they will not be overlooked.

If microcalcifications are present, it is sometimes useful to include magnification in addition to the standard radiograph. This provides additional information about further extremely small microcalcifications and their relationship to the margins (Fig. 3.**29**). In breast-conserving treatment of carcinoma, this is important for determining the extent of tumor and its proximity to the margin of the excised specimen.

Assessment of an excised lesion may not be possible by specimen radiography for areas removed because of asymmetry or a density in dense tissue. A repeat mammogram shortly after surgery is useful to confirm that the area in question was biopsied.

Mammography may be performed in the early postoperative period without causing any undue pain. However, only compression sufficient to stabilize the breast should be used.

Radiologic examination of the paraffin blocks is indicated whenever histopathologic examination of a biopsy performed for mammographically detected microcalcifications fails to reveal these calcifications since standard procedure involves microscopic examination of only representative sections of the biopsy. Radiologic examination of the paraffin block will reveal whether microcalcifications are present in the part of the biopsy that was not examined under the microscope, or if the microcalcifications were not excised.

Quality Factors

Hardware Factors that Influence Image Quality

The ACR has recommended specifications for new mammography equipment.[30]

These requirements and other important hardware factors that influence image quality are summarized and discussed in the following section. More detailed information is available in the applicable literature.[24, 20, 67, 68]

Generator and Tube Power

Adequate generator or tube output is required to achieve sufficiently short exposure times, particularly for thick and dense breasts and for magnification mammography. Most quality mammography units achieve 4–5 kW.

The required power also depends on the target and filter material used. When tungsten and rhodium targets are used, the change in radiation quality is enough to penetrate even thick and dense breasts using less power than conventional molybdenum tubes and filters.

Insufficient power requires excessively long exposures times (>2 seconds) that result in motion bluring. Moreover, insufficient power disproportionately increases the exposure time and radiation dose required for adequate optical density (reciprocity law failure). If the automatic exposure control system is unable to compensate for this effect enough, then an underexposed image will result.

Before installing a mammography unit, it is advisable to check the electrical system on the premises for voltage fluctuations. Mammography units cannot compensate for voltage drops; fluctuations in radiation quality will result, even when settings remain constant.

Because of the need to keep voltage constant over time and, furthermore, because of the short exposure times required for low-dose film–screen systems, newer units are equipped with high-frequency generators.

Resolution

ACR requires measurement of a bar pattern 45 mm above the breast support surface of the unit, within 1 cm of the chest wall and centered laterally. At this point resolution should be 11 line-pairs/mm when the pattern is oriented with the bars perpendicular to the cathode–anode axis of the X-ray tube, and 13 line-pairs/mm when parallel to this axis.

Magnification Technique

Magnification mammography has become increasingly important. Studies have demonstrated that magnification mammography permits better analysis of microcalcifications, better visualization of the extent of carcinomas, and more reliable exclusion of malignancy. Most importantly, magnification mammography can reduce the number of unnecessary diagnostic biopsies. For this reason, breast imaging facilities, which are used for problem solving, must be able to perform magnification mammography. This requires an additional focus with a rated size less than or equal to 0.1–0.15 depending on the magnification factor, an insert for positioning the breast at a distance from the cassette, and a collimator. Magnification should be between 1.5–2.0×. Greater magnification may result in blurring due to long exposure times and increased geometric blurring. The dose also may become excessive.

Radiation Quality

The requirement that voltage must be regulated emphasizes the importance of radiation quality adapted to match the thickness and density of the breast.

The voltage settings required to achieve a certain desired radiation quality will vary depending on the mammography unit, target, filter, and generator, and thus are not necessarily comparable.

The ACR recommends that the X-ray source assembly include a molybdenum target, a beryllium window of 1.5 mm thickness or less, and a molybdenum filter. Alternate combinations can be used if they can achieve comparable diagnostic quality with equal or reduced radiation dose.

The newest mammography units offer a choice of various target/filter combinations to achieve the ideal radiation energy for the breast thickness and density to be penetrated. An autoselect mode is provided to aid in selecting the optimum parameter combination.

The distribution of calcifications should be described as:

- Grouped or clustered: occupying less than 2 cm^3 of breast volume
- Segmental: occupying more than 2 cm^3 but less than regional
- Regional: occupying a large volume of the breast, not in a ductal distribution, and not the entire breast
- Diffuse or scattered, distributed throughout the breast in a random fashion
- Linear, corresponding to a ductal pattern

Furthermore, a lobular distribution according to Lanyi[70] describes the presence of multiple punctate, generally round calcifications within a small area (2–3 mm). Such calcifications are usually located within the lobule and are arranged like a small morula or flower (rosette).

■ Associated Changes

These can be added to descriptions of masses or calcifications or can be used independently. They include:

- skin retraction
- skin thickening
- trabecular thickening
- nipple retraction
- axillary adenopathy
- architectural distortion
- increased vascularity

Additionally, the mammogram can show a diffuse increase in breast density. If previous studies are available, whether or not a finding represents an interval change, a new or increasing finding should be reported.

The final diagnosis should be categorized as:

- No pathologic findings, normal mammogram (BI-RADS category I)
- Focal benign findings for which nothing further is required (II)
- Indeterminate findings for which a short interval, e. g., 6-month, mammographic follow-up is recommended (III)
- Indeterminate lesion for which biopsy is recommended (IV)
- Highly suggestive of malignancy and requiring biopsy (V)

If the mammogram is normal or benign findings are diagnosed, a recommendation should be made regarding the interval for routine follow-up (1 or 2 years). Whenever the findings are indeterminate, the report should recommend either a follow-up examination for probably benign lesions (specifying the interval and examination method) or further diagnostic studies (sonography, MRI, additional views).

Any supplemental studies required should be specifically recommended. When a biopsy is indicated, this should be stated in the report. It should also be directly communicated to the referring physican and the patient. It is advisable to document this communication in the written report.

■ Interpreting and Documenting Screening Findings

To reduce costs and save time, screening findings can be documented in a brief form to facilitate computer processing. The following scale (such as the BIRADS scale recommended in the United States for documenting findings) should be used: 1 = no pathologic findings, 2 = benign, 3 = indeterminate probably benign, 4 = suggestive, and 5 = highly suggestive.

Categories 1 and 2 require only the standard follow-up examinations (in 1 or 2 years). Category 3 requires early follow-up examination (usually within 6 months). Category 4 means that a malignant process may be present and biopsy should be performed. Category 5 necessitates biopsy.

Cost–benefit analysis is an important factor in evaluating screening mammography. A positive biopsy rate of 1 in 10 (malignant to benign), (i. e., positive predictive value of a biopsy recommendation of 10%) involves many unnecessary biopsies, i. e., biopsies of benign findings, which represent unacceptable costs. The other extreme, a rate of 1 : 1 (100% malignancies among the recommended biopsies), involves a significant risk of overlooking carcinomas, which would result in a high incidence of interval carcinomas because many indeterminate lesions, some of which are cancers, are not being sent for biopsy.

Screening involves more than documenting findings. It also requires documentation and evaluation of histologic results, of interval carcinomas and critical assessment of the positive predictive value, which should be in the 25–40% range, and of the accepted rate of so-called interval carcinomas. To assure that small cancers are appropriately diagnosed and not just large cancers for which diagnosis will not change the outcome, cancers diagnosed in a screening population should consist of more than 50% of diagnosed cancers as DCIS or invasive cancers ≤ 1 cm and less than 25% lymph node positive cancers.[71]

Example Reports

The asymptomatic patient: Compared to the previous examination of (date), the glandular tissue remains dense and nodular without evidence of focal lesions, calcifications, or structural changes.

Diagnosis: No mammographic evidence of malignancy. Follow-up examination in 1 year is recommended.

The patient with palpable findings: Corresponding to the palpable lesions is an ill-defined mass measuring 18 mm with pleomorphic microcalcifications in the left upper outer quadrant in the 2 o'clock axis in the mid-third of the breast. No associated findings.

Diagnosis: Highly suspicious mammographic findings corresponding to the palpable findings. Biopsy is required.

Another patient with a palpable mass: Dense and nodular parenchyma. Mammographic assessment is limited. Additional ultrasound examination of the suspected mass is required for further evaluation.

Digital Mammography

Detection and diagnosis of breast disease with mammography is possible because of its ability to resolve and image fine structures with only slight differences in density. Conventional mammography uses steeply graded films that produce high-contrast details. The disadvantage of such films is that they only can visualize a limited dynamic range (a maximum of about 1 : 50) and are sensitive to overexposure and underexposure. This is particularly limiting in dense breasts.

In digital mammography, images are recorded and reproduced in separate processes that can be independently optimized. For recording images, the exposure range (dynamic range) should be as wide as possible and have a linear curve so as to eliminate underexposed and overexposed images. One example of such an image recording system is a phosphor storage screen, which can record an exposure range of about 1 : 40 000. With suitable postprocessing and windowing techniques, the image data can be processed so that all areas of the image are shown with optimum contrast when the image is recorded on a laser film.

In addition to current research into improvement of storage phosphor screens, other technical approaches are being developed. These include solid state image recorders (CCD sensors), which convert the optically minified image of a phosphor screen into an electric signal. Since the field of view that can be achieved with such a system is currently only 5 × 5 cm, this technique is limited to stereotaxic applications. Better resolution can be attained using this technique than with storage phosphor screens. Latest research concerns the development of CCD-arrays that will allow visualization of the complete breast.

Furthermore, systems are being developed that use selenium as an image intensifier. This material was applied in xeromammography. In contrast to toner development, digital systems electronically read the stored image to achieve high sensitivity and image quality. Systems employing this technology are already available for chest radiography. Units for diagnostic, full breast digital mammography should be commercially available in the near future.

Although both can be labelled as digital imaging, there is a difference between digital mammography involving digital acquisition and storage of information and techniques for subsequent digitization of conventional mammographic images. The brightness and contrast of this secondary digitalized image can be processed, and the image can be stored and undergo digital postprocessing. However, its information content is no higher than the original screen–film mammogram.

Frequently cited advantages of digital mammography include:

- Minimizing repeat images due to poor radiographic technique
- Digital storage

- Digital data transfer
- Computer-assisted image interpretation
- Rapid availability of the image for interpretation
- No need for cassettes, dark room, processor, and film

Due to still significant limitations of the existing monitors and due to their limited availability, however, even digital images are presently read from points and are often taken with different window settings. Therefore film and processing have so far not been replaced as initially expected.

Given the greater dynamic range, repeat exposures are usually not required even in situations that would have been difficult in conventional mammography. Moreover, appropriate image postprocessing can visualize high-density parenchymal areas with high contrast, which is particularly important in detecting microcalcifications in this tissue. However, the spatial resolution with some systems may not be sufficient for analyzing their shape and for resolution of very fine mircocalcifications.

Obvious advantages of digital mammography include the time and spacc saved in archiving and retrieving digital mammograms. The possibilities for digital data transfer (for example in resident training and continued education) could open up a number of opportunities in the future.

Computer-assisted image interpretation might in the future assist the physician in detecting pathology. Diagnostic systems with high sensitivity can aid the physician's eye by preselecting suggestive areas. Such programs have already been used to detect microcalcifications. At present, efforts are focusing on expanding the process to include focal densities and parenchymal changes. However, differential diagnosis will remain the responsibility of the physician for the foreseeable future.

Summary

Digital mammography appears particularly promising for the future. At present, however, screen–film mammography is still superior to available digital techniques, particularly digital luminescence radiography, in clarity of detail. The limiting factor here is both the limited spatial resolution in line pairs per millimeter and the increased radiographic noise of the storage phosphor screens. It is expected that detectors with an improved signal-to-noise ratio and a reduced pixel size (about 50 μm) that achieve the clarity of detail of screen–film systems will become available in the future.

Appendix

Further possibilities for improving existing technology currently under research include:

- **Magnification mammography** in combination with digital technology. It is hoped that the increased dynamic range will permit sufficient dose reduction to overcome limitations of the receptor system by use of magnification technique. The issue of feasibility must still be addressed.
- **Microfocus mammography:** Electronic focusing now visualizes extremely small foci. This may be of interest for spot compression with magnification and if routine mammography is combined with a magnification technique, which allows one to achieve higher resolution and overcome limitations of the image receptor. Of course, this means adjusting all factors influencing resolution. At present, the reduced output of the microfocus requires longer exposure times, which appear to be a limiting factor for making this technique suitable for standard mammography.
- **Slit mammography:** This technique produces an image by exposing only part of the breast through a slit. The image is read behind the breast by an image receptor collimated to the slit. Scanning the breast from right to left with this slit reduces scattered radiation and eliminates the increased dose that compensates for the absorption of a grid.

Galactography

■ Definition

Galactography refers to the examination of lactiferous ducts using a contrast medium.

Injecting a water-soluble contrast medium permits mammographic imaging of the lactiferous duct system belonging to the excretory duct into which the needle is introduced. After the duct is filled with contrast medium, the breast is imaged in the craniocaudal and mediolateral planes. Oblique views or magnification mammograms may also be required. Galactography should only be performed in the presence of pathologic secretion, which itself makes it possible to detect the opening of the excretory duct. Absence of secretion precludes any ductal probing.

■ Indications

Galactography is indicated for the workup of pathologic discharge.

Pathologic discharge includes:

- Spontaneous, nonmilky discharge (clear serous, cloudy, or brownish green) from a single or several ducts, usually unilateral. This does not include discharge that is expressed under firm pressure, since such a discharge can be provoked in many women.
- Bloody discharge.
- Discharge with suggestive, cytologic findings (Groups IV or V).

Galactography is not indicated in the presence of:

- Galactorrhea, i. e., milky discharge that is not due to pregnancy or breast feeding. Galactorrhea is always a sequelae of primary and/or secondary hyperprolactinemia and may occur bilaterally or unilaterally.
- Bilateral, bloodless discharge from multiple ducts (serous or brownish green) without cytologic abnormality. This too can be the result of hormonal imbalance or duct ectasia with chronic inflammation.

■ Contraindications

Galactography is contraindicated in the presence of inflammation, which can exacerbate the process.

Hypersensitivity to contrast medium is a relative contraindication. The indication should be reviewed and the galactography only performed when clearly indicated and appropriate precautionary measures are taken (adrenaline, antihistamines, corticosteroids, or anesthesia standby). The physician may also consider intraoperative probing of the duct or, after injecting methylene blue, excision of the lactiferous duct without galactography.

■ Side Effects

Since a pathologic discharge is usually associated with duct ectasia, galactography can lead to *galactophoritis* or mastitis. This has only be observed in rare cases since the introduction of water-soluble contrast media.

Allergic reactions to contrast media are rare with galactography. Prophylactic antihistamine therapy may be considered in patients with known allergies to contrast media. Furthermore, the indication should be checked and appropriate precautionary measures taken (see previous section).

If a mild, acute reaction occurs, it can be treated with antihistamines. Severe reactions should be treated with intravenous cortisone and, in applicable cases, intravenous epinephrine, as with other contrast reactions.

If the injection pressure is too high or if too much contrast medium has been instilled, extravasation of contrast medium can occur, with contrast medium seen outside the duct system in breast parenchyma. In this setting lymphatic vessels may be imaged. The patient will usually perceive this as *pain*, although this has no serious effects other than insufficient or obscured visualization. The galactogram needs to be terminated, if this occurs. Contrast medium will be reabsorbed and the procedure can be repeated after a few days.

■ Procedure

Comfortable patient positioning and good lighting are important for this procedure. A magnifying lens or an eyepiece mounted on an eyeglass frame can be helpful in locating the excretory duct.

- Cytologic smears of the discharge may be taken before galactography.

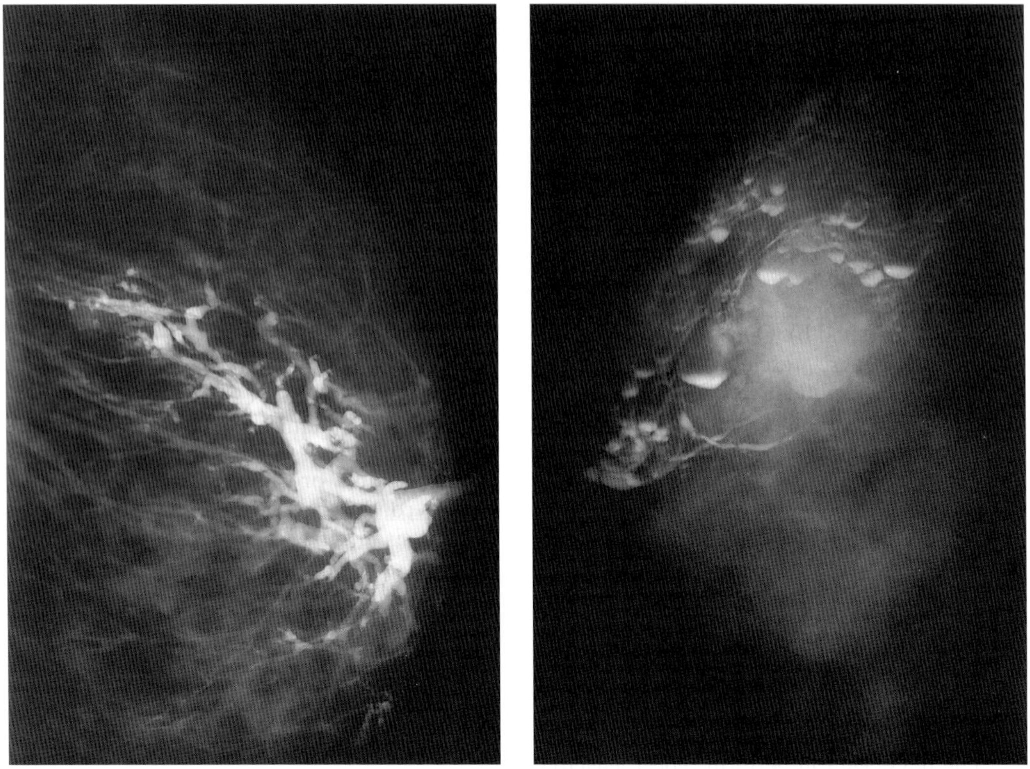

a b

Fig. 3.**34 a** and **b**
a Duct ectasia. No evidence of an intraductal mass
b Duct ectasia with multiple cystic distensions

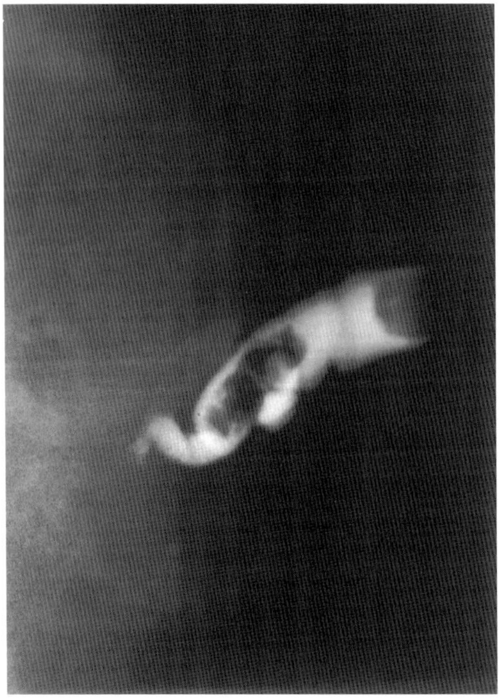

Fig. 3.**35 a** and **b**
a Intraductal masses lead to isolated or multiple filling defects, i. e., the contrast medium flows around the intraductal mass in an arc-shaped pattern
b Multiple round filling defects in a distended lactiferous duct, histologically confirmed papillomatosis. The small, smooth-contoured, focal lesion in the parenchyma also corresponds to a papilloma

Fig. 3.**35 b**

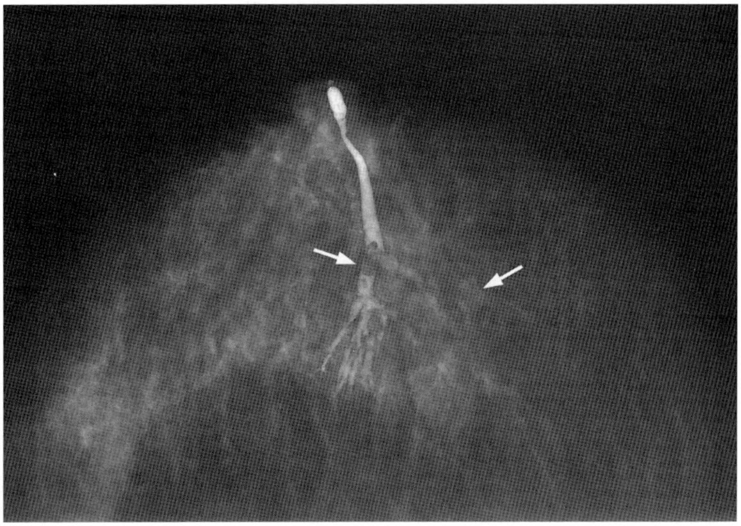

■ Appendix: Sonographic Imaging of Lactiferous Ducts

Initial work has been done in using high-frequency ultrasound transducers in diagnosing intraductal masses. The higher resolution permits better sonographic imaging of ducts, particularly those located close to the nipple, than before. Sometimes it is possible to detect even small intraductal masses (Figs. 3.**36**–3.**40 a** and **b**). However, since sonography as a cross-sectional imaging modality cannot reliably visualize every segment of a winding duct and since it will not allow the necessary overview of the complete tree of a secreting ductal system, it cannot replace galactography.

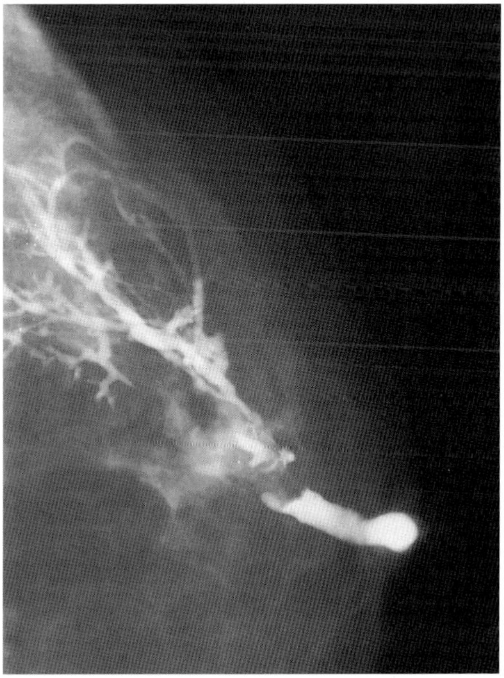

Fig. 3.**36** Where an intraductal mass completely blocks the respective lactiferous duct, the galactogram will show a filling defect with partial truncation of the duct

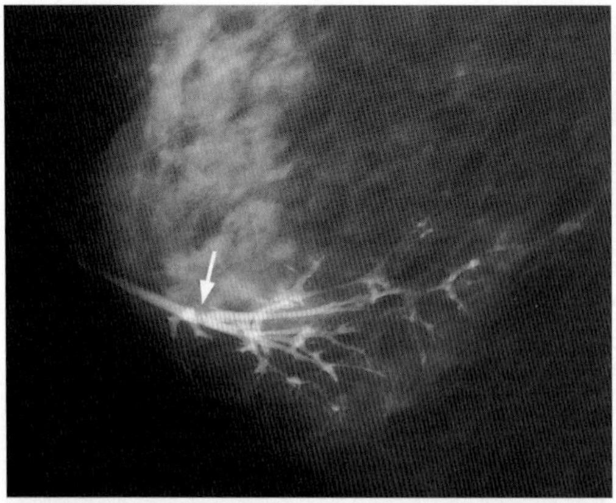
a

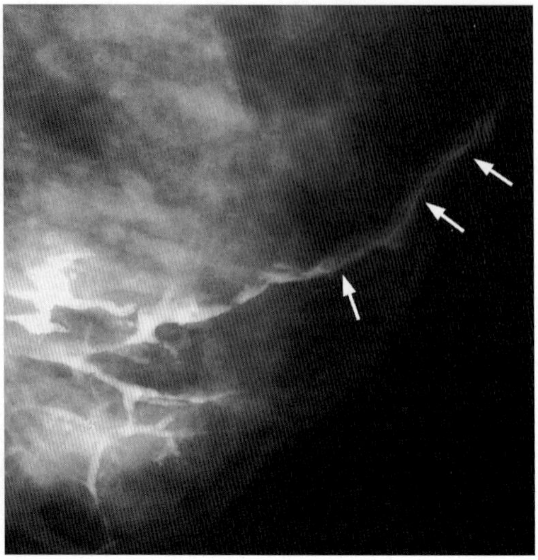
b

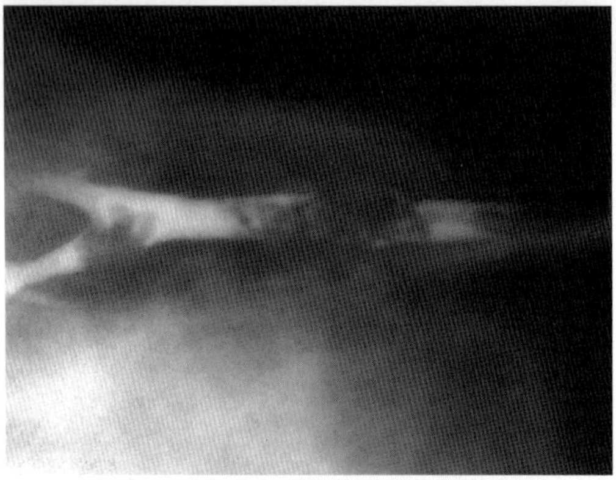
c

Fig. 3.**37 a–c** Various intraductal processes are shown
a Marginal filling defects that interrupt the contour of the wall: ductal carcinoma in situ (DCIS)
b Tiny round filling defects arranged like a string of beads in a main excretory duct: DCIS
c Multiple irregular filling defects with loss of the contour of the wall: papillomatosis in transition to an invasive carcinoma

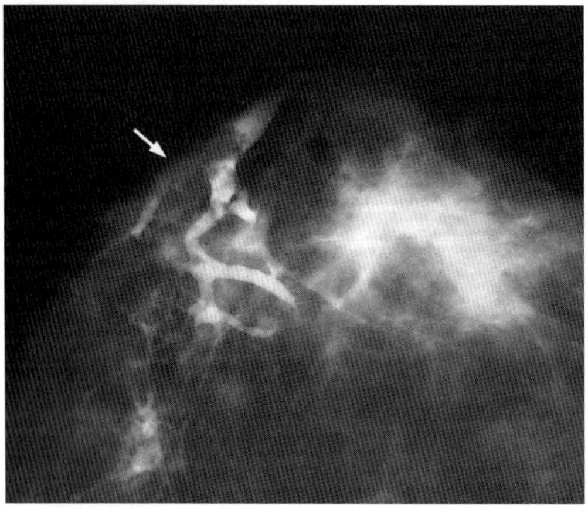

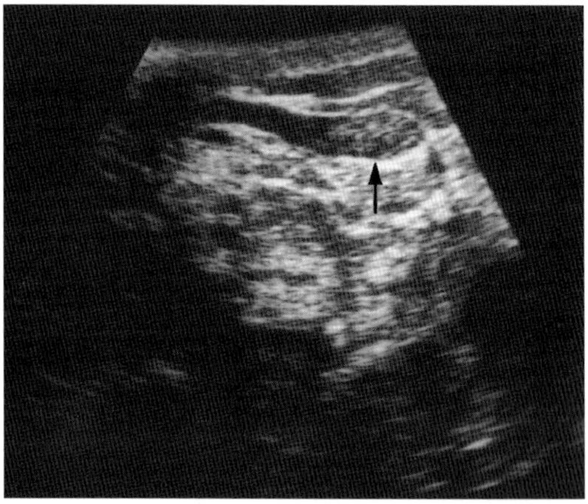

Fig. 3.**38 a** and **b**
a Lobulated filling defect in an ectatic lactiferous duct: papillomatosis

b Good sonographic image (13.5-MHz technique) of a distended duct containing a tiny hyperechoic mass

Fig. 3.**39** Extravasation of constrast medium (short ▷ arrow) and several fine winding lymph vessels (long arrow)

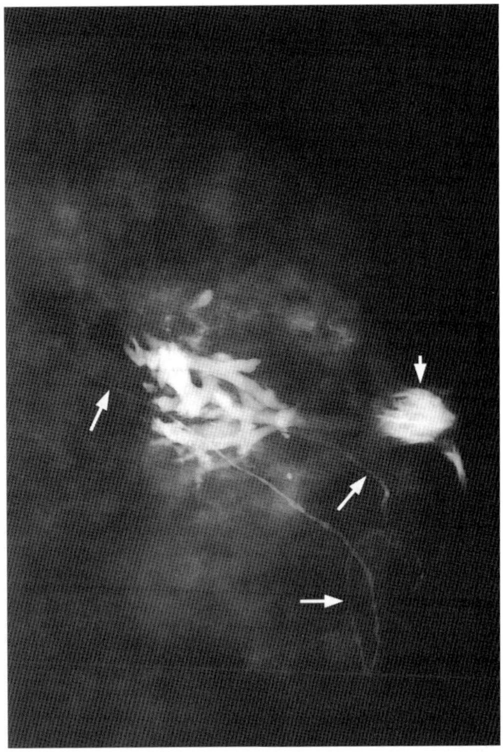

Fig. 3.**40 a** and **b**
a Lobulated focal density in the superior half of the breast was normal sonographically
b Galactography revealed this to be a small convoluted cyst. Air bubbles in the lactiferous duct system can be identified by their uniform round shape and their varying localization on several views. On the mediolateral view, they can be identified by their localization along the superior wall of the ducts (arrow). Leakage of contrast is seen in the inferior aspect of the breast
▽

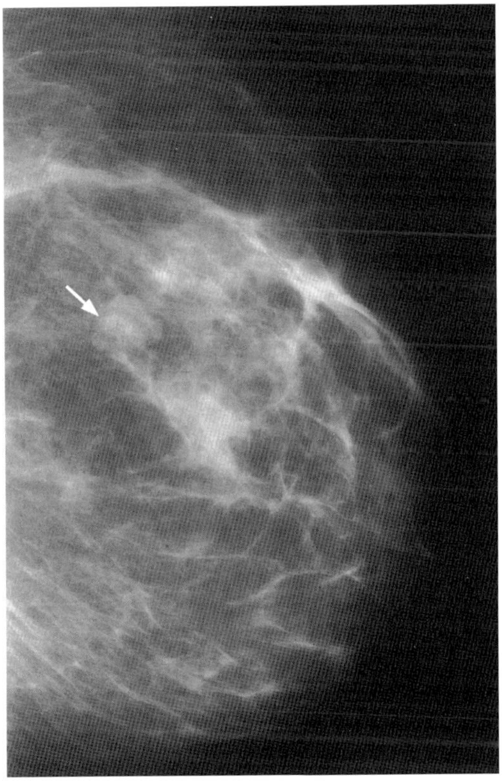

a

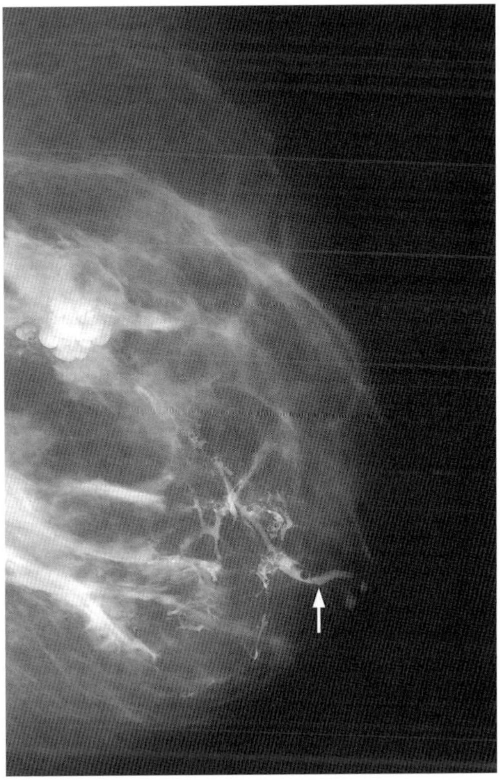

b

Pneumocystography

■ Definition

Pneumocystography refers to mammographic imaging of an aspirated cyst that has been filled with air. It has been used to diagnose and to treat cysts, i. e., bring about its involution.

■ Indications

As indications for pneumocystography decrease, some investigators apply it for treatment of *symptomatic cysts*. Since large cysts can cause a sensation of pressure and pain, decompressing the cyst will relieve these symptoms.

With increasing capabilities of ultrasound, the application of pneumocystography for workup of *sonographic findings that are suspicious but inconclusive for cysts* decreases (uncertain differentiation between hyperechoic debris in the cyst, intracystic mass, and a hypoechoic solid mass). If a solid mass is suspected, core biopsy or excisional biopsy are indicated instead.

■ No Indications

- Cysts with sonographically detected *irregularities in their walls* or intracystic masses. For these cases, pneumocystography has been replaced by biopsy.
  Aspirating a cyst containing a small intracystic mass can even be detrimental since surgery may become impossible if the mass is no longer palpable or visible in mammographic and sonographic images after aspiration and air absorption. However, this sort of complicated cyst will generally fill again if a papilloma or carcinoma is actually present, and the cyst will then again become visible for preoperative marking (possibly even palpable) in about 2 to 4 weeks.
- Unequivocal sonographic diagnosis of *asymptomatic* cysts. These cysts need no further assessment.

■ Contraindications

- Acute inflammation.
- Coagulopathies or anticoagulant therapy.

■ Side Effects

- Puncturing the skin is only slightly painful. Puncturing a hardened, chronically inflamed cyst wall may be painful. Filling the cyst with air sometimes causes painful tension in the breast.
- Inflammatory reaction after aspiration is extremely rare when the skin has been properly disinfected and sterile procedure has been observed.
- Hematomas due to injury of a vascular structure are rare but possible. The indication must be carefully checked in patients with coagulatory disorders or on anticoagulant therapy or aspirin.
- Pneumothorax has been observed in very rare cases in which the pleura was perforated while attempting to aspirate a deep cyst. For this reason, the needle should always be introduced parallel to the chest wall and never perpendicular to it. Perform the aspiration under sonographic guidance.

■ Procedure

- Palpable lumps can be aspirated without guidance.
- Aspiration under sonographic guidance is recommended for nonpalpable or confluent cysts. Aspiration under sonographic guidance is generally performed with the patient supine. In some cases with large palpable cysts, it is also possible to aspirate the cyst while the patient is seated. The fluid will collect at the bottom of the cyst and thus can be completely aspirated.
- Aspirate after disinfecting the skin. Select a needle that is not too thin (a 20-gauge needle will usually be sufficient) since the contents of the cyst may vary in viscosity.
- Empty the cyst completely. With the needle still in place, attach a new syringe and insufflate the cyst with a slightly smaller volume of air than the volume of fluid that was removed (note that the air will expand at body temperature).

In the presence of large septated cysts, pressing the cyst in the final phases of aspiration will facilitate emptying. When doing so, the needle should not be dislocated to avoid perforating the opposite wall with the needle outside the cyst during subsequent insufflation. The contents of the cyst can be clear and serous, or it can be greenish, brownish, black, or cloudy, or tinged with blood following aspiration. If the cyst contains older blood (as opposed to fresh blood from an iatrogenic injury), excision should be considered to determine its cause.

- The rarely performed diagnostic pneumocystography (to differentiate between intracystic debris or masses, which is only used in sonographically inconclusive studies) should be performed in two imaging planes since smaller wall irregularities may not be visible when projected en face.

The lateral view is sufficient for therapeutic pneumocystography since absence of an air–fluid level confirms that the cyst is completely empty.

■ Findings

When the cyst is completely empty, it will appear as a well-circumscribed round or lobulated, thin-walled transparency (Figs. 3.**41 a–c**). Air inadvertently injected into the parenchyma will appear as transparent strips or bubbles of varying length on the mammogram (Fig. 3.**42**).

If the cyst is not completely empty, an air–fluid level may be visible (Fig. 3.**43**) or foam may appear showing up as multiple transparent bubbles. While this is not a pathologic sign, it may interfere with the diagnostic process.

Pneumocystography cannot reliably distinguish between benign and malignant intracystic masses. Overall, intracystic carcinomas are less frequent than papillomas. Like papillomas, they mammographically project into the lumen of the insufflated cyst (see Chapter 10).

Any suspicious intracystic mass is an indication for biopsy. Negative cytologic examination of the aspirated fluid should not prevent biopsy because false negative results are possible in the presence of necrotic material.

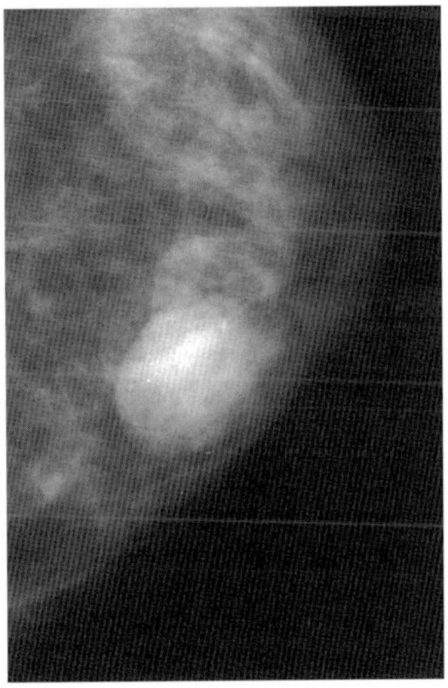

a

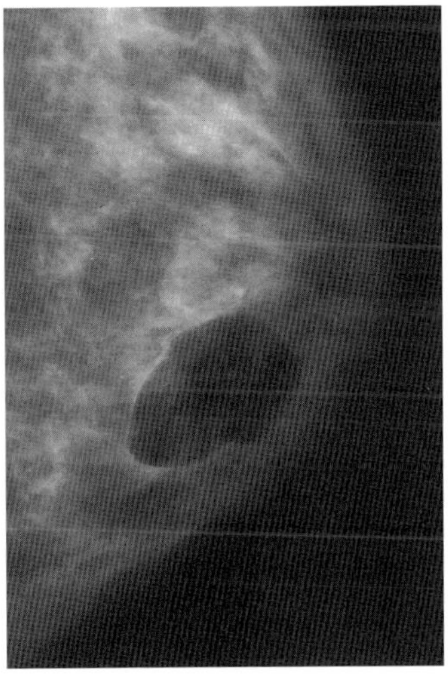

b

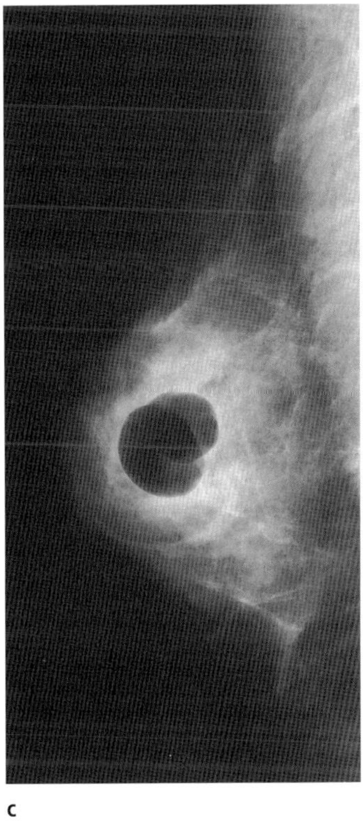

c

Fig. 3.**41 a–c**
a Mammography: Oval focal lesion with a halo, in the inferior half of the breast
b Pneumocystography: After aspiration and air insufflation, an oval, lobulated bright area with a faint halo is visible
c Pneumocystography of two communicating cysts

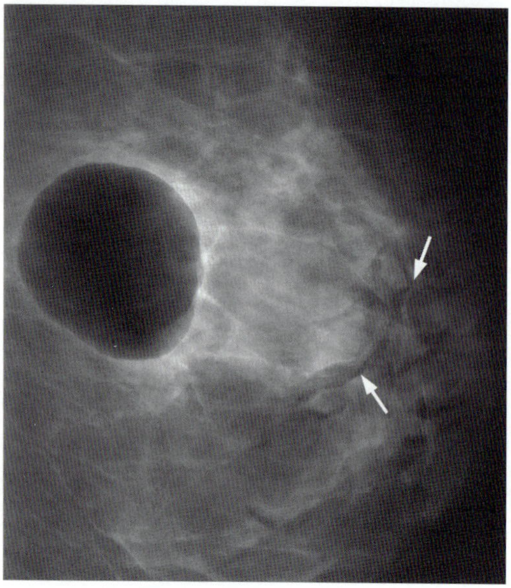

Fig. 3.**42** Curvilinear radiolucencies (arrow) in the parenchyma after pneumocystography, caused by caused by interstitial air

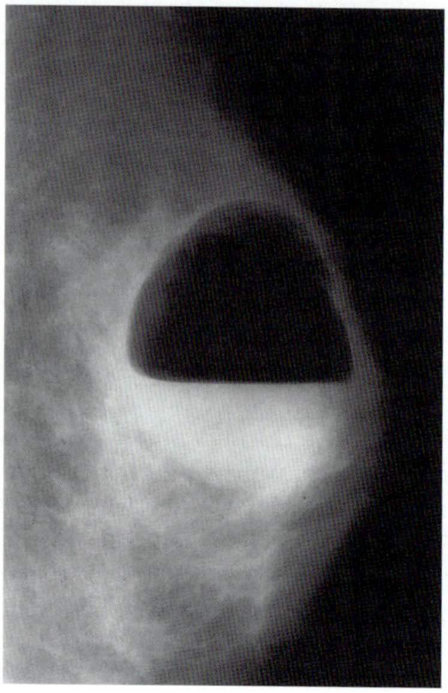

Fig. 3.**43** An air–fluid level is visible in the cyst that has not been completely emptied

Summary

If applied diagnostically, pneumocystography is used to verify the diagnosis of a cyst by aspirating it in the rare case of sonographically inconclusive findings. It may sometimes be used to decompress a painful cyst.

The introduction of air is believed by some to prevent refilling of the cyst by facilitating shrinkage of the cyst walls. If pneumocystography shows no pathologic findings, standard follow-up examinations will be sufficient.

When bloody fluid is aspirated from the cyst yet cytologic results are negative and pneumocystography shows no pathologic findings, a short interval (e. g., 3 months) follow-up sonographic examination may be desirable.

References

1 Kopans DB. Mammography screening for breast cancer. Cancer. 1993;72:1809

2 Moskowitz M. Restructured data comparing screening approaches. Radiology. 1980;134:262

3 Bird RE, Wallace TW, Yankaskas BC. Analysis of cancers missed at screening mammography. Radiology. 1992;184:613

4 Van Dijck JAAM, Verbeek ALM, Hendricks JHCL, Holland R. The current detectability of breast cancer in a mammographic screening programm. Cancer. 1993;72:1933

5 Sickles EA, Ominski SH, Sollitto RA et al. Medical audit of a rapid throughput mammography screening practice: methodology and results of 27 114 examinations. Radiology. 1990;175:323

6 Homer MJ. Breast imaging: pitfalls, controversies and some practical thoughts. Radiol Clin North Am. 1985;23:459

7 Page DL, Winfield AC. The dense mammogram. AJR. 1986;147:487

8 D'Orsi CJ. To follow or not to follow, that is the question. Radiology. 1992;184:306

9 Knutzen AM, Gisvold JJ. Likelihood of malignant disease for various categories of mammographically detected nonpalpable breast lesions. Radiology. 1993;189:927

10 Bjurstam N. Early carcinoma: the great mimick. Report of the Nicer Breast Imaging Course, Scandinavian Society of Mammography, August 24-28, 1994

11 Meyer J, Timothy J, Stomper P, Sonnenfield M. Biopsy of occult breast lesions: analysis of 1261 abnormalities. JAMA. 1990;263:2341

12 Moskowitz M. The predictive value of certain mammographic signs in screening for breast cancer. Cancer. 1983;51:1007
13 Sickles EA. Mammographic features of 300 consecutive nonpalpable breast cancers. AJR. 1986;146:661
14 Rubin E. Critical pathways in the analysis of breast masses. Radiographics. 1995; 15:925
15 Dershaw DD, Eddens G, Liberman L, Deutch BM, Abramson AF. Sonographic and clinical findings in women with palpable breast disease and negative mammography. Breast Dis. 1995;8:13–17
16 Boyd NF, Jong RA, Yaffe MJ et al. Critical appraisal of the Canadian National Breast Cancer Screening Study. Radiology. 1993;189:661
17 Aichinger H, Dierker J, Säbel M, Joite-Barfuß S. Bildqualität und Dosis in der Mammographie. Electromedica. 1994;62:7
18 Küchler A, Friedrich M. Fortschritte in der Mammographiethechnik – Bimetall-Anodenröhre und selektive Filtertechnik. Fortschr Rontgenstr. 1993;159:91
19 Christensen EE, Curry TS, Dowdey JE. An introduction to the physics of diagnostic radiology. Philadelphia: Lea Febinger 1978
20 Kimme-Smith C, Bassett LW, Gold RH. Workbook for quality mammography. Williams & Wilkins: Baltimore; 1992
21 Barnes GT, Brezovich IA. Contrast: effect of scattered radiation. In: Logan W W, Muntz EP eds. Reduced dose mammography. New York; Masson: 1979
22 Teubner J, Lenk JZ, Wentz KV, Georgi M. Vergrößerungsmammographie mit 0,1 mm Mikrofokus. Radiologe. 1987;21:155
23 Ranallo FN. Physics of screen–film mammography. In: Peters ME, Voegeli DR, Scanlan KA, eds. Handbook of breast imaging. New York: Churchill Livingstone; 1989:25
24 Friedrich M. Technik und Ergebnisse der Mammographie. Radiologe. 1993;33:243
25 Frederick EE, Squillante MR, Cirignano LJ et al. Accurate automatic exposure controller for mammography: design and performance. Radiology. 1991;178:393
26 McKinney WE. Radiographic processing and quality control. Philadelphia: JB Lippincott; 1988
27 Yaffe MJ. Physics of mammography: image recording process. Radiographics. 1990;10:341
28 Kimme-Smith C, Rothschild PA, Bassett LW et al. Mammography film processor temperature, development time and chemistry; effect on dose, contrast and noise. AJR. 1989;152:35
29 Haus AG. Effects of geometric unsharpness in mammography and breast xeroradiography. In: Logan WW, Muntz WW, eds. Reduced dose mammography: New York: Massone; 1979
30 American College of Radiology. Recommended specifications for new mammography equipment. Screen-film x-ray systems, image receptors and film processors. Reston: American College of Radiology; 1995
31 Aichinger H, Joite-Barfuß S, Marhoff P. Die Belichtungsautomatik in der Mammographie. Electromedica. 1990;58:61
32 Barnes GT. Mammography equipment: compression, scatter control and automatic exposure control. In: Haus AG, Yaffe MJ, eds. Syllabus: A categorical course in physics: Technical aspects of breast imaging, 3rd ed. Oak Brook: RSNA Publications; 1994:75
33 Friedrich M. Neue Entwicklungstendenzen der Mammographietechnik: Die Rastermammographie. Fortschr Rontgenstr. 1978;128:207
34 Dershaw DD, Masterson ME, Malik S, Cruz NM. Mammography using an ultrahigh stripdensity, stationary, focused grid. Radiology. 1985;156:541–544
35 Barnes GT, Moreland RF, Yester MV, Witten DM. The scanning grid: a novel and effective bucky movement. Radiology. 1980;135:765
36 Laubenberger T. Technik der medizinischen Radiologie. 6. Aufl. Köln: Dt Ärzteverlag; 1990
37 Yaffe MJ. Digital mammography. In: Haus AG, Yaffe MJ, eds. Syllabus: A categorical course in physics. Technical aspects of breast imaging. Oak Brook: RSNA Publications 1994:275
38 Baral E, Larrson LE, Mattson B. Breast cancer following irradiation of the breast. Cancer. 1977;40:2905–10
39 Boice JD, Land CE, Shore RE, Norman JE, Tokunaga M. Risk of breast cancer following low-dose radiation exposure. Radiology. 1979;131:589–97
40 Howe GR, Miller AB, Shermann GJ. Breast cancer mortality following fluoroscopic irradiation in a cohort of tuberculosis patients. Cancer Detect Prev. 1982;5:175–8
41 Howe GR. Epidemiology of radiogenic breast cancer. In: Boice JD, Fraumeni JF, eds. Radiation carcinogenesis: epidemiology and biological dignificance. New York: Raven; 1984:119–30
42 Hrubec Z, Boice JD, Monson RR, Rosenstein R. Breast cancer after multiple chest fluoroscopies: second follow-up of Massachusetts women with tuberculosis. Cancer Res. 1989;49:229–34
43 Mettler FA, Hempelmann LH, Dutton AM, Pofer JW, Toyooka ET, Ames WR. Breast neoplasms in women treated with x-rays for acute postpartum mastitis: a pilot study. J Natl Cancer Inst. 1969;43:803–11
44 Miller AB, Howe GR, Sherman, GJ et al. Mortality from breast cancer after irradiation during fluoroscopic examinations in patients being treated for tuberculosis. N Engl J Med. 1989;321:1285–9
45 Shore RE, Hempelmann LH, Kowaluki E et al. Breast neoplasms in women treated with x-rays for acute postpartum mastitis. J Natl Cancer Inst. 1977;59:813–22
46 Shore RE, Hildreth N, Woodard ED, Dvoretsky P, Hempelmann L, Pasternack B. Breast cancer among women given x-ray therapy for acute postpartum mastitis. J Natl Cancer Inst. 1986;77:689–96
47 Kato H, Schull WJ. Studies of the mortality of A-bomb survivors. 7. Mortality, 1950–1978: I. Cancer mortality. Radiat Res. 1982;90:395–432
48 McGregor DH, Land CE, Choi K et al. Breast cancer incidence among atomic bomb survivors, Hiroshima and Nagasaki, 1950–1969. J Natl Cancer Inst. 1977;59:799–811
49 Preston DL, Kato H, Kopecky KJ, Fujita S. Studies of the mortality of A-bomb survivors. 8. Cancer mortality, 1950–1982. Radiat Res. 1987;111:151–78
50 Preston DL, Pierce DA. The effect of changes in dosimetry on cancer mortality risk estimates in atomic bomb survivors. Radiat Res. 1988;114:437–66
51 Shimizu Y, Kato H, Schull WJ. Life span study report 11. II. Cancer mortality in the years 1950–1985 based on the recently revised doses (DS86): Radiation Effects Research Foundation Treatise 5–88. Hiroshima: Radiation Effects Research Foundation; 1988
52 Shimizu Y, Kato H, Schull WJ, Preston DL, Fujita S, Pierce DA. Studies of the mortality of A-bomb survivors. 9. Mortality, 1950–1985: I. Comparison of risk coefficients for site-specific cancer mortality based on DS86 and T65 DR shielded kerma and organ doses. Radiat Res. 1989;118:502–24
53 Tokunaga M, Norman JE, Asano M. Malignant breast

tumors among atomic bomb survivors, Hiroshima and Nagasaki, 1950–1974. J Natl Cancer Inst. 1979;62:1347–59

54 Tokunaga M, Land CE, Yamamoto T et al. Breast cancer among atomic bomb survivors. In: Boice JD, Fraumeni JF, eds. Radiation carcinogenesis: epidemiology and biological significance. New York: Raven; 1984:45–56

55 Tokunaga M, Land CE, Yamamoto T et al. Incidence of female breast cancer among atomic bomb survivors, Hiroshima and Nagasaki, 1950–1980. Radiat Res. 1987;112:243–72

56 Feig SA, Ehrlich SM. Estimation of radiation risk from screening mammography: recent trends and comparison with expected benefits. Radiology. 1990;174;638–47

57 Kopans DB. Breast imaging. Philadelphia: JB Lippincott; 1989

58 Tabar L, Dean PB. Optimum mammography technique: the annotate cookbook approach. Admin Radiol. 1989;54

59 Bassett LW, Bunnell D, Jahanshahi R et al. Breast cancer detection: one versus two views. Radiology. 1987;165:95

60 Muir BB, Kirkpatrick A, Roberts MM, Duffy SW. Oblique view mammography: adequacy for screening. Radiology. 1984;151:39

61 Eklund GW, Cardenosa G. The art of mammographic positioning. Radiol Clin North Am. 1992; 30:21

62 Logan WW, Janus J. Use of special mammographic views to maximize radiographic information. Radiol Clin North Am. 1987;25:953

63 Sickles EA. Practical solutions to common mammographic problems: tailoring the examination. AJR. 1988; 151:31

64 Berkowitz JE, Gatedwood OMB, Gayler BW. Equivocal mammographic findings: evaluation with spot compression. Radiology. 1989;171:369

65 Sickles EA. Magnification mammography. In: Basett LW, Gold RH, eds. Breast cancer detecion: Mammography and other methods in breast imaging. Orlando: Grune & Stratton; 1987:111

66 Eklund GW, Busby RC, Miller SH et al. Improved imaging of the augmented breast. AJR. 1988; 151:469

67 Strauss KJ, Rossi RP. Specification, acceptance testing and quality control of mammography imaging equipment. In: Haus AG, Yaffe MJ, eds. Syllabus: A categorical course in physics. Technical aspects of breast imaging. Oak Brook: RSNA Publications; 1994:275

68 Yaffe M, Hendrick RE et al. Recommended specifications for mammography equipment. Reston: American College of Radiology; 1993

69 Gray JE. Mammographic quality control for the technologist and the medical physicist as consultant to the technologist. In: Haus AG, Yaffe MJ, eds. Syllabus: A categorical course in physics. Technical aspects of breast imaging. Oak Brook: RSNA Publications; 1994:275

70 Lanyi M. Diagnostik und Differentialdiagnostik der Mammaverkalkungen, 2nd ed. Berlin, Heidelberg, New York: Springer; 1989

71 Linver MN, Osuch JR, Brenner RJ, Smith RA. The mammography audit: a primer for the mammography quality Standards act (MQSA). AJR. 1995;165:19–25

72 Kindermann G. Diagnostic value of galactography in the detection of breast cancer. In: Zander J, Baltzer J, eds. Early breast cancer. Berlin: Springer; 1985:136–9

73 Bässler R. Pathologie der Brustdrüse. Berlin, Heidelberg, New York: Springer (Spezielle Pathologische Anatomie, vol. 11); 1978

■ Suggested Reading

Beahrs OH, Smart CR. The breast cancer detection demonstration projects as viewed by, the clinician. In: Feig SA, McLelland R eds. Breast carcinoma: current diagnosis and treatment. New York: Masson; 1983: 307

Ciatto S, Bravetti P, Berni D, Catarzi S, Bianchi S. The role of galactography in the detection of breast cancer. Tumori. 1988; 74: 171–81

Fajardo LL, Jackson PJ, Hunter TB. Interventional procedures in diseases of the breast: needle biopsy, pneumocystography, and galactography. Am J Radiol. 1992; 1231-8

Harvey JA, Fajardo LL, Innis CA. Previous mammograms in patients with impalpable breast carcinoma: retrospective versus blinded interpretation: AJR. 1993; 161: 1167

Hoeffken W, Hintzen C. Die Diagnostik der Mammazysten durch Mammographie und Pneumozystographie. Fortsch Röntgenstr. 1970; 9–18

Linver MN, Osuch JR, Brenner RJ, Smith RA. The mammography audit: a primer for the Mammography Quality Standards Act (MQSA). AJR. 1995; 165: 19–25

Neugefaßte Qualifikationsvoraussetzungen für die Radiologie, Nuklearmedizin und Strahlentherapie: Dtsch Arztebl. 1993; 90 (B 331): 45

Rose A Osborne J, Wright G, Billson V. Is what you see what you get?

Breast specimen handling revisted: Australas Radiol. 1991; 35: 145

Samuels T, Kerenyi N, Taylor G. Practical aspect of mammographic pathological correlation: experience with needle localisation. Can Assoc Radiol J. 1990; 47: 127

Tabar L, Dean PB, Pentek Z. Galactography: the diagnostic procedure of choice for nipple discharge. Am J Radiol. 1983; 149: 31-8

Tabar L, Pentek Z, Dean PB. The diagnostic and therapeutic value of breast cyst puncture and pneumocystography. Radiology. 1981; 141: 659-63

4. Sonography

Purpose, Accuracy, Possibilities, and Limitations

At present, sonography is the most important adjunctive breast imaging modality. It is used for:

- Diagnosing cysts
- Identifying lesions in mammographically dense tissue
- Guided preoperative marking and percutaneous biopsy (see Chapters 6 and 7)

Diagnosing Cysts

Diagnosis of cysts and their differentiation from other masses is the domain of sonography. With proper technique and diligent evaluation, ultrasound is able to distinguish between cystic and solid masses with almost 100% accuracy and for this reason has largely replaced diagnostic pneumocystography.[1–3]

Therefore sonography should be used to diagnose any palpable findings, mammographic densities, or dense or asymmetrical structures that could be the result of cysts. If ultrasound reveals one or more cysts that explain the findings in question, further diagnostic procedures will not be necessary. Avoiding unnecessary biopsies of simple cysts is a most significant advantage of ultrasound.

Differentiating Solid Lesions

Sonography may be helpful as an additional imaging modality for assessing the characteristics of masses that are partially or completely obscured by dense tissue on the mammogram. Palpable lesions detected in radiodense tissue that cannot be clearly or completely visualized mammographically can often be further characterized by ultrasound.

If all typical criteria of a benign tumor including compressibility and excellent mobility are met, then it is highly probable that the lesion is benign. However, exceptions have been reported.[4–7]

Sonography should be used in the following context:

- For lesions that are not simple cysts, mammography should be performed for further evaluation.
- Benign sonographic findings in the presence of suspicious mammographic findings do not exclude malignancy.
- If any clinical (history, patient age), sonographic, or mammographic doubts exist concerning the benignity of a solid lesion, further diagnostic studies (i. e., needle core biopsy, MRI, or excision) are required.

Diagnosing Carcinomas

Various factors influence sonographic visualization of carcinomas:

1. Most carcinomas are hypoechoic. However, some carcinomas are isoechoic with breast tissue and may not be identifiable sonographically.
2. Fat in the breast usually appears hypoechoic (as do most malignancies). Normal anatomic structures, therefore, can sometimes mimic cancers if care is not taken during the sonographic examination.
3. Glandular tissue and fibrocystic changes are usually, but not always, hyperechoic compared to fat.

In terms of accuracy, this means:

- Sonography *may be limited at detecting hypoechoic carcinomas in fatty tissue.* This problem has decreased with modern equipment. Diagnostically, this fact is not important, be-

cause mammography provides excellent resolution in fatty breasts.
The differentiation between solid and cystic masses usually succeeds in both fatty and dense breasts.

- *The hypoechoic carcinomas that represent the majority of carcinomas are easily recognized, when surrounded by homogenously hyperechoic tissue.* This is an advantage because, in the presence of suggestive palpable findings, ultrasound can complement mammography by providing information about radiodense areas in which the diagnostic value of mammography is limited.
  Even in hyperechoic tissue, excluding a malignant process by sonography requires caution, because some carcinomas may be isoechoic. For this reason, excluding a malignant process *always requires using sonography combined with mammography. Mammographic or clinical signs of a suspected malignant process will require further diagnostic studies, even if sonography is negative.*
- *Many dense breasts contain numerous interspersed hypoechoic fat lobules.* The experienced sonographer can usually recognize fat lobules interposed in the glandular tissue as such by rotating the transducer and by their good compressibility. However, multiple, deep-lying fat lobules in large breasts may *make this distinction difficult. In some patients hypoechoic foci* and, occasionally, acoustic shadows may be caused by normal breast parenchyma. Here detection and exclusion of malignancy are quite difficult.
- Since small hypoechoic tumors may be difficult to distinguish from fat lobules, since hypoechoic areas may occur within fibrocystic areas, and since small and preinvasive carcinomas in particular can be isoechoic with breast parenchyma, *ultrasound has limited sensitivity in diagnosing small lesions.* This applies to high-resolution transducers as well.[7–12]

Summary

Sonography is the most important adjunctive imaging modality. Its excellent accuracy in the diagnosis of cysts reduces the number of unnecessary biopsies.
If a poorly demarcated solid mass in radiodense tissue can be visualized with ultrasound and it shows typical features of a benign lesion (see p. 88, Interpreting Sonographic Findings), then sonography supports the diagnosis. If, however, any doubts exist concerning the benignity of a hypoechoic lesion (based on clinical findings, patient history, mammographic, or sonographic criteria), biopsy is recommended to confirm the diagnosis.
Sonography can provide important information to confirm the presence of palpable carcinomas in radiodense tissue. The accuracy of ultrasound in detecting malignant processes depends both on the surrounding tissue (homogeneous, hyperechoic tissue is best) and on the lesion itself. Accuracy is limited for small carcinomas and, in particular, preinvasive carcinoma.
For this reason, sonography should never be used to rule out a malignant process without corresponding mammographic studies. Benign sonographic findings in the presence of mammographic or clinical signs of a suspected malignant process do not exclude malignancy. In view of these restrictions, the known examiner-dependent accuracy, and its high physician time requirements, ultrasound is also not suitable as a screening modality.

Equipment Requirements

Sonography of the breast is generally performed by hand, and not automated, using high-frequency transducers.

Selecting the Transducer

To achieve sufficient visualization of the glandular tissue even in the near field, *linear transducers* are used for the evaluation of the breast. Since the breast is a superficial structure and resolving power increases as wavelength decreases (i.e., with increasing ultrasonic frequency), frequencies of 7.5 MHz or higher should be used for optimal resolution.

The maximum useful frequency is limited by penetration depth, which decreases as ultrasonic frequency increases. To create a useable image that offers a comprehensive view of all tissue structures down to the chest wall for routine diagnostic studies, *transducers with frequencies of at least 7.5 MHz are the best suited.* This frequency achieves an axial resolution between 0.3 and 0.4 mm. Sound attenuation at 7.5 MHz is about 50% per centimeter of tissue thickness.

Recently developed high-resolution transducers with frequencies up to 13 MHz permit higher resolution, but they can only be used for supplemental evaluation of small sections of tissue.

Image Quality

Factors determining the image quality of a breast sonography unit are resolving power, image quality in the near field, and slice thickness.

Resolution

Resolving power is determined by axial resolution, lateral resolution (Figs. 4.**1 a–c**), and contrast resolution.

1. Axial resolving power (resolution along the direction of sound travel) is determined by the length of the ultrasound pulse, which is generally from 2 to 3 wavelengths. The minimum axial resolution is half of this value (reflection mode imaging). That means that at 7.5 MHz, resolution is approximately 0.3–0.4 mm.
2. Lateral resolution (the width of the ultrasound pulse) is determined by the size of the transducer element (aperture), the ultrasonic frequency, and the type of focus. Focusing can be achieved by:
   - Concave arrangement of the transducer elements or use of an acoustic lens (fixed focus).
   - Alternatively, an electronic focusing can be used, the standard method used today. The degree of focusing and the distance of the focal point from the transducer is determined by electronically controlling the excitation of individual elements of an array system over time (Figs. 4.**1 a–c**). Depending on the delay (in excitation of the central elements compared with the respective outer ones), the focal surface can be moved closer to or farther away from the transducer. This technique of electronic focusing allows the emitted ultrasound beam to be focused on a desired depth of tissue.

   A particular advantage of electronic focusing is that it can sequentially bring different depths into focus. By extending the transmission time, an image can be created with simultaneous *sharp focus in several depth ranges (multifocus).* The same principle is used to bring different depths into focus during *reception of echoes (dynamic focusing).*

   Electronic focusing during transmission (*multifocus*) and reception (*dynamic focusing*) makes it possible to *improve lateral resolution over a wide range of depths.*

   The image can be further optimized by electronically adjusting the aperture (the area of the active piezoelectric element array).

   The quality of focus depends on the transducer. If it does not have multifocus ability, the examiner must adjust the depth of focus to match the distance of the tissue in question from the transducer.
3. *Contrast resolution* is a major factor in determining the quality of the image. Among other things, it is a measure of the sharpness of the lateral definition of the pulse and of how well a weak echo can be discerned next to a strong echo. Contrast resolution also depends on the transducer and sonographic unit.

a

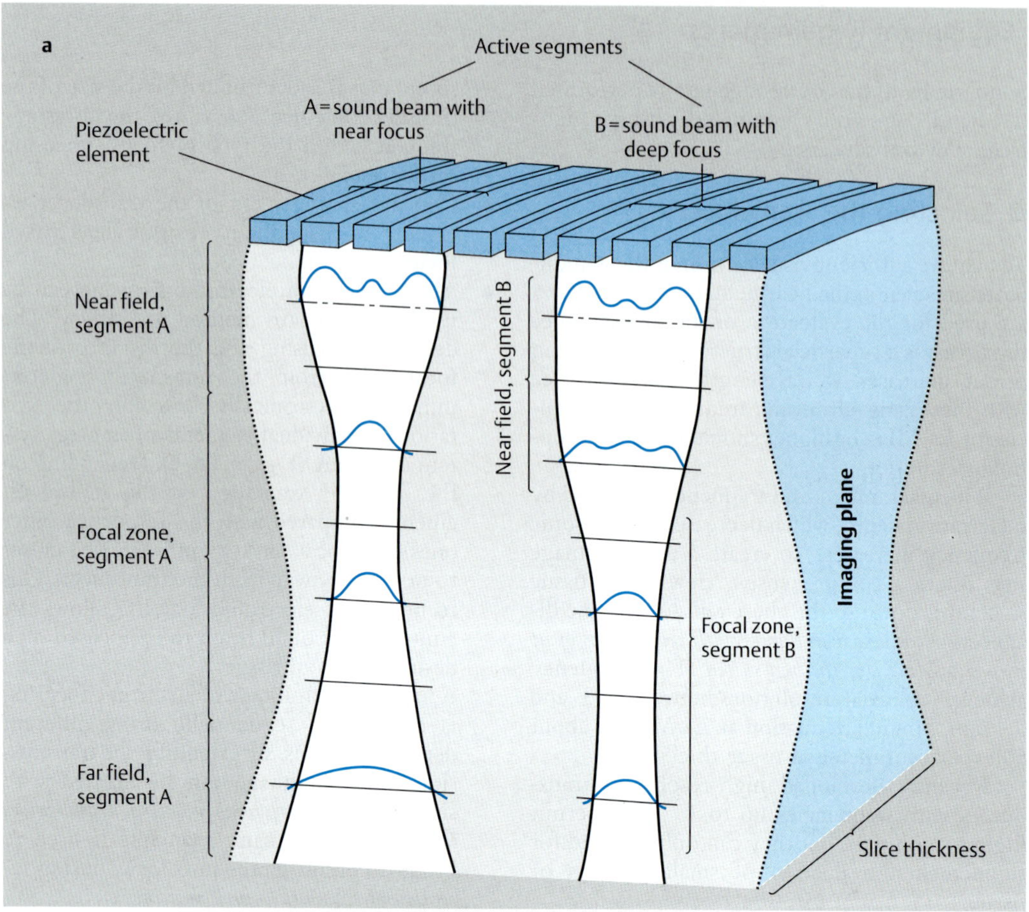

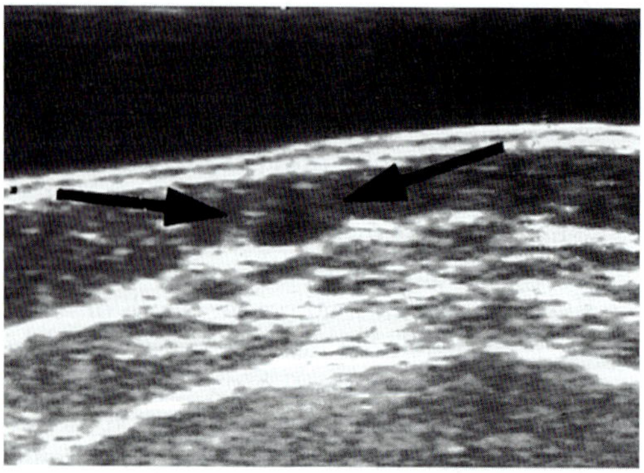

b

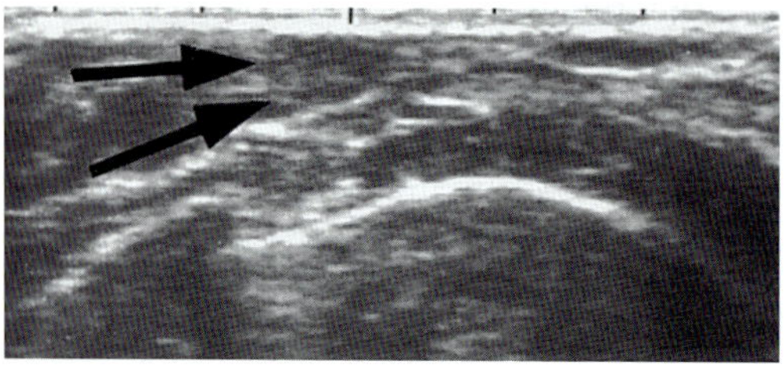

c

Fig. 4.**1 a–c**

a Schematic diagram showing the ultrasound beam emitted by a transducer.

The depth of focus (shown here for segments A and B) is set by delaying the excitation of the respecitve central transducer element accordingly. The ultrasound signal (depicted in the diagram as individual echoes in the ultrasound beam) shows artifacts in the near field due to interference. A fixed focus can be achieved by a concave arrangement of the piezoelectric elements

b and **c** A small subcutaneous fibroadenoma illustrates the effect of near-field interference

b When a stand-off pad is used, the small subcutaneous fibroadenoma is clearly visible over the fascia at the inferior margin of the breast (arrow) as a hypoechoic structure in the subcutaneous tissue

c Although the fibroadenoma is palpable directly under the transducer, it is scarcely discernible without stand-off (arrow). Note that the echoes close to the transducer are significantly wider and more blurred than in **b**

■ Image Quality in the Near Field

Aside from the optimal overall resolution, the image quality in the *near fields* is important for breast sonography. The near field is particularly critical since the short distance to the transducer makes focusing more difficult.

This area can be subject to significant interference that can degrade image quality and interfere with the interpretation (Figs. 4.**1 a–c**).

This interference results from the different paths of the ultrasound signals to and from the individual piezoelectric elements in the near field. This not only broadens the echo but also leads to artificial superimposition and cancellation of the signal.

This interference may significantly compromise the image quality in the near field. A variety of technical measures and optimizations result in decreasing the length of the near field that is of limited diagnostic quality; image quality in the near field will vary with the equipment.

Only some of the ultrasound units achieve diagnostic image quality in subcutaneous tissue. For the other units a stand-off pad between the transducer and the breast is necessary to achieve good quality images of the subcutaneous tissue.

When using a *stand-off* pad filled with water, it should not contain any gas bubbles to ensure efficient sound transmission. For all stand-off pads be sure to use enough gel between the transducer and the offset and the offset and the skin. Reverberation echoes can occur with insufficient acoustical coupling or significant differences in impedance (depending on the material of the stand-off). Reverberation echoes may be the result of repeated reflection between stand-off and transducer (Fig. 4.**2**). They produce lines of echoes that run parallel to the transducer and that repeat at 1, 2, 3, or more times a given distance from the transducer. They compromise image quality.

Gel stand-off pads applied directly to the breast work well. The transducer above the gel-plate and the breast below it are coupled to the plate with usual ultrasound gel, and both can be moved over the breast.

■ Slice Thickness

Slice thickness is the third major factor that determines image quality in all sonographic procedures. It is a function of quality and design of the transducer. For this reason, one should consider the effects of slice thickness in the image when selecting the transducer.

If the slice is too thick, accurate imaging of anechoic cysts may not be possible, due to insufficient exclusion of signal from neighbouring slices, which contain solid tissue. This will produce echoes within the cyst and can thus lead to problems with the differential diagnosis.

■ Other Factors

Compared with earlier sonographic units, newer units provide significantly finer gray-scale definition (4–8 bits, corresponding to 16–256 shades of gray). These units can produce high-contrast images of the varying echo intensities occurring in tissue and will elicit echoes within the cyst.

Special phantoms are available for assessing relevant image quality parameters for breast sonography.

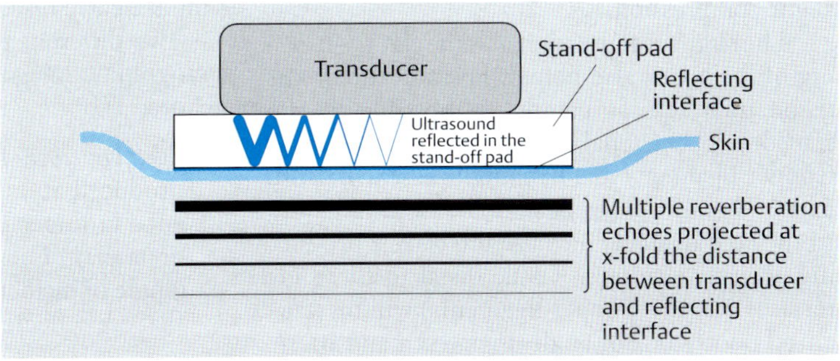

Fig. 4.**2** Reverberation echoes resulting from insufficient contract between stand-off pad and skin

■ **Summary**

Linear transducers with a nominal frequency of at least 7.5 MHz should be used for breast sonography. Very high frequency transducers may not be suitable for routine studies but only for additional examination of limited areas of tissue.

Image detail is determined by axial, lateral, and contrast resolution. Lateral resolution is significantly influenced by focusing. The optimum combination is multifocus transmission with a dynamic focusing receiver system. If these features are not available, the examiner must match the focus to the depth of the lesion.

In addition to resolution, slice thickness and image quality in the near field influence the quality of the image.

Slice thickness depends on the design of the transducer and is important for diagnosing small cysts.

Many units provide poor image quality in the near field that must be compensated for by using a stand-off pad. When using a stand-off, every attempt should be made to minimize reverberation echoes in the image.

Examination Technique

Sonography of the breast should be performed with the patient *supine*. When the breast is being examined, the patient should extend her ipsilateral arm over her head and turn slightly toward the contralateral side. Place a cushion under the ipsilateral shoulder to help the patient maintain this position. This positioning helps the *breast to lie as flat as possible* on the chest wall (which reduces the penetration thickness) and reduces breast mobility.

When examining the outer quadrants in a large breast, it helps to have the patient turn slightly more toward the contralateral side. When the inner quadrants are being examined, it is helpful to position the patient straight supine.

A *sufficient amount of gel* must be used between the transducer and stand-off pad and between the stand-off pad and the skin. This is important for minimizing reverberations at the interfaces. The transducer should be applied with slight compression.

The slight compression and the flat positioning of the breast also help to position the breast tissue interfaces as parallel as possible to the transducer. Diagonal tissue interfaces such as Cooper ligaments in a hanging breast will cause part of the ultrasound beam to be reflected away from the transducer at these interfaces, producing acoustic shadows. Tissue distal to these interfaces (usually Cooper ligaments) will be visualized poorly or not at all (Figs. 4.3 **a** and **b**).

■ Time-gain Compensation

Attenuation compensation (depth compensation, time-gain compensation) is necessary since ultrasound energy is absorbed in tissue (at 7.5 MHz, a little over 50% per centimeter of tissue thickness). This means that the gain must increase with the distance of the echo from the transducer (i.e., with depth). The time-gain compensation should be adjusted so that echoes from comparable tissue (i.e., glandular tissue compared with glandular tissue or fat compared with fat) appear at approximately equal intensity regardless of the distance from the transducer (Fig. 4.**4**).

The time-gain compensation must be adjusted to match the specific ultrasound absorption of the skin and breast tissue.

The total gain must be set so that the difference between stronger and weaker echoes and between fat, fibrotic tissue, glandular tissue, and skin is clearly discernible.

Two different types of echoes appear in the sonographic image, specular echoes and scatter echoes:

– *Specular echoes* are strong echoes, which are produced at interfaces with sufficient difference in impedance (wall of a cyst, ligament, or fascia). These are mirror-like reflections (angle of incidence equals angle of reflection) that are reflected back to the transducer after

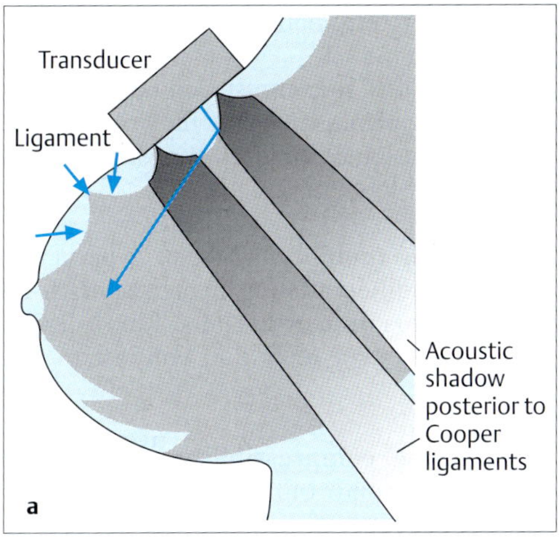

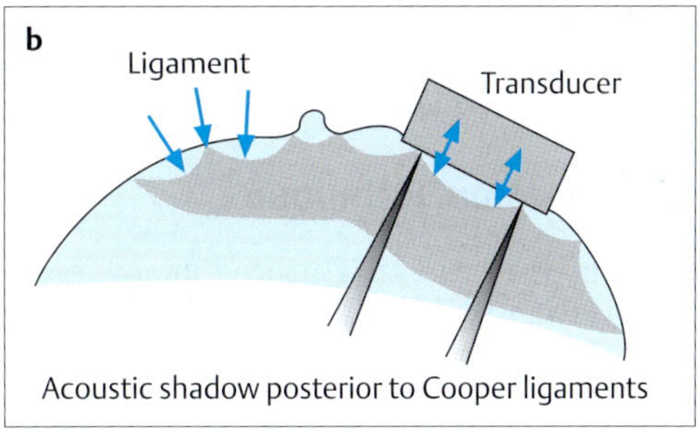

Fig. 4.3 **a** and **b** Positioning the patient supine and applying slight compression helps to orient the interfaces parallel to the transducer (**b**). Less ultrasound energy is reflected away from the transducer than in a hanging breast (**a**)

striking an interface perpendicular to the direction of sound propagation. Echoes striking diagonal interfaces can be reflected away from the transducer.

– *Scatter echoes* occur at small interfaces with irregular surfaces. The size of these small interfaces is of the same order of magnitude as the wavelength. The ultrasound beam is scattered in every direction at these interfaces. This means that the echo returned to the transducer will be significantly weaker since it represents only part of the ultrasound energy. Most echoes in glandular and fatty tissue are produced along microscopic interfaces of this type and are thus scatter echoes.

■ Stand-off

The physical limitations in the near field and the varying ability of ultrasound units to compensate for them mean that many units require a stand-off pad for imaging the near field (see p. 85). The examiner should verify that good coupling is achieved.

■ Focusing

The areas of interest must lie in the focal zone. Lesions whose echogenicity differs only slightly from the surrounding tissue can be overlooked outside the focal zone. To minimize this problem when using an older unit, the appropriate focal setting (proximal, mid-range, or distal focus) should be selected according to the location of the lesion relative to the transducer.

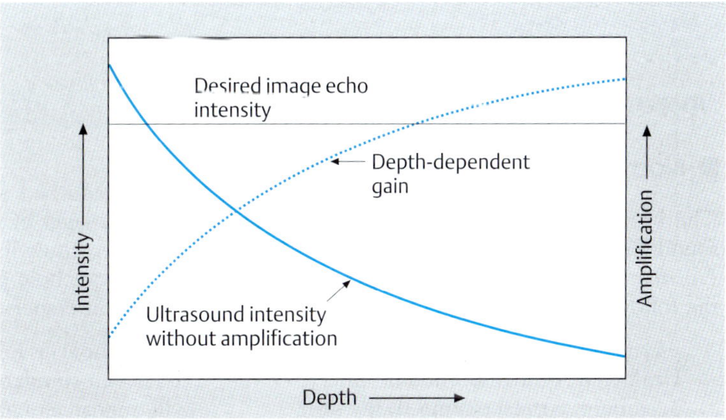

Fig. 4.4 Time-gain compensation

Modern units can do this automatically with multifocus transmission and dynamic focusing of the received signal.

Examination Technique

Glandular tissue can be visualized in any imaging plane (transverse, sagittal, or radially toward the nipple). A comprehensive overview of the tissue is usually easier to obtain in the *transverse* or *sagittal* plane. Imaging the breast in a *radial plane* is helpful for imaging ducts, which often can be traced to the nipple as tubular structures.

If an overview of all of the glandular tissue is desired, it should be kept in mind that isolated glandular tissue can be found anywhere between the clavicle and the inframammary fold or in the axillary tail. Sonography is often better able to image peripheral areas of glandular tissue than mammography.

As a rule, *sonography* should be used for the additional assessment of selected areas or findings. At present, sonography is *not recommended* for routine breast screening.

Examining Lesions

1. Imaging in multiple planes: Any suspicious or questionable finding must be imaged in multiple planes. With real-time scanning the entire lesion should be examined completely in multiple planes including two orthogonal planes. In this way fat lobules that simulate hypoechoic tumors in one plane can usually be correctly identified in the second plane. They typically appear as elongated structures in the second plane. Often the image will reveal a connection to subcutaneous or retromammary fat (Figs. 4.5 **a** and **b**).

Real lesions, in contrast, can be identified in two imaging planes and generally prove to have a three-dimensional extent as opposed to the flat extent of fat lobules.

2. Assessing mobility: Mobility is particularly helpful for differentiating benign smooth-contoured tumors from malignancy. Fibroadenomas are generally very mobile in contrast to carcinomas.[13]

3. Assessing compressibility: The examiner can assess compressibility by vertically compressing the lesion with the transducer or with a finger inserted beneath the transducer.[13, 14] Compressing the lesion between the thumb and index finger during ultrasound inspection provides more reliable information. The compression test helps to differentiate fat lobes from hypoechoic masses more reliably. Most cysts are compressible, as well. Published studies have reported a compressibility of at least 20% of fibroadenomas and less compressibility of malignant lesions.[12] Our results only partially confirm these findings. Only a small proportion of the fibroadenomas we examined could be compressed at least 20%. Since some lymphomas and certain infrequent types of carcinomas can also have a soft consistency, ultrasound-guided aspiration provides a more reliable information and can contribute to the differential diagnosis.

For obvious reasons, this test is unreliable in large breasts and small, deep lesions (Figs. 4.5 **e–f**).

Interpreting Sonographic Findings

Normal Sonographic Findings

The broad range of variation in normal ultrasound findings makes them difficult to define. Normal findings are basically characterized by the following features:

- *Absence of a focal sonographic lesion*
- Uniformly echogenic double line, 2–3 mm maximum, corresponding to the skin
- Undisturbed subcutaneous and retromammary layer of fat interrupted only with thin hyperechoic liagments
- Hyperechoic glandular body that may contain interspersed fat lobules

Hypoechoic fat lobules surrounded by glandular tissue can simulate focal lesions. Many of them will appear elongated in other imaging planes,

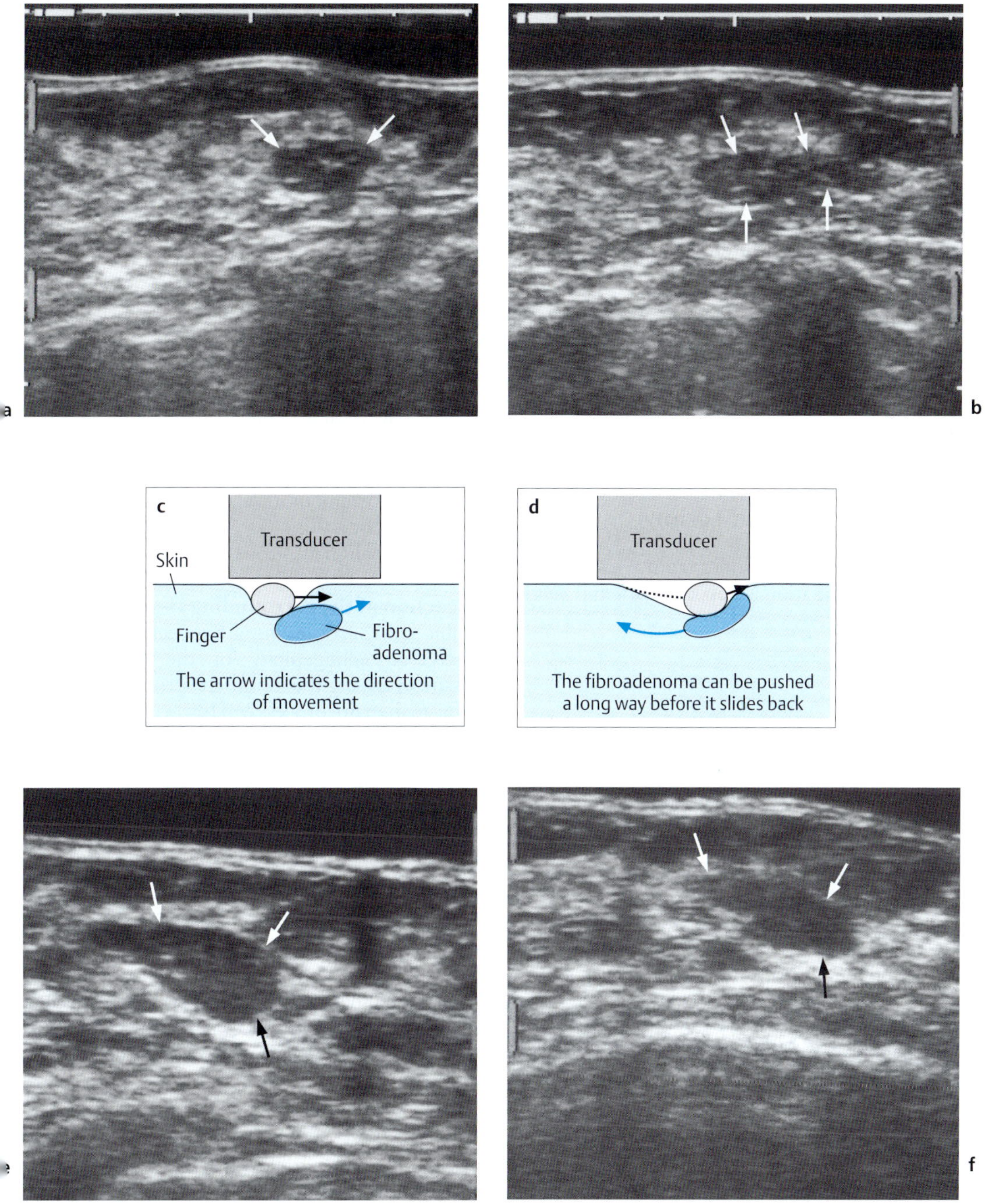

Fig. 4.**5 a–f**

a and **b** Imaging in two planes:

a Interspersed fat lobules can simulate a hypoechoic tumor

b As the transducer is turned, the same fat lobule appears as an elongated structure (arrow). The image in this plane also reveals that the fat lobule is connected to subcutaneous fat

c and **d** Assessing mobility (diagram). To assess mobility, insert a finger underneath the transducer. Fibroadenomas usually are far more mobile than carcinomas

e and **f** Assessing compressibility:

Fat lobes are usually easily compressed, in contrast to tumors.

e Fat lobe (arrows) before compression

f compressing the fat lobe (arrows) with the transducer

and therefore rotating the transducer and assessing compressibility are important methods for differentiating fat from focal lesions (see Figs. 4.5 **a** and **b**).

Normal utlrasound findings cannot rule out carcinoma in the presence of questionable or suggestive mammographic findings.

The reason for this is that the sensitivity of ultrasound decreases with the size of the focal lesion. The sensitivity for detecting carcinomas in situ is low.[7–11] The same applies to suggestive palpable findings.

In the presence of inconclusive palpable findings, negative sonographic examination, and negative mammographic examination, the physician may elect follow-up examination in 6 months, needle core biopsy, or surgical excision, depending on the clinical suspicion.

Focal Ultrasound Lesions

In describing focal sonographic lesions, the major differentiation is between *cystic* and *noncystic findings.*

Cysts

Simple cysts are characterized as:

- An anechoic mass (usually oval, sometimes septated), in some cases, additional information can be obtained by varying the gain of the unit (see p. 86)
- A focal lesion with a smooth contour and thin wall
- A focal lesion with good posterior enhancement
- Good compressibility

When sonography can clearly identify a mammographic density or a palpable finding as a simple cyst, no further workup is necessary.

If these cirteria are not completely fulfilled, then the physician may elect follow-up examination, aspiration, core biopsy or surgical excision, depending on the size and morphology of the lesion. Sedimentation can be identified by changing the patient's position. Biopsy is indicated whenever sonography reveals an intracystic mass.

Solid (Non-cystic) Masses

The following features should be considered in the differentiation between benign and malignant lesions:

- contour of the focal lesion
- acoustic absorption
- internal echo pattern
- orientation (parallel to the transducer or "upright")
- compressibility
- mobility

Contour: An irregular contour suggests malignancy, yet can occur in some benign tumors (e. g., fibrosed fibroadenomas and papillomas). A smooth contour sugests a benign lesion, but this criterion is not conclusive.[5, 7, 12, 14, 15] Poor definition of part of the contour suggests a process with invasion into adjacent tissues or surrounding inflammation.

When a solid, oval lesion orients with its longitudinal axis parallel to the transducer, this is a sign of a fibroadenoma (rare exceptions are known). A round or lobulated smooth contour is suggestive of a fibroadenoma, although this can occur in malignant processes.

Reaction of the surrounding tissue: A hyperechoic halo surrounding a hypoechoic mass and increased echogenicity of the subcutaneous tissue overlying the lesion are strong indications of a malignant process.[12] However, when these signs are absent, a malignant process is not excluded.

Acoustic absorption: An acoustic shadow posterior to the entire lesion or posterior to a part of the lesion is a strong indication of a malignant process if a calcified fibroadenoma or a calcified oil cyst has been excluded.

Indifferent absorption (i. e., absence of both shadowing or posterior enhancement) does not exclude a malignant process. Homogeneous acoustic enhancement is mostly a sign of a benign lesion. Thin lateral shadows are generally seen with benign tumors but are not conclusive.[5, 7, 14, 15]

Internal echo pattern: A homogeneous echo pattern tends to indicate a benign lesion, whereas a heterogeneous echo pattern is strongly suspicious for malignancy. However, findings frequently deviate from this rule.[4, 7, 9, 10, 13] Anechoic areas can be seen centrally in a tumor with regions of necrosis or cyst formation.

Orientation: If the longitudinal axis of the lesion is perpendicular to the transducer, this is a strong indication of a malignant process.

An oval lesion with its longitudinal axis parallel to the transducer is a sign of a benign lesion, although this criterion is not conclusive.[4, 5, 16]

Compressibility: Superficial fat lobes and cysts can easily be differentiated from superficial tumors by compressing them. Easily compressible solid focal lesions are mostly benign lesions, such as fibroadenomas.[13, 14]

These criteria can overlap in either direction, i. e., fibroadenomas may be only slightly compressible, whereas some types of hyperechoic carcinomas or lymphomas may be more compressible.

Mobility: Good mobility is a strong indication of a benign lesion such as a fibroadenoma. Poor mobility is a sign of a carcinoma.[13, 14]

It is important to remember the following points:

- *No ultrasound criterion permits differentiating between benign and malignant hypoechoic focal lesions with 100% certainty.*
- *The examiner must compare mammographic, clinical findings, and information from patient history and age to sonographic findings when assessing the possibility of malignancy.*
- Depending on the combination of characteristics observed in a solid sonographic lesion, the physician has the following options:

– Follow-up sonography may be performed in the presence of a highly mobile lesion when all other sonographic criteria, patient history, and breast examination indicate a fibroadenoma, and when mammography shows no evidence of malignancy.
– Further diagnostic studies (needle core biopsy, excision, or, in rare cases, MRI; see Chapters 11–14) are indicated for indeterminate findings.

Exception: *Small hypoechoic foci only detected by sonography* are quite frequent. To avoid too many unnecessary biopsies of such hypoechoic areas, which are mostly due to benign breast disease, sonographic follow-up should be considered if these lesions are felt to be worthy of further study.

References

1 Barth V, Prechtel K. Atlas der Brustdrüse und ihrer Erkrankungen. Stuttgart: Enke; 1990
2 Hackelöer BJ, Duda V, Hüneke P et al. Ultraschallmammographie: Entwicklung, Stand und Grenzen. Ultraschall. 1982;3:94
3 Stavros AT, Dennis MA. An introduction to breast ultrasound. In: Parker SH, Jobe WE. Percutaneous breast biopsy. New York: Raven Press; 1993
4 Adler DD, Heyde DL, Ikeda DM. Quantitative sonographic parameters as means of distinguishing breast cancers from benign solid masses. J Ultrasound Med. 1991;10:505
5 Fornage BD, Lorigan JG, Andry E. Fibroadenoma of the breast: sonographic appearance. Radiology. 1989;172:671
6 Heywang SH, Dunner PS, Lipsit ER, Glassmann LM. Advantages and pitfalls of ultrasound in the diagnosis of breast cancer. J Clin Ultrasound. 1985;13:525
7 Pamilo M, Soiva M, Anttinen J et al. Ultrasonography of breast lesions detected in mammography screening. Acta Radio. 1991;32:220
8 Balu-Maestro C, Bruneton JN, Melia P et al. High frequency ultrasound detection of breast calcifications. Eur J Ultrasound. 1994;3:247
9 Bassett LW, Kimme-Smith C. Breast sonography AJR. 1991;156:449
10 Ciatto S, Roselli-del-Turco M, Catarzis M et al. The diagnostic role of breast echography. Radiol Med (Torino). 1994;88:221
11 Potterton AJ, Peakman DH, Young IR. Ultrasound demonstration of small breast cancers detected by mammographic screening. Clin Radiol. 1994;49:808
12 Teubner J, Behrer M, von Kaick G, Georgi M. Echomorphologie des Mammakarzinoms. Radiologe. 1993;33:277
13 Tohno E, Cosgrove DO, Sloane UP. Ultrasound diagnosis of breast diseases. Edinbourgh: Churchill Livingstone; 1994
14 Leucht D, Madjar H. Lehratlas der Mammasonographie. 2. Aufl. Stuttgart: Thieme; 1995
15 Jackson VP, Rothschild PA, Kreipke D et al. The spec-

benign require further workup, usually percutaneous biopsy. If they are *detected* only by MRI, if no peripheral enhancement or early washout exists, and if no significantly increased risk of malignancy exists, we recommend a *follow-up MRI examination* after a period of 6 and 12–18 months. This procedure is necessary to avoid unnecessary biopsies of small otherwise asymptomatic fibroadenomas, which are discovered with very high sensitivity by c.e. MRI.

- *MRI does not provide diagnostic information in the presence of diffuse enhancement.*

The high sensitivity of MRI is certainly its most important advantage. To make use of it, we recommend that a low threshold is selected above which the level or speed of enhancement will be regarded as significant. Sufficient specificity should be achieved by integrating information from mammography and clinical examination, follow-up examination, or needle core biopsy of indeterminate lesions.

Whether specificity can be improved by quantitative or semiquantitative evaluation that includes enhancement dynamics is still under investigation.[8, 31] However, we must warn against improving specificity at the cost of sensitivity. Further research is required regarding the extent to which quantitative data from one unit may be transferred to another.

Unenhanced MRI

Knowledge of normal findings with a breast implant is an important prerequisite for correct diagnosis of implant failure.

Normal Findings in the Presence of a Breast Implant

The single-lumen implant consists of the very thin silicone plastic envelope containing either liquid silicone (silicone implant) or a saline solution (saline implant).

Double-lumen implants have a second smaller implant within the outer implant (which is generally filled with saline solution, rarely with silicone). The smaller inner implant is generally filled with silicone, rarely with saline solution. Some temporary implants have a valve through which the implant can be filled. Since this is magnetic, it will generally cause a larger artifact.

The outer envelope of the implant is surrounded by a capsule of connective tissue that forms as the wound heals. Usually, the outer envelope will be in direct contact with the capsule of connective tissue so that a thin strip of low signal intensity (1–2 mm wide) will surround the implant.

In rare cases, fluid can accumulate between the outer envelope of the implant and the capsule of connective tissue (especially in folds). This fluid will appear as an area of high signal intensity in T2-weighted images and must be carefully distinguished from silicone leakage from the envelope of the implant (see below). Both the inner and outer implant envelopes can form folds.

Capsular Fibrosis

In capsular fibrosis, the capsule of connective tissue surrounding the implant contracts. This produces a sensation of tension and causes the implant to assume a balloon-like shape. The diagnosis of capsular fibrosis is made clinically.

This balloon-like configuration is also seen by MRI. Thickening of the connective-tissue capsule only may be observed in some of these patients.

Implant Rupture

Rupture of a silicone-filled single-lumen implant or a silicone-filled outer implant envelope is recognizable by one of the following characteristic features:

- Silicone is present outside of the connective-tissue capsule *(extracapsular rupture)*. Such extracapsular silicone depots are best visualized with a so-called "silicone-only" sequence or with a T2-weighted water saturation sequence, where they present as an area of high signal intensity outside the capsule (Fig. 5.**1 a**).
- Silicone is present outside the implant folds but still within the connective-tissue capsule *(intracapsular rupture)*. With the aid of this sign (described in the literature as the *"keyhole sign"* or *"reverse C sign"*; Fig. 5.**1 a**), the examiner can detect even small implant defects.
- The outer envelope of the silicone implant or the silicone part is completely ruptured and collapsed. It then appears as a thin folded

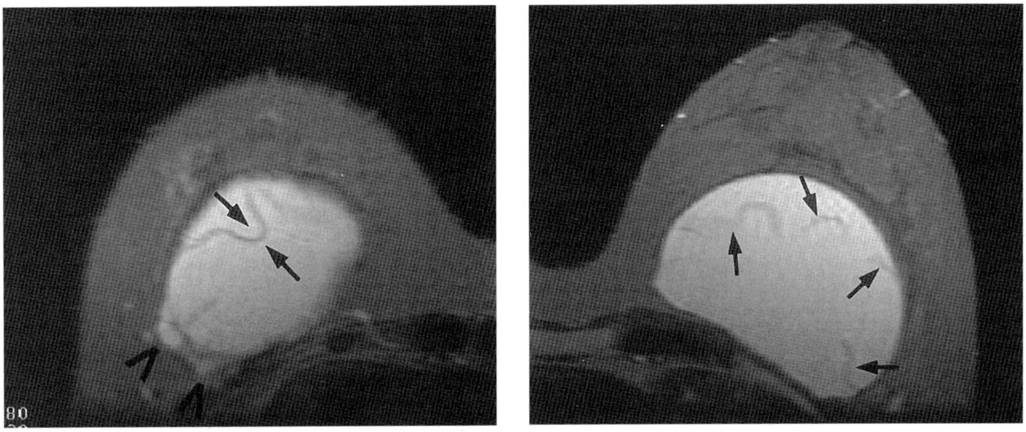

a b

Fig. 5.**1 a** and **b** Implant rupture
a Extracapsular rupture (open arrowheads) and intracapsular rupture (arrows). In the intracapsular rupture, silicone is present on both sides of the fold marked with the arrows. This is the "reverse C sign" referred to by Dr R Patt, Georgetown University
b "Linguini sign" in an intracapsular rupture. The torn outer envelope floats in the puddle of silicone fluid (similarly to linguini noodles) surrounded by the fibrous capsule

linear structure floating in the puddle of silicone fluid, which is only surrounded by the connective-tissue capsule (so-called "*linguini sign*").

If a saline-filled implant or the saline-filled outer envelope of an implant ruptures, it can usually be diagnosed clinically from the sudden loss in volume.

If only the inner envelope of a double-lumen implant ruptures, the silicone and saline solutions will mix. This will produce droplets within the implant fluids as found when salad oil is mixed with vinegar (so-called "salad oil sign").

■ References

1 Heywang-Köbrunner SH, Viehweg P. Sensitivity of contrast-enhanced MR imaging of the breast. MRI Clin North Am. 1994;2(4)527
2 Heywang-Köbrunner SH, Beck R. Contrast-enhanced MRI of the breast. 2nd ed. Berlin: Springer; 1996
3 Allgayer B, Hauck W, Jänicke F et al. MRT-Diagnostik von Mammakarzinomen mit einem nicht-ionischen Kontrastmittel in 2D- und 3D-Gradientenecho-FFE-Technik. Radiologe. 1995;35(4)
4 Fischer U, v. Heyden D, Vosshenrich R et al. Signalverhalten maligner und benigner Läsionen in der dynamischen 2D-MRT der Mamma. Fortschr Rontgenstr. 1993;158:287
5 Flickinger FW, Allison JD, Sherry R et al. Differentation of benign from malignant breast masses by dynamic time-intensity evaluation of contrast-enhanced MRI. Book of Abstracts. Berkeley: Society of Magnetic Resonance Publ. 1992:955
6 Gilles R, Guinebretiere JM, Shapeero LG et al. Assessment of breast cancer recurrence with contrast-enhanced subtraction MR imaging: Preliminary results in 26 patients. Radiology. 1993;188:473
7 Hewang-Köbrunner SH. Diagnosis of Breast Cancer with MR-review after 1250 patient examinations. Electromedica. 1993;61:43
8 Klengel S, Hietschold V, Neumann U et al. Quantitative dynamic mamma MRI: Value of early and late phase parameters. In: Proceedings of the 11th annual meeting of the European Society of Magnetic Resonance in Medicine and Biology. Vienna; 1994:117
9 Kuhl CK, Elevelt A, Kreft BP. Comparative study of diagnostic accuracy of dynamic MR mammography at 0,5 T versus 1,5 T. In: Proceedings of the 11th annual meeting of the European Society of Magnetic Resonance in Medicine and Biology. Vienna; 1994:122
10 Schnall MD, Orel S, Muenz L. Analysis of time intensity curves for enhancing breast lesions. In: Proceedings of the annual meeting of the Society of Magnetic Resonance in Medicine. Berkeley, California; 1993:120

11 Harms SE, Flamig DP, Hesley KL et al. MR imaging of the breast with rotating delivery of exitation off resonance: Clinical experience with pathologic correlation. Radiology. 1993;187:493

12 Kaiser WA. MRM promises earlier breast cancer diagnosis. Diagn Imaging. 1992;11:44

13 Oellinger H, Heins S, Sander B et al. Gd-DPTA enhanced MR breast imaging: The most sensitive method for multicentric carcinomas of the female breast. Eur Radiol. 1993;3:223

14 Gilles R, Guinebretiere J, Lucidarme O et al. Nonpalpable breast tumors: diagnosis with contrast-enhanced subtraction dynamic MR imaging. Radiology. 1994; 191:625–31

15 Dresel V, Bühner M, Schulz-Wendtland R, Bauer M. Intraduktale Karzinome der Mamma – ist eine Diagnose in der Kernspintomographie möglich? der Radiologe 1995; 35/4:87

16 Fischer U, Westerhof JP, Vosshenrich R et al. Das präinvasive duktale Mammakarzinom in der MR Mammographie. Zentralbl Radiol. 1995. In press

17 Brem RF, Tempany CMC, Zerhouni EA. MR detection of breast implant rupture. xxx 1992;16:157

18 De Angelis GA, de Lange EE, Miller LR, Morgan RF. MR imaging of breast implants. Radiographics. 1994;14:783

19 Ferrari G, Giovanni G, Lauro F et al. Nuclear magnetic resonance in the follow-up after augmentation mammoplasty. Riv Ital Chir Plast. 1994;26:295

20 Gorczyca DP, Sinha S, Ahn CY et al. Silicone breast implants in vivo: MR imaging. Radiology. 1992;185:407

21 Mund DF, Farria DM, Gorczyca DP et al. MR imaging of the breast in patients with silicone gel implants: spectrum of findings. AJR. 1993;161:773

22 Boné B, Aspelin P, Isberg B et al. Contrast-enhanced MR imaging of the breast in patients with breast implants after cancer surgery. Acta Radiol. 1995;36:111

23 Heywang SH, Hilbertz T, Beck R et al. Contrast-material enhanced MRI of the breast in patients with postoperative scarring and silicone implants. J Comput Assist Tomogr. 1990;14:348

24 Heywang-Köbrunner SH, Schlegel A, Beck R et al. Contrast-enhanced MRI of the breast after limited surgery and radiation therapy. J Comput Assist Tomogr. 1993;17:891–900

25 Lewis-Jones HG, Whitehouse GH, Leinster SJ. The role of MRI in the assessment of local recurrent breast carcinoma. Clin Radiol. 1991;43:197

26 Fischer U, Vosshenrich R, Probst A et al. Preoperative MR mammography in patients with breast cancer – useful information or useless extravagance. Fortschr Rontgenstr. 1994;16:300

27 Heywang-Köbrunner SH, Deimling M, Kösling S. KM-MRT der Mamma: technische Besonderheiten und Pitfalls. Zentralbl Radiol. 1994;150(13):52

28 Heywang-Köbrunner SH, Haustein J, Pohl C et al. Contrast enhanced MRI of the breast: Comparison of two dosages. Radiology. 1994;191:639

29 Beck R, Heywang-Köbrunner SH, Untch M. Contrast-enhancement of proliferative dysplasia in MRI of the breast due to the menstruation cycle. ECR '93 Book of Abstracts. Berlin, Heidelberg, New York: Springer 1993:151

30 Kuhl CK et al. Focale und diffuse KM-anreichernde Läsionen in der MR-Mammographie bei gesunden Probandinnen: Bandbreite des Normverhaltens und Zyklusphasenabhängigkeit. Radiologe. 1995;35(4):86

31 Boetes C, Barentsz JO, Mus RD et al. MR characterization of suspicious breast lesions with gadolinium-enhanced Turbo FLASH subtraction technique. Radiology. 1994;193:777

6. Percutaneous Biopsy Methods

Purpose, Definitions, Accuracy, Indications, Contraindications, and Side Effects

■ Purpose

The increasingly widespread use of mammography has seen a corresponding increase in the number of incidentally discovered mammographic findings requiring further diagnostic studies. While mammographic screening allows a reduction in the mortality of breast cancer, the increased use of mammography has also resulted in an increase in mammographically indicated excisional biopsies, of which only a small number reveal malignant findings. Mammographic, sterotaxic, or ultrasound-guided percutaneous biopsy is a minimally invasive diagnostic step before or instead of surgical excision. Percutaneous biopsy methods are less expensive, less time-consuming, and involve less morbidity than surgical intervention.

■ Definitions

In *fine-needle aspiration cytology*, cells are aspirated with a fine needle for cytologic examination.

In a *core-needle biopsy*, small cores of tissue are removed for histologic examination.

■ Accuracy

■ Fine-needle Aspiration Cytology

■ Possibilities

Recently, several institutions have used fine-needle aspiration cytology in diagnosing palpable breast tumors. This method has achieved a sensitivity of 53–99% and specificity of 96–100% [1,2,3,4]. Data from published studies of aspiration cytology of incidentally discovered mammographic or sonographic lesions are still limited. Swedish research groups have the greatest experience in this area. They achieve a sensitivity of 71–100% and specificity of 91–100% under stereotaxic guidance. These sensitivity and specificity rates are unique in that the patient population is preselected, and diagnostic accuracy is verified by subsequent biopsy. Caution must be exercised in applying these results to other patient groups. A critical issue is whether the incidence of nondiagnostic aspirations enters into the calculation. If aspiration cytology is exclusively used on lesions with unequivocal mammographic evidence of suspected malignancy, then its sensitivity and specificity will appear unrealistically high. If surgical biopsies are performed only in the presence of malignant findings on fine-needle aspiration, then the study will fail to include false negative cytologic results.

At highly specialized facilities, such as the Karolinska Hospital in Stockholm, regular use of stereotaxic fine needle aspiration cytology has reduced the incidence of surgical intervention to only 22% of all incidentally discovered mammographic findings suggestive of malignancy. These impressive results have only been reproduced in referral institutions with highly trained radiologists and, above all, cytologists.

■ Limitations

Outside specialized referral centers, significant fluctuations may occur. Differences in the rate of false negative findings and inadequate tissue samplings pose the biggest problems. This

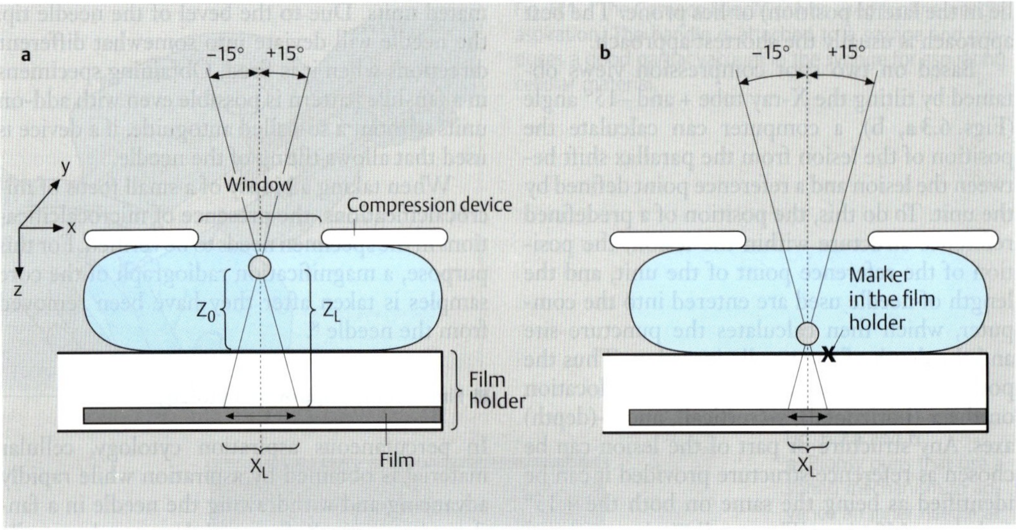

Fig. 6.**3 a** and **b** Principle of depth localization
a First, the breast is compressed with a fenestrated compression plate. The opening needs to be precisely above the lesion to be sampled. Spot compression views are obtained by tilting the X-ray tube + 15° and – 15° out of the center
b Lesions closer to the film (**b**) will appear with less of a shift (X_L) on the film than lesions farther from the film (**a**). The mammography unit can calculate the depth of the lesion from the parallax shift of the lesion (X_L). The depth of the lesion (Z_L) is calculated using the following formula:

$$\frac{X_L}{2} = Z_L \cdot \tan \mathrm{Ih}^\circ$$

or

$$ZL = \frac{XL_2}{2 \cdot \tan 15^\circ}$$

The formula can be adapted accordingly to determine the depth of the lesion with respect to the film holder. To do so, a reference point on the film holder is used and the formula is changed accordingly. This reference point is also used as a reference point for the lateral shift, since the film cassette is also moved manually between the + 15 and – 15 views to avoid exposing it twice

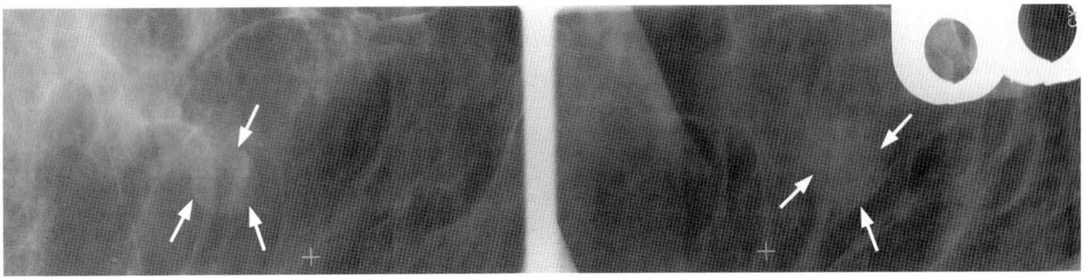

a

Fig. 6.**4 a–c**
a Two test views of a small focal lesion prepared with the tube tilted at + and – 15°
b Sonography
c Documentation views to verify correct needle positioning after biopsy

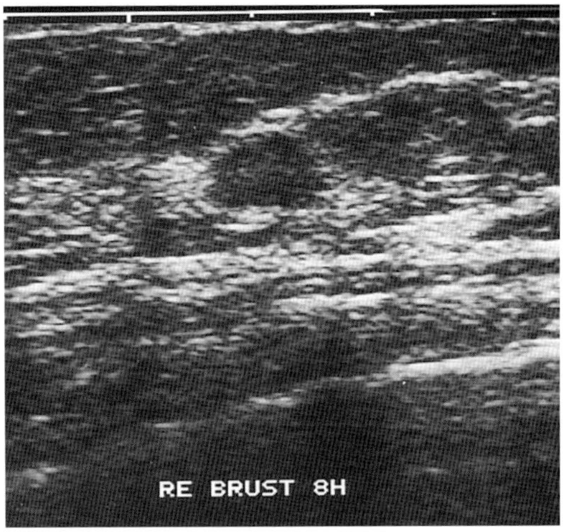

b

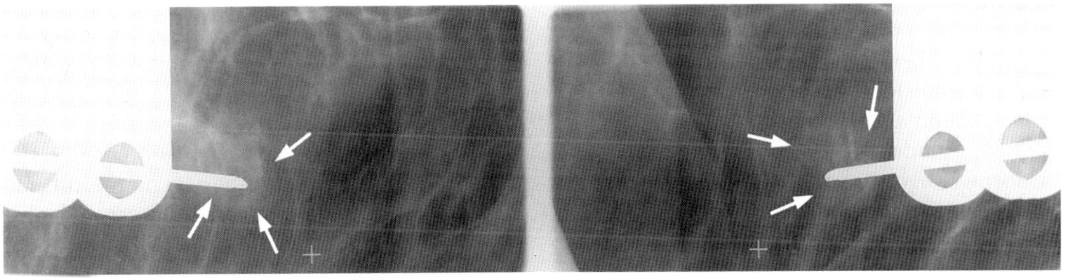

c

the initial localization view represent possible sources of severe error. If the needle and gun are not correctly positioned in the needle holder, the needle tip will not be in the position calculated by the computer. Careful technique should minimize these errors.

■ Problems and Their Solutions

Stereotaxic biopsy takes some time. The time needed depends on whether conventional films (≥ 15–20 min) or digital technique (≤ 10 min) is used. The longer the time required, the more likely patient motion may degrade the precision of needle positioning.

Not all patients and not all lesion localizations are suitable for mammographic stereotaxic examination.

- The compression device may not be able to reach lesions located extremely close to the chest wall or in the axilla, particularly with prone table and stereotaxic devices.
- Needle deviation is a source of error that should not be overlooked. It is a problem particularly in dense breast tissue. This problem is considerably greater when using thin cytology needles. However, even the beveled edge of large-core biopsy needles can be deflected several millimeters in dense tissue and can fail to reach the targeted location. The following techniques can minimize needle deflection:

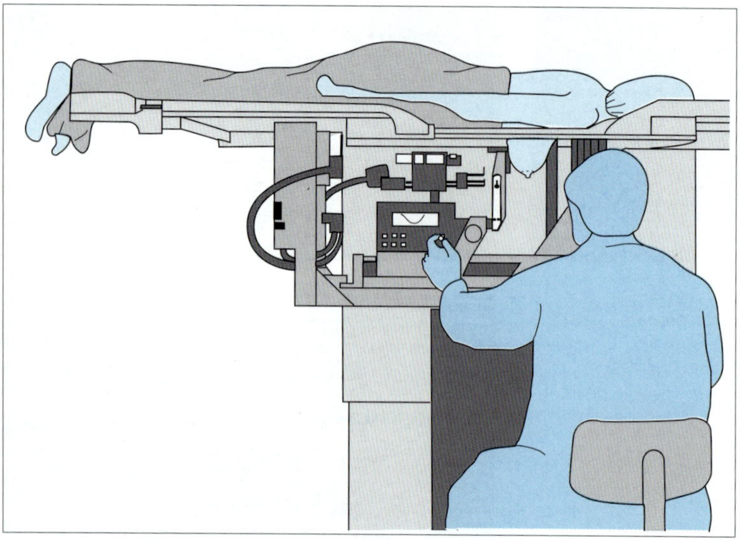

Fig. 6.**5** Dedicated unit for localizing a lesion and performing a stereotaxic needle biopsy with the patient positioned prone

- Selecting the stiffest possible needle
- Rotating the needle while inserting it
- Inserting the core or cytology needle through a heavy straight bevel needle or cannula to minimize the risk of deflection

- In some ill-defined lesions, it is extremely difficult or even impossible to identify the same structure in the two stereotaxic localization views. If this is not possible with certainty, other localization procedures (mammographic localization with a grid and depth correction using a second plane[9] or ultrasound-guided localization) should be performed, because incorrect identification of a reference structure will lead to incorrect calculation of the depth.
- In a few cases with multiple fine microcalcifications, it may also be difficult to define exactly the same microcalcification in the stereotaxic localization views. If this appears to be impossible, stereotaxic localization may be tried in another plane or a different mammographic localization technique (see above) has to be chosen.
- In thin breasts or for lesions in thin parts of the breast (retroareolar), there may not be enough tissue to accomodate the 1.5–2.3 cm throw of the needle in core biopsies.

■ Ultrasound-guided Needle Biopsy

Ultrasound-guided needle biopsy enables the diagnosis of focal lesions. This technique requires that a lesion originally detected at mammography be *clearly* identifiable by ultrasound. The advantage of ultrasound-guided biopsy is that the correct position of the needle tip can be verified before aspirating the lesion, as opposed to verifying only the correct *projection of the needle* in the lesion using stereotaxis. With sufficient practice, ultrasound-guided needle biopsy can achieve the same accuracy as stereotaxis for those lesions that are visible sonographically.

■ Procedure

First choose the best approach and position the patient comfortably with the arm on the affected side placed behind her head. Next, carefully disinfect the skin. Inject local anesthetic under sonographic visualization. Be certain that the anesthetic is instilled without air, as air can obscure the lesion or needle tract. Make a skin incision.

Two persons are often needed to perform the biopsy. The first person holds the ultrasound transducer, while the examiner immobilizes the breast tissue that contains the lesion with his or her nondominant hand in a sterile glove, and performs the biopsy with the dominant hand. If the needle is difficult to visualize in the sonographic image, moving it slightly may help. The movement of the surrounding tissue helps identify the needle, which will appear in cross section as a hyperechoic spot, and longitudinally as a hyperechoic line (Figs. 6.**6 a** and **b**, and 6.**7 a** and **b**). In fine-needle aspiration, superficial lesions can be aspirated in the direction of sound propagation. When per-

Fig. 6.**6 a** and **b** Schematic diagram of ultrasound-guided biopsy (from [10])
a The needle is advanced toward the lesion under the transducer within the plane of the ultrasound-beam. Thus its entire length is visible. Anterior view
b Lateral view, i. e., in the direction of the biopsy

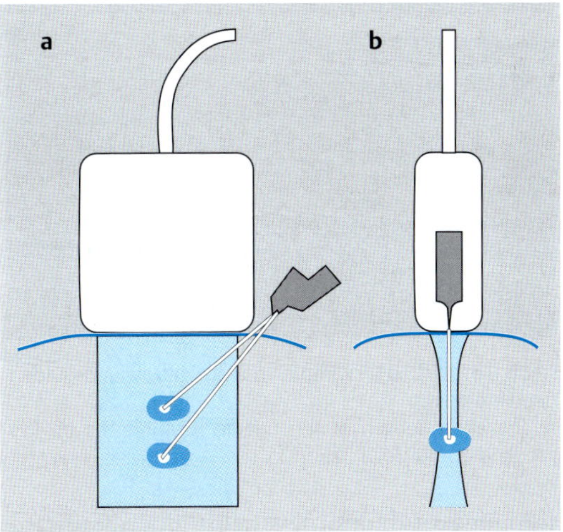

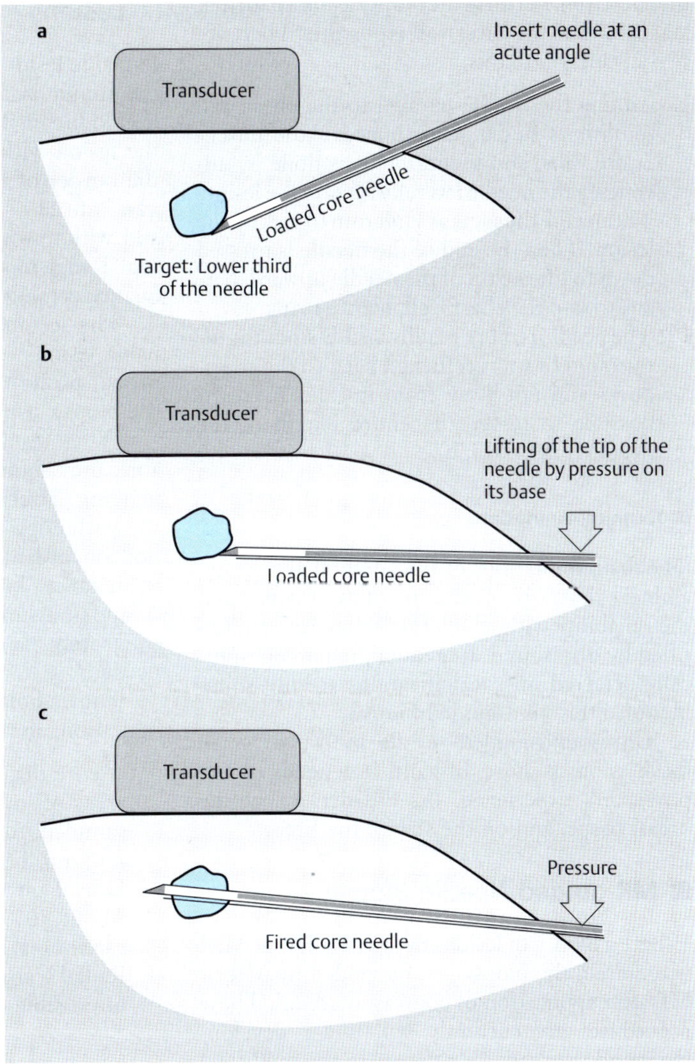

Fig. 6.**7 a–c** Procedure for ultrasound-guided needle biopsy:
a The needle is held at an acute angle to the surface of the breast. The needle points at the lower third of the lesion
b Pressing on the base of the needle lifts the tip of the needle upward
c This prevents injury to the chest wall when the device is fired

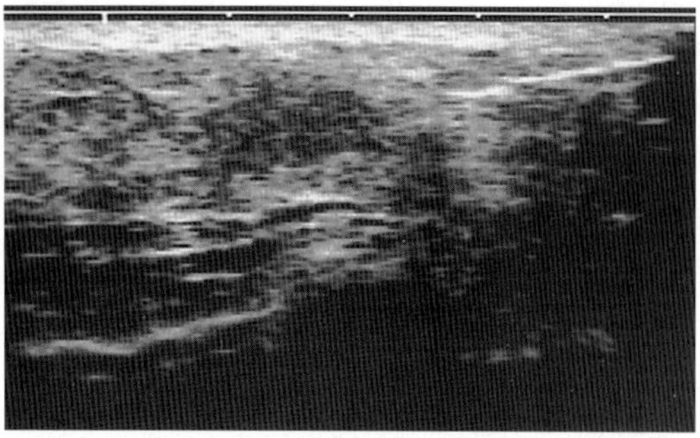

a

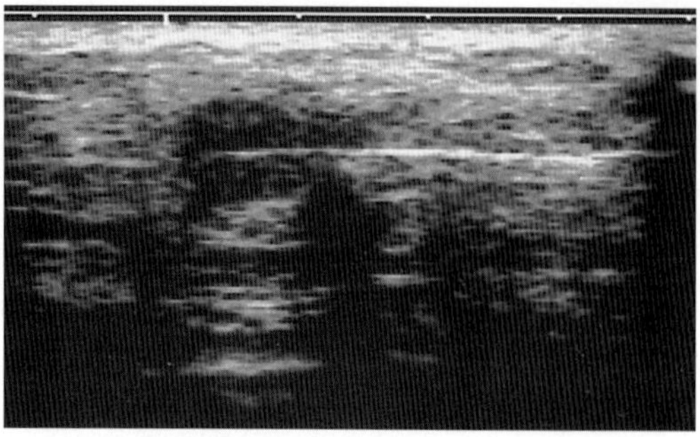

b

Fig. 6.**8 a** and **b** Example of an ultrasound-guided needle biopsy.
a The entire length of the needle is visible. Its tip lies proximal to the focal lesion,
b Documenting a correct biopsy. The entire length of the needle passing through the lesion must be visible

forming a core biopsy, never aim the needle toward the chest wall. Perform the biopsy using a path that is as parallel to the chest wall as possible. There are two advantages to this:

1. Aiming the needle parallel to the chest wall minimizes the danger of injuries to the musculature, ribs, and pleura. This is done by advancing the needle laterally *beneath* the lesion. The needle thus acts as a fulcrum to pick up the lesion. Then the end of the needle is pressed down to lift the tip of the needle upward, i. e., away from the chest wall, before firing.
2. The needle is more readily visible since the ultrasound beam is reflected back to the transducer and not away from it. This makes it possible to image the entire length of the needle (Figs. 6.**8 a, b**).

Technical Limitations

The main limitations of this method are the examiner's dexterity (a function of experience) and the reliability with which the lesion can be identified by ultrasound. In general, mammographically detected microcalcifications are not suitable for ultrasound-guided biopsy.

Ultrasound-guided needle biopsy of small focal lesions is more difficult. It depends on the physician's experience, on the density of the breast tissue, and on the size of the breast.

MR-guided Needle Biopsy

Where a biopsy of lesions detected solely at MRI is required, the biopsy can be guided by MR or CT after application of contrast medium. These procedures are currently still under development and the reader is referred to the published results.[11, 12, 13, 14]

Percutaneous Biopsy of Palpable Lesions

Palpable lesions can be aspirated by hand. After the tumor is immobilized with the examiner's nondominant hand, the needle is inserted into the lesion with the dominant hand, directly to the border of the lesion. Then the core biopsy gun is fired or the cytology needle is advanced and withdrawn several times in a fan-like fashion. Rapid motion is necessary to obtain good quality cytology material.

The accuracy of percutaneous biopsy of palpable lesions can be improved by verifying the proper position of the needle and documenting the biopsy, using ultrasound.

When results of biopsy or cytology are available, they should always he correlated with the imaging pattern that has prompted the biopsy. If the pathology results and imaging findings are not concordant, i. e., the mammogram looks like malignancy but the pathology is benign, it should be assumed the lesion in question was not adequately sampled, and a repeat biopsy is needed.

The radiologist should be aware of certain limitations in histologic assessment:

- A core diagnosis of DCIS does not exclude areas of invasion in parts of the tumor not sampled. About 20% of these lesions will be found to be invasive at surgery.[16]
- Ductal atypia requires surgical excision. About 50% will be found to have areas of carcinoma, usually DCIS, at surgery.[17]
- Radial scar requires surgical excision because of possible coexistant carcinoma.[18]

Summary

In contrast to aspiration cytology, core biopsy methods are characterized by significantly improved reproducibility and permit complete histologic examination.

Based on existing studies, core biopsy is a method of high accuracy. Even though long term follow-up on large numbers of patients is not yet available, present data show that an accuracy comparable to that of open biopsy can be achieved. Since with traditional needles—even when from 5 to ten 2 mm thick cores were removed—the accuracy was generally higher for masses than for microcalcifications, the final diagnosis and therapeutic decision based on the correlation of imaging findings and the histopathology of the cores has to be made with special care. New needles, which work with a vacuum and allow percutaneous removal of contiguous areas of tissue, may help to solve this problem.

At present we recommend the following procedure:

- Follow-up diagnostic imaging studies appear sufficient in the presence of benign findings or findings with a very high probability of benignity (> 98%).
- Lesions that are indeterminant should be confirmed by percutaneous biopsy (i. e., guided by ultrasound or stereotaxis), and follow-up examinations should be performed at regular intervals.
- For any suspected malignant lesions that core biopsy yields a negative result, surgical biopsy remains necessary.
- In the presence of positive histologic examination following needle biopsy, the surgeon may elect to perform mastectomy immediately without obtaining an open biopsy.

References

1 Azavedo E, Svane G, Auer G. Stereotactic fine-needle biopsy in 2594 mammographically detected non-palpable lesions. Lancet. 1989;I:1033–6

2 Dent DM, Kirkpatrick AE, McGoogan E, Chetty U, Anderson TJ. Stereotaxic localisation and aspiration cytology of impalpable breast lesions. Clin Radiol. 1989;40:380–2

3 Dowlatshahi K, Yaremko ML, Kluskens LF, Jokich PM. Nonpalpable breast lesions: Findings of sterotaxic needle-core biopsy and fine-needle aspiration cytology. Radiology. 1991;185:639–40

4 Dempsey P, Rubin E. The roles of needle biopsy and periodic follow-up in the evaluation and diagnosis of breast lesions. Semin Roentgenol. 1993;28:252–8

5 Fajardo LL, Jackson VP, Hunter TB. Interventional procedures in diseases of the breast: Needle biopsy, pneumocystography and galactography. AJR. 1992;158:1231–8

6 Kopans DB. Review of stereotaxic large-core needle biopsy and surgical biopsy results in nonpalpable breast lesions. Radiology. 1993;189:665–9

7 Parker SH, Burbank F, Jackman RJ et al. Percutaneous large-core breast biopsy: A multi-institutional Study. Radiology. 1994;193:359–64

8 Liberman L, Evans WP III, Dershaw DD, Hann LE, Deutsch BM, Abramson AF, Rosen PP. Radiography of microcalcifications in stereotaxic mammary core biopsy specimens. Radiology. 1994;190:223–5

9 Viehweg P, Heywang-Köbrunner SH, Beck R et al. Mammographische Stereotaxie: Fallstricke und Lösungsmöglichkeiten. Radiologe. 1995;35/4:79

10 Fornage BD, Coan JD, David CL. Ultrasound-guided needle biopsy of the breast and other interventional procedures. Radiol Clin North Am. 1992;30:167

11 Heywang-Köbrunner SH, Requardt H, Huynh AT et al. MRI of the breast: first experiences with a new localisation device. Eur Congr Radiol. 1993;93:204

12 Heywang-Köbrunner SH. Work in progress: Prototype breast coil for MR-guided needle localization – first experiences. J Comput Assist Tomogr. 1994;18:876–81

13 Heywang-Köbrunner SH, Beck R. Contrast-enhanced MRI of the breast. 2nd ed. Berlin: Springer; 1996

14 Greenstein-Orel SG, Schnall MD, Newman RW et al. MR imaging-guided localization and biopsy of breast lesions: Initial experience. Radiology. 1994;193:97–102

15 Fischer U, Vosshenrich R, Keating D et al. MR-guided biopsy of suspect breast lesions with a simple stereotaxic add-on device for surface coils. Radiology. 1994;192:272–3

16 Liberman L, Dershaw DD, Rosen PP, Giess CS, Cohen MA, Abramson AF, Hann LE. Stereotaxic core biopsy of breast carcinoma: accuracy at predicting invasion. Radiology. 1995;194:379–81

17 Liberman L, Cohen MA, Dershaw DD, Abramson AF, Hann LE, Rosen PP. Atypical duct hyperplasia at stereotaxic core breast biopsy as a predictor of carcinoma. AJR. 1995;164:1111–13

18 Dershaw DD, Morris EA, Liberman L, Abramson AF. Non-diagnostic stereotaxic breast biopsy: results of rebiopsy. Radiology. 1966;198:323–5

Suggested Reading

Dershaw DD, Moris EA, Liberman L, Abramson AF. Non-diagnostic stereotaxic breast biopsy: results of rebiopsy. Radiology. 1996; 187: 323–325

Fornage BD, Faroux MJ, Simatos A. Breast masses: US-guided fine-needle aspiration biopsy. Radiology. 1987; 162:409-14

Liberman L, Evans WP III, Dershaw DD, Hann LE, Deutsch BM, Abramson AF, Rosen PP. Radiography of microcalcifications in sterotaxic mammary core biopsy specimens. Radiology. 1994; 190: 223–225

Liberman L, Dershaw DD, Rosen PP, Giess CS, Cohen MA, Abramson AF, Hann LE. Stereotaxic are biopsy of breast carcinoma: accuracy at predicting invasion. Radiology. 1995 a, 194: 379–381

Liberman L, Cohen MA, Dreshaw DD, Abramson AF, Hann LE, Rosen PP. Atypcial duct hyperplasia at sterotaxic core breast biopsy as a predictor of carcinoma. AJR. 1995; 164: 1111–1113

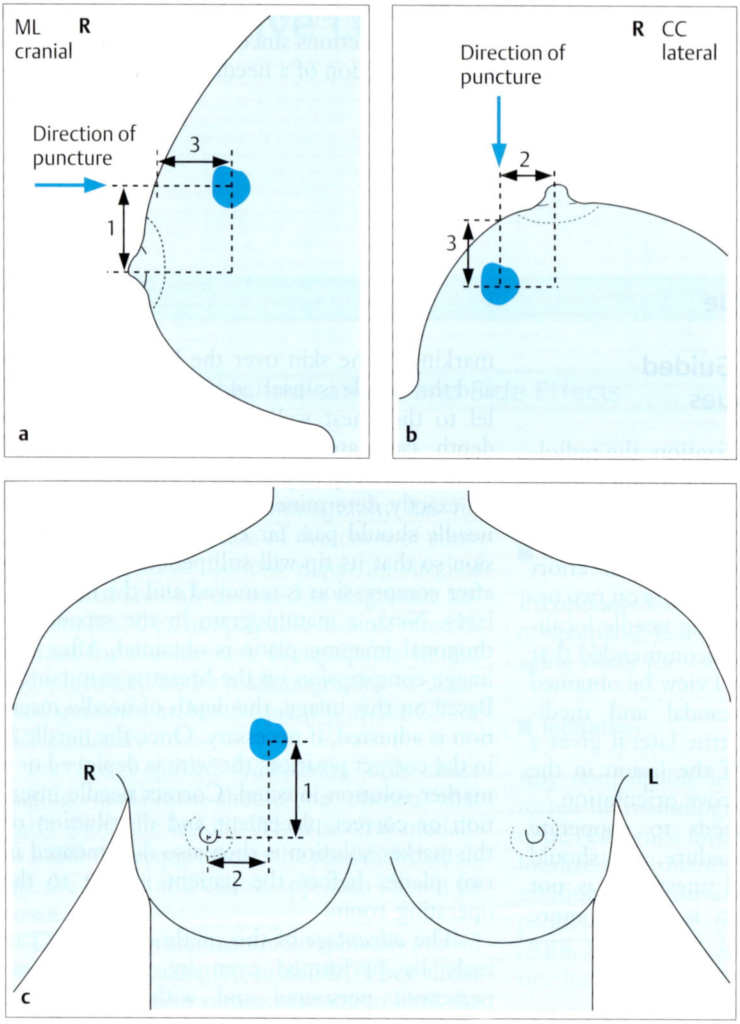

Fig. 7.**1 a–c** Schematic diagram of manual localization: The coordinates of the lesion in the horizontal (CC view) and vertical (ML view) direction (**a** and **b**) with reference to the nipple are marked on the skin of the breast and the depth of the lesion from the skin surface is measured

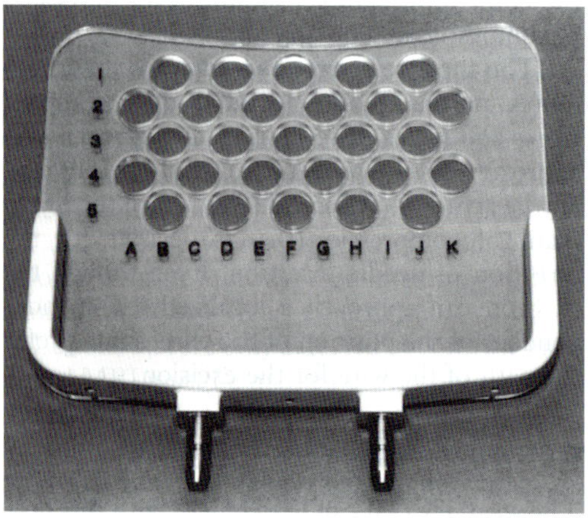

Fig. 7.**2** Perforated compression plate for localizing breast lesions

possible pitfalls exists and the procedure is performed very diligently. This is due to various hazards (see below) and the failure to readjust the needle depth on a second, orthogonal view before final deployment. The procedure is the same as in a stereotaxic biopsy (see p. 108). Once the correct position of the needle is verified, a marker wire is placed or a contrast solution injected. The needle usually just acts as a guide for the wire and needs to be removed before releasing the compression on the breast. If the needle is to stay in place, an appropriate opening in the needle holder is necessary to allow detaching of the needle from it.

First the needle is placed in the same manner as for stereotaxic percutaneous biopsy. After the wire is placed, the proper position is first documented in the usual stereotaxic views (+ 15° and – 15°). After compression is released we strongly recommend that the correct wire placement be further documented in another plane perpendicular to the primary imaging plane (for example, in the mediolateral plane, if the first plane was the CC plane; Figs. 7.2 a–e). This is important because, particularly in dense breasts, tissue elasticity can cause the tip of the needle to lie above the lesion, not readily apparent in the stereotaxic views. A positioning error of a few millimeters in a compressed breast can correspond to a large positioning error (> 1 cm) in the relaxed breast.

To minimize the upward displacement of the needle that often occurs as a result of tissue elasticity, the needle may be placed 3–6 mm deeper than the calculated target point. This compensates for tissue elasticity, and once compression is relieved, the needle will usually lie at the desired location.

For localization procedures the stereotaxic method is comparable to localization using a perforated compression plate. The major importance of stereotaxy is its use for percutaneous biopsy (see Chapter 6).

The following special problems can occur in stereotaxic needle localization:

- Due to the geometry of stereotaxy, slight deviations in the position of the needle in the targeting or documentation views can correspond to a significant deviation in depth localization. Localization errors can occur if the patient moves (in nondigital systems significant time may elapse for development of the localization views and for depth determination), or if the targets chosen on the + and – 15° stereotaxic views prove not to be identical. This may occur with ill-defined lesions, for which it is difficult to identify the same structure on the + and – 15° views or with multiple microcalcifications showing minimal pleomorphism.
- Even with the tip of the needle in the correct position, inserting the marker wire will usually push the denser breast tissue forward a few millimeters. The resulting positioning error in the compressed breast can result in a final positioning error in the relaxed breast of over 1 cm.

To minimize these problems, the following steps are recommended:

- Exercising extreme care in selecting the target point and in verifying it in the + 15° and – 15° views.
- Switching to another localization method if identical target points cannot be clearly located on the compression views.
- Always advancing the needle a few millimeters deeper than the target point to compensate for tissue elasticity.
- Always verifying the final result in two perpendicular planes.
- Always (with this method) using localization needles that can be repositioned in case of an unsatisfactory position.

■ Manual Localization

Manual localization was the first and simplest method for advancing a needle to a lesion under mammographic guidance. In most institutions in the USA, it has been replaced by the grid technique since an approach parallel to the chest wall is preferred. In the hands of an experienced radiologist it may, however, allow a fast approach to superficial lesion.

The *advantages* are the simplicity and the fact that the point of entry lies directly anterior to the lesion, which often corresponds to the approach preferred by the surgeon.

Disadvantages are that it is generally not as precise as localizing with add-on devices with the necessity for corrections in a certain percentage of lesions, and it requires more practice and skill in three-dimensional visualization than other methods of localization. Finally, the axis of the needle is perpendicular to the chest wall, increasing the risk of injury to the chest wall when a lesion is located posteriorly.

Procedure: Figure 7.3 shows how the point of entry on the skin is selected based on the mammograms and how the depth of the lesion is measured. When transferring the coordinates of the lesion with respect to the nipple, the assistant must be careful to hold the breast in the same position as it was in the original mediolateral view. When inserting the needle, the physician places his or her other hand around the tissue into which the needle is to be inserted. This minimizes the risk of injury to the chest wall and brings the breast into a shape similar to that on the mediolateral view. The position of the needle is then verified in mammograms in two planes (CC and 90° mediolateral) and corrected if necessary. After verification of the correct

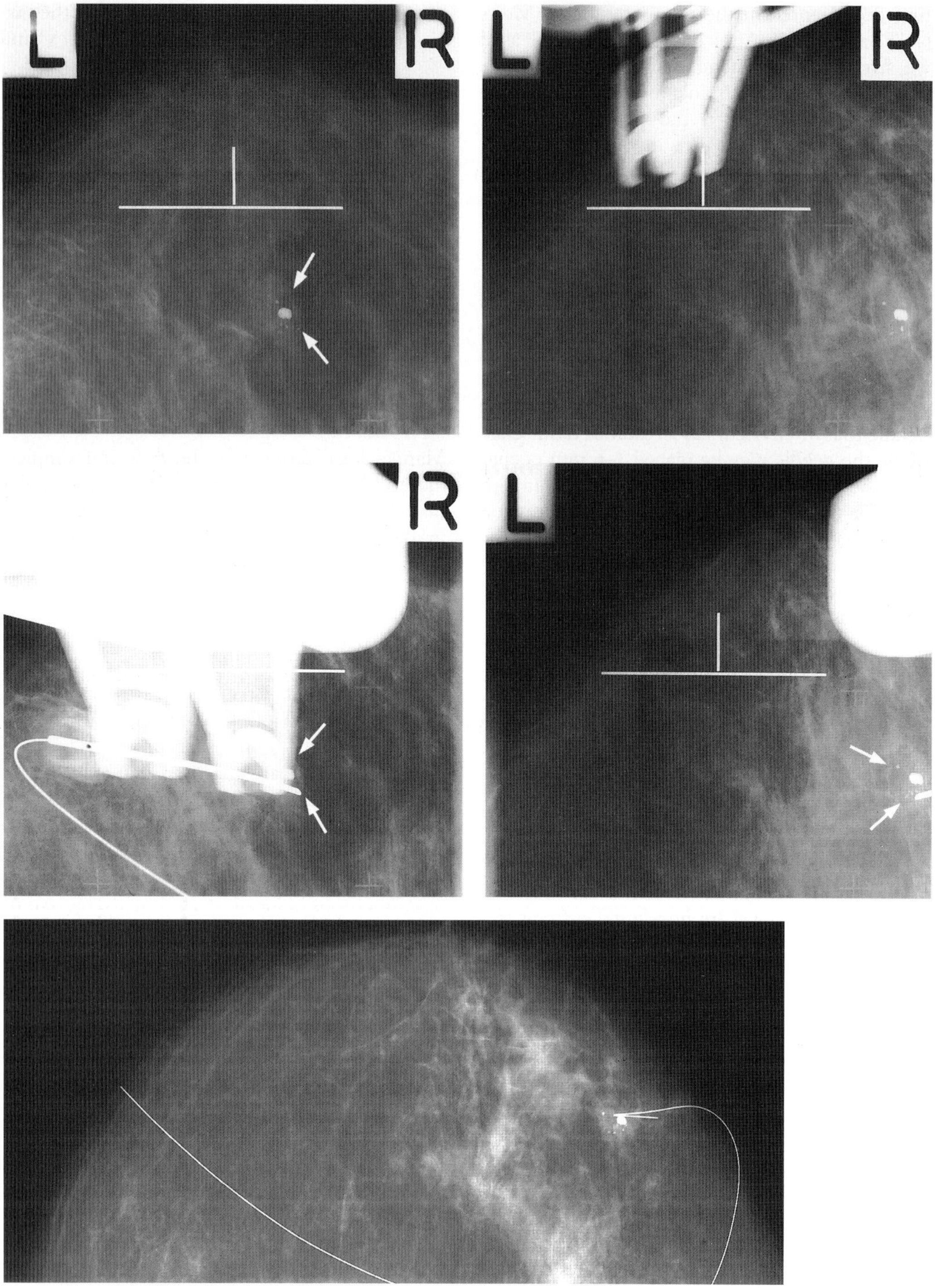

a

b

c

Fig. 7.**3 a–e**
a Two partial views with the tube tilted – 15° and + 15° reveal a small focal lesion requiring localization or biopsy
b Demonstrating the tip of the needle in the center of the focal lesion
c and **d** Documentation view demonstrating correct positioning of the localization wire
e Specimen radiography

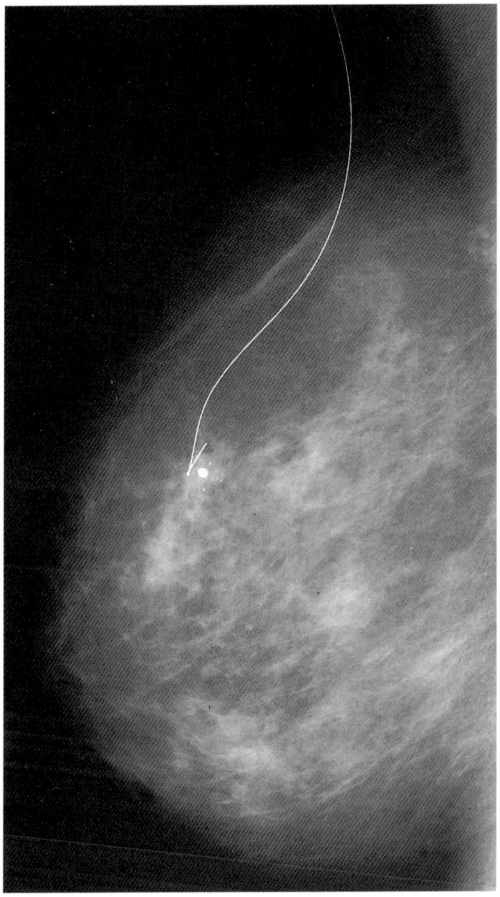

d

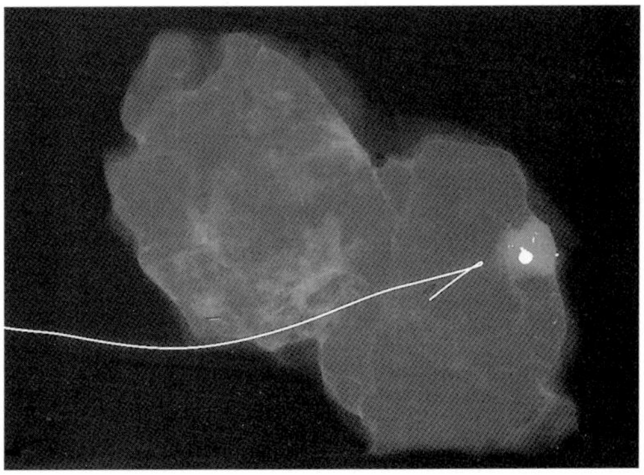

e

needle position, a contrast solution is injected or a wire is placed through the needle.

■ Ultrasound-guided Localization

Ultrasound-guided localization requires that the lesion be visualized via sonography. This means that it cannot be used with microcalcifications, yet it is very effective in localizing focal lesions. The procedure is similar to the ultrasound-guided percutaneous biopsy (see p. 108). Instead of aspirating or performing a core biopsy, the radiologist deploys a marker wire through the needle. Contrast solutions are not generally used in ultrasound-guided localization. Sonographic verification of the correct needle position is mandatory (Fig. 7.4).

The *advantage* of ultrasound-guided localization over other methods of localization is that it takes the least amount of time. A *disadvantage* is that visualization of small or preinvasive lesions may be uncertain or impossible. Furthermore, it

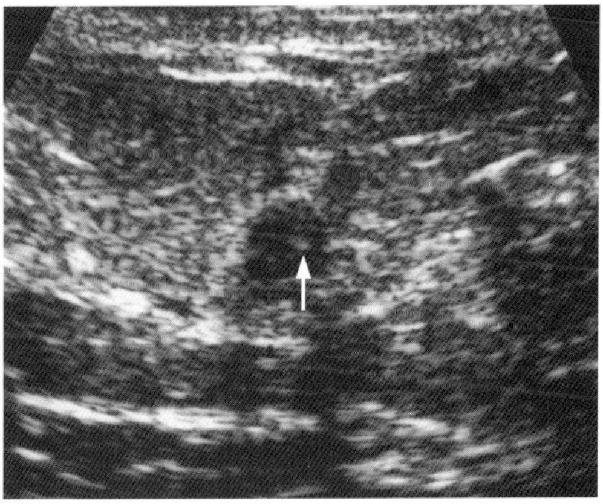

Fig. 7.**4** Documenting correct positioning of the needle after ultrasound-guided localization. The tip of the needle is visible as a hyperechoic point in the center of the lesion. Definite localization of the needle-tip position requires visualization of the needle in its long axis

may sometimes be difficult to identify the lesion in a subsequent specimen sonogram.

MR-guided Localization

Lesions detected by MRI alone must be preoperatively marked using contrast-enhanced MRI or contrast-enhanced CT. Ultrasound-guided localization by a physician experienced in both sonography and MRI is recommended only where subsequent sonograms unequivocally demonstrate a lesion correlating with the detected by MRI. Due to respiratory motion, a lesion detected by MRI can be localized with an accuracy of ± 1 cm using a CT or MRI unit without a special biopsy coil. Highly precise preoperative marking (and localization for core biopsy) is possible through the use of special "biopsy" or "localization" coils. Since these special coils for MR-guided localization are still undergoing development, the reader is referred to published studies [1, 2, 3, 4, 5].

Galactographically Guided Localization

If a lesion is only detected at galactography, repeat galactography will be required for preoperative localization of the lesion.

Technique

Several options for galactographically guided localization are available:

1. After galactography (see Chapter 3, p. 69) in the craniocaudal and mediolateral planes, the galactographic findings are localized using the standard mammographic localization techniques (i. e., manually, using a perforated plate, or by means of stereotaxy).
2. If only a single duct is involved, the duct may be galactographically visualized and delineated immediately preoperatively using a combination of contrast medium and patent blue. The blue-dyed ductal system must be excised immediately after instillation of contrast medium.
3. In the presence of significant duct ectasia, the lactiferous duct itself will sometimes be visible at mammography or sonography. In this case, mammographic or ultrasound localization is possible without the use of contrast media.

Localization Materials

The selection of localization materials depends on the interval between localization and surgery. Usually, localization is performed shortly before surgery.

In this case, the physician may elect to use low-cost *dye marking* with patent blue immediately preoperatively. Having verified correct needle position, the radiologist injects 0.2–0.3 mL of blue dye, such as methylene blue or patent blue, after which the surgeon removes the blue-stained parenchymal tissue. For mammographically guided localization, the radiologist adds 0.2–0.3 mL of a nonionic radiographic contrast medium. This is necessary for subsequent documentation of proper dispersion of the contrast solution on the two-view mammogram done after the localization has been completed. It is important to perform the operation as quickly as possible after injecting the blue solution because within a few hours the solution can diffuse throughout large areas of the breast or even the entire breast, rendering precise localization impossible. If the interval between administration of the contrast solution and operation cannot be limited to a few hours, the radiologist should choose a different localization procedure. Further disadvantages are that diffusion renders it impossible for the pathologist to identify the exact injection site, and in addition to contrast allergies, severe allergies to patent blue, although rare, have been known to occur.

A more suitable procedure, and one that is equally simple and inexpensive, is to use a *carbon solution for marking the lesion*. This can be performed several days preoperatively since the carbon remains at the injection site until the surgeon removes it along with the lesion. However, even though inert and harmless, carbon solution is not approved in some countries (USA) for use in the breast.

This method is particularly suitable for CT- and MR-guided localization since in these cases it is often difficult to coordinate the scheduling of the examination and surgery.

The sterile carbon solution, which can be prepared by most pharmacies (4 g of activated charcoal in 100 mL of 0.9% saline solution), in injected into the center of the lesion to be excised or directly proximal to it. Approximately 1–1.5 mL of solution have to be injected to achieve sufficient dispersion and visualization.

For mammographically guided localization, 0.2–0.3 mL of nonionic radiographic contrast medium should be added to the solution for subsequent image documentation of correct dispersion. Then a fine line of carbon extending all the way to the skin is injected as the needle is withdrawn, to permit the surgeon to locate the lesion after the needle or wire has been removed. A particular advantage of this method is that the carbon also enables the pathologist to locate the injection site in the specimen.

Some surgeons prefer to have the needle left in place (suitable only if the mammography suite is close to the operating room) or have a marker wire placed through the localization needle to facilitate locating the lesion, which may be stained with dye or unstained.

In contrast to needles, *localization wires* have the advantage of being more flexible and better anchored in the tissue. This minimizes the risk of wire migration.

There are various types of localization wires (Fig. 7.**5**). The tenacity of staying in place varies with their shape and the type of breast tissue. Dislocation can occur particularly in soft fatty tissue, whereby dislocation primarily occurs in the soft, fatty tissues. In rare cases, wires have been observed to migrate distally. This usually occurs only in wires whose form predisposes them to migrate in a certain direction, such as a simple 1-shaped hookwire. The so-called twist marker (which can also be retracted through tissue like a corkscrew), the Homer wire, and the Fixmarker (from BIP) are nondirectional. The particular advantage of these wires is that they can be withdrawn or retracted through the needle, making it possible to correct the position of the needle at any time.

Regardless of the wire chosen, the physician should ensure that the needle through which the wire is advanced is sufficiently stiff (it should not be too thin and flexible) because otherwise it can deviate considerably in dense tissue and seriously compromise the accuracy of localization. An adequate length of wire should extend beyond the skin and be securely taped to it to avoid retraction of the wire and its subsequent loss. During surgery, if the surgeon is dissecting along the length of the wire, he or she should be careful not to transsect it. It may then retract into the breast and be very difficult to locate.

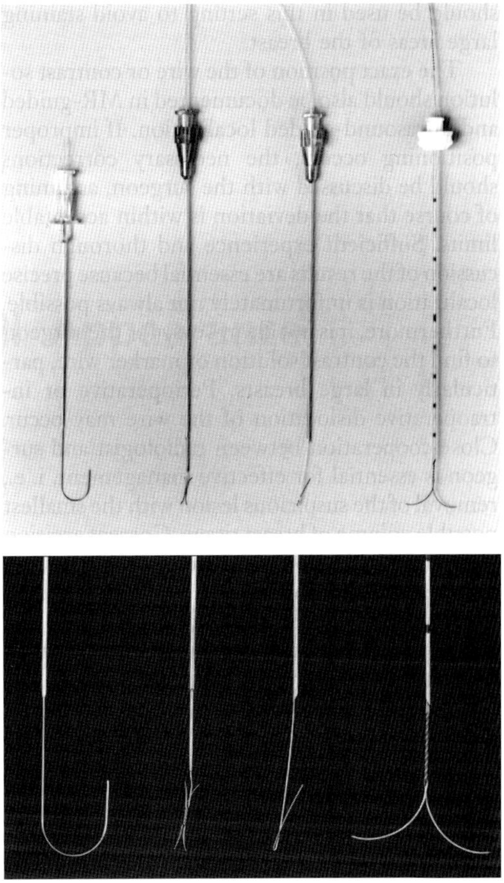

Fig. 7.**5** Various localization wires

Problems and Their Solutions

All methods require documentation of the final position of the localization wire or the contrast solution. This means that after mammographically guided localization, the position of the needle should be documented in two mammographic planes (craniocaudal and mediolateral; see p. 115). If the wire is improperly positioned but the distance between the tumor and the tip of the wire is still acceptable (i. e., does not exceed 10 mm), the radiologist may describe to the surgeon the exact position of the lesion in the image with respect to the tip of the wire. Large areas undergoing excision should have their margins marked with two wires. Multiple lesions can be needle localized for excision in one surgical procedure. Wires rather than dye

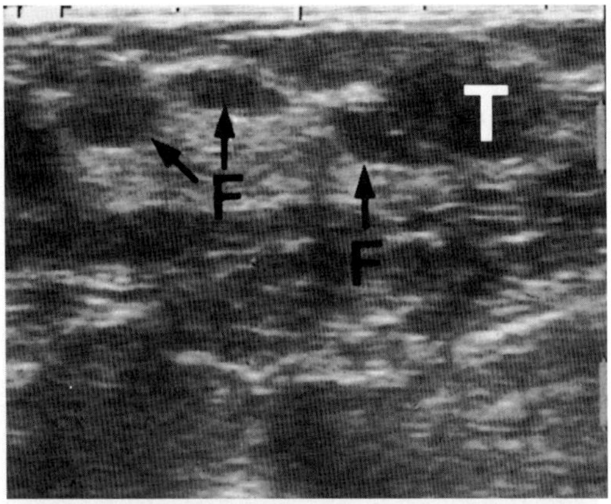

g

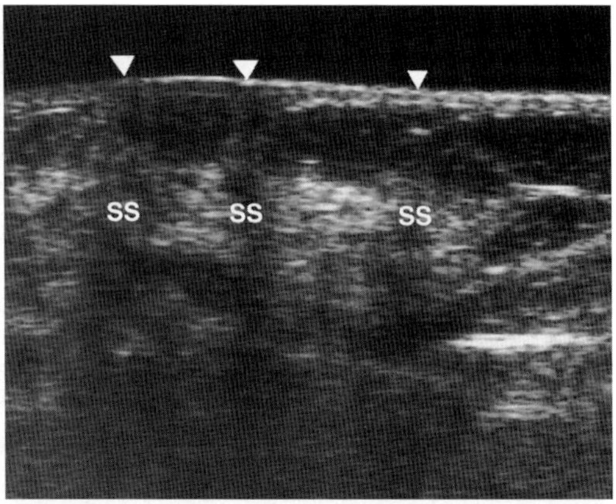

h

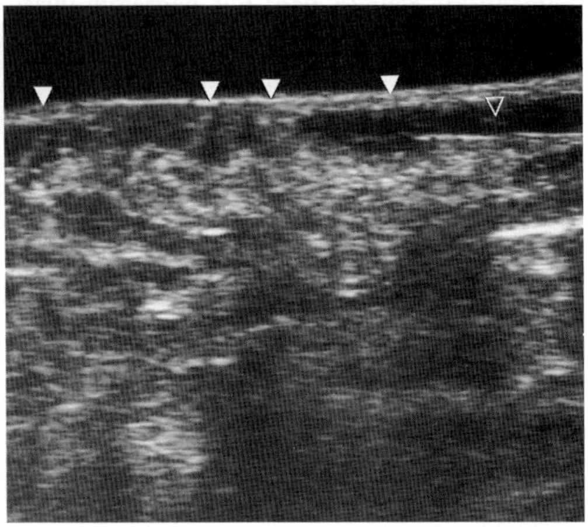

i

Fig. 8.**5g** If hypoechoic fat lobules (F) are interspersed in the glandular tissue, they may simulate a tumor (T). The shown tumor proved to be a fibroadenoma. It is surrounded by multiple interspersed fat lobules (F). The main criteria for differentiation include:

1. Fat lobules are easily compressible
2. In the vertical plane, the fat lobules will generally appear as long structures that often are connected to the subcutaneous fat (see also Fig. 4.**5**)

h Acoustic shadows (SS) can occur at Cooper's ligaments (arrowheads) if they are parallel to the direction of sound propagation. These shadows can be distinguished from pathologic shadows by their point of origin. These shadows also generally disappear when compression is increased or the transducer is tilted, i. e., they are not constant

i The same breast as in Figure 8.**5h** with increased compression applied. The open arrowhead shows a Cooper's ligament that does not cause an acoustic shadow regardless of whether compression is applied. The other Cooper's ligaments produce obvious acoustic shadows without compression, which disappear when compression is applied

Cooper's ligaments are hyperechoic and permeate the layer of fatty tissue, appearing as fine linear structures. Due to their orientation (almost parallel to the direction of sound propagation), Cooper's ligaments can produce acoustic shadows that occur when the sound is reflected away from the transducer. These acoustic shadows can be recognized by the fact that they originate from Cooper's ligaments. They can generally be eliminated by compression and do not represent a pathologic finding.

The skin itself appears as a hyperechoic line or, depending on the resolution of the transducer, as a double contour whose thickness generally does not exceed 3 mm except at the areola.

Since the retroareolar ducts run nearly parallel to the direction of sound propagation and periductal fibrosis is frequently present, the sound waves will often be reflected away from the transducer or absorbed behind the nipple. The acoustic shadow ("nipple shadow") thus produced does not represent a pathologic finding but a normal structure that can vary. This nipple shadow may impair visualization of the retroareolar region.

Magnetic Resonance Imaging (Fig. 8.6 a–d)

MRI is not necessary for imaging the normal breast. However, normal breast tissue will often be incidentally visualized on MR images, or normal tissue will be diagnosed after a suspected pathologic change has been ruled out.

In T1-weighted spoiled-gradient echo sequences (FLASH, T1 FFE, and SP GRASS),

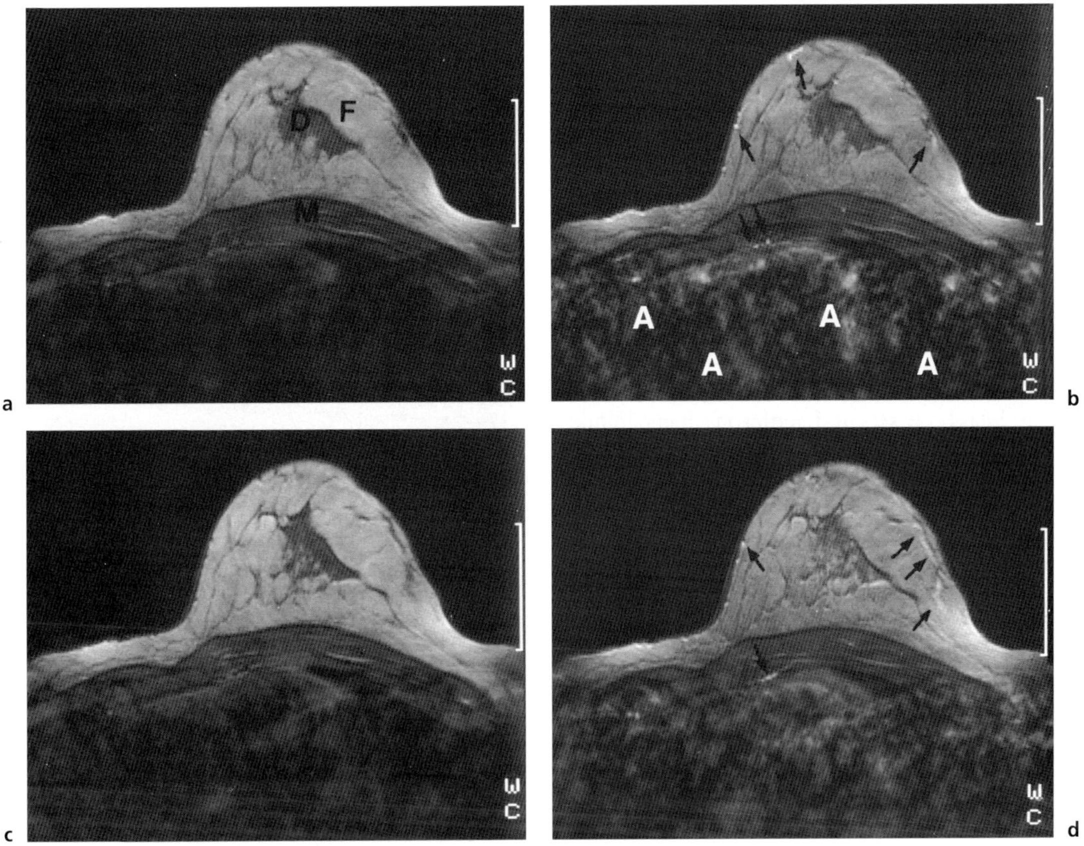

Fig. 8.6 **a–d** Contrast-enhanced MRI of a normal breast.
a On the T1-weighted transverse slice of the breast (FLASH 3D), glandular and connective tissue (D) are visualized with low signal intensity, as is muscle (M). Fat (F) shows moderate signal intensity.
b After application of contrast, normal glandular tissue and fatty tissue only enhance slightly at the beginning of the menstrual cycle (between the 6th and 16th days) and in the postmenstrual phase. This means that the signal intensity hardly changes at all in comparison to the plain image (**a**). Only the band of artifacts caused by blood flowing through the heart (A) significantly increases in signal intensity, as do the vessels (arrow) that can be traced through the images after contrast application as winding or punctiform structures of high signal intensity
c and **d** In the second half of the menstrual cycle, slight to intense diffuse or nodular enhancement patterns are often seen in normal glandular tissue
c Comparable image of the same breast as in Figure 8.**6 a** in the second half of the cycle before application of contrast
d After application of contrast in the second half of the cycle, moderate diffuse enhancement may be seen (arrows indicate vascular structures)

fat has moderate signal intensity, whereas all glandular and ductal structures and fibrous connective tissue (with Cooper's ligaments) are visualized with low signal intensity. After intravenous injection of the contrast medium gadolinium-DTPA, glandular, fatty, and connective tissue do not normally enhance, i. e., these structures appear identical in precontrast and postcontrast images. Only vascular structures can be traced through the images as small enhancing worm-like structures or punctate cross sections of high signal intensity. Contrast enhancement of the nipple itself occurs in approximately 50% of all patients and should not be regarded as pathologic in the absence of suggestive clinical findings. Occasionally, a milky or patchy diffuse enhancement, sometimes even focal enhancement, can appear in normal glandular tissue. This enhancement is probably due to hormonal changes and usually occurs in young patients with active glandular tissue or in postmenopausal patients receiving hormone therapy (particularly where preparations with a high progesterone content are used). It is usually transient and more pronounced before and during menstruation. Since this enhancement can interfere with the exclusion of malignancy and can lead to false positive findings, we recommend to perform contrast-enhanced MRI between day 6 to day 17 *of the menstrual cycle*, whenever possible. Also, it should be performed in young patients (those below the age of 30–35 years in whom the incidence of malignancy is typically very low and the glandular tissue tends to be metabolically more active) only if definitely indicated.[2, 3]

Involution

Histology

As ovarian function decreases, involution of the glandular body sets in. Lactiferous ducts, lobules and parenchyma become atrophic, and fatty and fibrous tissue dominate. Often ectasia of the large excretory ducts occurs.

Clinical Examination

The findings of the clinical examination vary considerably, depending on the extent of the parenchymal involution, the presence of structural changes due to benign breast disorders, and the extent of fibrosis.

Mammography

The formerly dense epithelial and mesenchymal parts of the glandular tissue that absorb radiation are replaced with fat as involution progresses. The body of the gland itself becomes considerably more radiolucent and fibrous tissue, vascular structures, and remaining glandular lobules become more readily discernible, as do the large retroareolar ectatic lactiferous ducts (Fig. 8.7).

Involution begins in the inner half of the breast and involves the upper outer quadrant and the retroareolar region later. Thus mammography in the older woman will reveal residual glandular tissue primarily in the retroareolar region and in the upper outer quadrant. Involution improves the visualization of the breast. *In a completely involuted fatty breast, the sensitivity of mammography approaches 100%.*

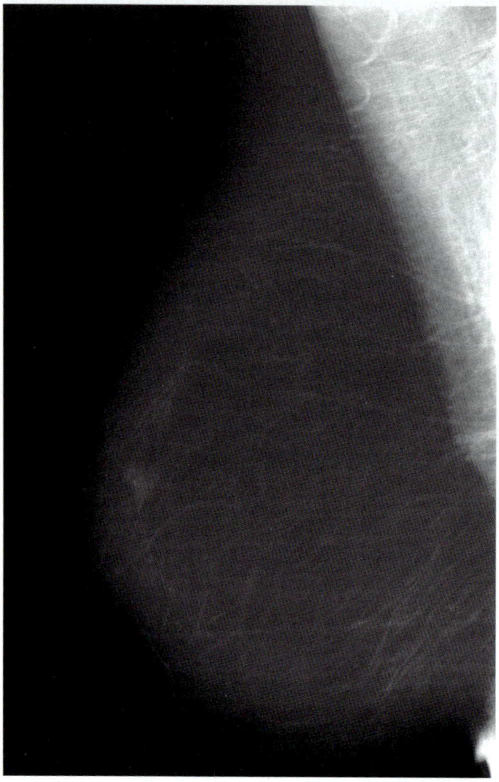

Fig. 8.7 Involution. Radiolucent glandular body only delineating Cooper ligaments and vascular structures (ML view)

Sonography

The fatty involuted breast appears hypoechoic on sonographic examination (Fig. 8.5 e). Only remaining islands of hyperechoic connective tissue and Cooper ligaments traverse the hypoechoic fatty tissue. Residual parenchyma generally appears as moderately echogenic islands in hypoechoic fat.

Over 90% of breast carcinomas are hypoechoic (similar to fatty tissue). Only some breast carcinomas have a distinctive posterior acoustic shadow or a hyperechoic peripheral rim. This comprises the *sensitivity of ultrasonography in the fatty breast.* Islands of fatty tissue with or without posterior shadowing due to fibrous septa can also be mistaken for tumors. To avoid both false positive and false negative calls the sonogram should generally be read in conjunction with mammography.

With the excellent sensitivity of mammography applied to the involuted breast, sonography is not necessary for detecting or excluding malignancy. *However, it is indicated for differentiating cysts from solid masses* since simple cysts can reliably be diagnosed even in the fatty breast.

Magnetic Resonance Imaging

In MR images, fatty tissue has high signal intensity before and after intravenous administration of contrast medium, whereas residual parenchyma and connective-tissue structures have low signal intensity. Due to the high sensitivity of mammography, contrast-enhanced MRI is not generally needed in the fatty breast.

Summary

The breast of an asymptomatic patient over the age of 40 is generally examined clinically and mammographically. In the presence of uncertain palpable and mammographic findings, ultrasound can provide additional information. Ultrasound as the first diagnostic imaging procedure is only indicated in younger women.

The physician should verify the clinical absence of:

- Palpable pathologic findings
- Asymmetry
- Skin or nipple retraction
- Pathologic discharge

In diagnostic imaging studies, special attention should be given to:

- Uniform skin thickness
- Visualization of fine Cooper's ligaments
- Visualization of an undisturbed subcutaneous and retromammary layer of fat
- Symmetrical distribution of the body of the gland
- Regular configuration of ductal structures converging at the nipple

Furthermore, imaging studies serve to verify the absence of:

- Masses and densities
- Architectural distortion
- Suspected microcalcification

Comparison with the contralateral breast is important both in light of the immense variety in size, arrangement, and density of the parenchyma among patients, and because clinical, mammographic, and sonographic detection of abnormality will depend on the recognition of sometimes subtle structural abnormalities. Comparison with previous diagnostic imaging studies (where available) is even more important.

Abnormalities

Definition

Breasts may vary considerably with respect to size, shape, and consistency. The following conditions are regarded as abnormalities:

- Asymmetry
- Macromastia
- Polymastia (for example in the axillary tail or axilla)
- Inverted nipple

Accessory Breast Tissue (Polymastia)

Circumscribed development of glandular parenchyma in the axilla is the most common site of accessory breast tissue. This tissue is either completely separate from the rest of the parenchyma (Figs. 8.**8a–d**) or connected with the parenchymal tissue in the axillary tail. Glandular tissue extending far into the axillary tail can occur on one or both sides. Since breast cancer can also occur in ectopic glandular tissue, this tissue should always be carefully examined.

Supernumerary mammary glands are found along the milk line (mamma accessoria) and may or may not have an associated nipple (mamma aberrata). Polythelia refers to the presence of supernumerary nipples without mammary tissue.

■ Clinical Examination

Palpation will reveal what appears to be a soft tumor in the axilla, which may be isolated or adjacent to the glandular tissue in the axillary tail or at other locations. Sometimes the patient will report tenderness and fluctuations in size related to her menstrual cycle. Swelling may also occur during pregnancy and lactation.

■ Mammography

Corresponding parenchymal densities can be visualized mammographically with an oblique view in the axillary tail or in the axilla on an axillary view (Figs. 8.**8a** and **b**). The criteria for assessment are the same as those for glandular tissue within the breast.

■ Sonography and Magnetic Resonance Imaging

Sonography (Figs. 8.**8c** and **d**) also visualizes the asymmetrical configuration of normal or mastopathic glandular tissue. The same applies to MRI, where normal tissue and benign proliferative breast disorders normally will not enhance.

Due to its high sensitivity in detecting malignancy, MRI may be used for differential diagnostic problems cansed by asymmetric tissue.

Inverted Nipple

(Fig. 8.**9a–d**)

■ Clinical Examination

Unilateral or bilateral inverted nipples may represent normal variants. It is, however, important that the inversion exists since birth or is longstanding (unchanged for years). Recently occurring retraction and/or inversion can be the result of chronic inflammatory or malignant processes. Therefore, careful history is required to determine the need for workup of this finding.

■ Mammography

Depending on the projection, the inverted nipple can appear as a round, smooth-contoured mass mammographically. However, in most cases, the skin will be clearly seen to dip into this mass. The risk of confusing this condition with a lesion is minimal if the examiner is familiar with the clinical findings. Failure to image the nipple in profile may result in a false mammographic picture of nipple inversion.

■ Sonography

The inverted nipple itself can appear as a hypoechoic nodule with or without an acoustic shadow. Here, too, the risk of confusion is minimal if one knows the clinical findings and is familiar with the typical sonographic findings.

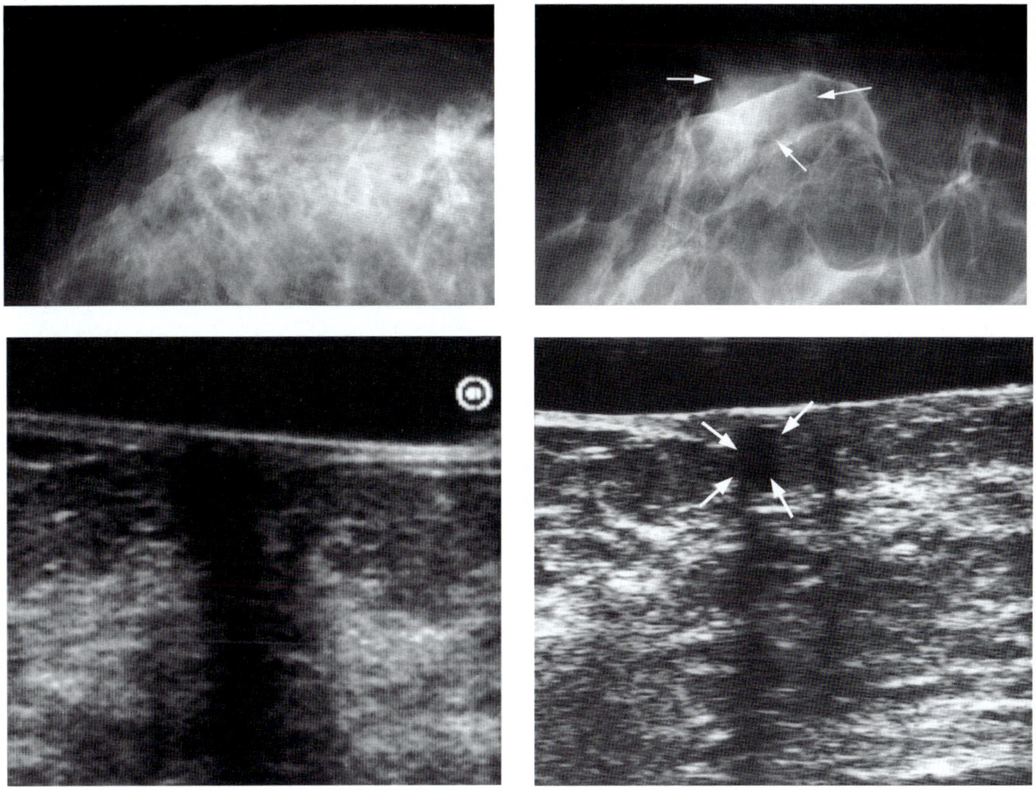

a b c d

Fig. 8.**9 a–d** Inverted nipple
a and **b** Mammographically, the inverted nipple typically appears as a funnel-shaped density (**a**) or a nodule (**b**)
c and **d** Sonographically, the inverted nipple can produce a pronounced nipple shadow (**e**) or it may appear as a hypoechoic nodule (**d**)

Magnetic Resonance Imaging

In MR imaging studies, the examiner should bear in mind that the normal inverted nipple can enhance.

Summary

Asymmetry and polymastia are congenital conditions that will generally be identified with a careful history. The examiner must exclude significant changes that are not due to hormonal influences (i. e., pregnancy or menstrual cycle). If the breast examination is normal (revealing just increased glandular tissue, but no change in consistency, and no retraction) and mammographic appearance is normal (composition corresponds to normal glandular tissue), then it is highly probable that the condition represents a normal variant.

In the presence of uncertain densities, further diagnostic studies (mammography, ultrasound, MRI, and/or percutaneous biopsy) are indicated (see also Chapter 19).
Congenital inverted nipple is another normal variant which cannot be confused with a mass if the examiner is aware of the history and physical examination. This condition should be distinguished from recently occurring nipple inversion. Here, particular care should be taken to exclude malignancy.

Pregnancy and Lactation

Histology

During pregnancy, proliferative changes occur, with lobular hyperplasia, hyperemia, and fluid retention in breast tissue. Lactogenesis, the milk synthesis in the glandular cell, begins in the second half of pregnancy. Toward the end of pregnancy, the alveoli begin to secrete and parenchyma largely displaces the stromal tissue.

Clinical Examination

During pregnancy, the breast increases in size and acquires a firmer consistency, accompanied by hyperpigmentation of the areola and nipple and by prominent veins. The firmer consistency of the breast makes palpation more difficult.

The proliferative stimulation can cause existing fibroadenomas to increase rapidly in size, typically leading to smooth-contoured, mobile, and round or oval palpable findings with a firmer consistency than that of the surrounding glandular tissue (see p. 168). Nevertheless malignancy, which can occur during pregnancy, needs to be excluded with great care.

Milk retention can develop during lactation. This can lead to focal thickening, inflammation, or formation of a galactocele (see p. 164).

Mammography (Fig. 8.**10a**)

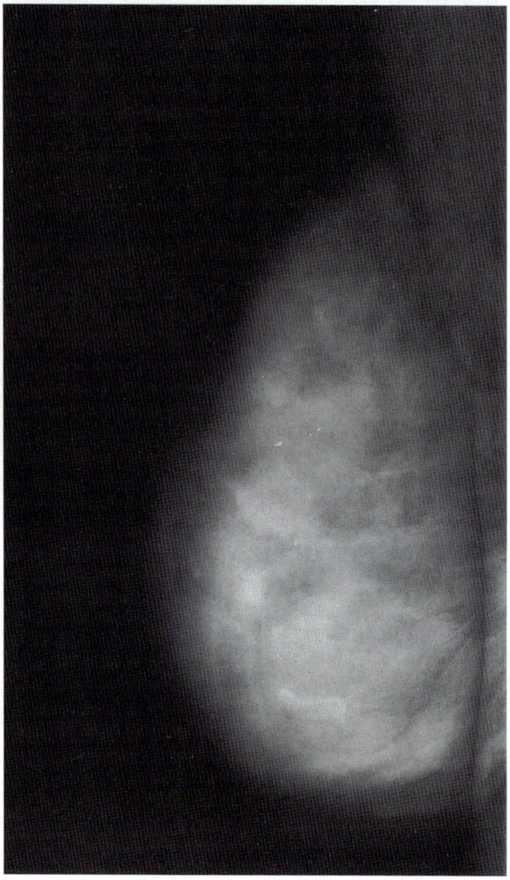

Fig. 8.**10a–e** Lactating breast
a Mammography reveals an extremely dense, heterogeneous, coarse, nodular parenchymal structure. Mammographic evaluation is impaired

Mammographically, the body of the gland appears very dense with heterogeneously coarse, nodular, confluent densities and minimal fatty tissue. This severely limits the diagnostic value of mammography. If clinical examination and mammography become necessary during the nursing period, the examination should be performed after breast feeding or pumping since the breast then has a softer consistency and is less radiodense. Screening mammography is usually not performed during pregnancy or lactation. It should be delayed for 3 to 6 months after the cessation of lactation to allow the breast density to decrease. Diagnostic mammography may be indicated during pregnancy or lactation if clinical suspicion exists. Although mass lesions may not be discernible because of the increased radiodensity of the breast tissue, microcalcifications typical of malignancy can be detected even in extremely dense breasts (Figs. 8.**10b, c**).

When mammography is performed during pregnancy, the abdomen should be shielded with lead aprons despite the fact that most of the extremely soft radiation will be absorbed in soft tissues of the abdomen and almost no radiation will reach the child.

b A 34-year-old pregnant patient with a highly suspicious palpable finding in the left upper inner quadrant, which core biopsy confirmed as a carcinoma. Mammography on the second day after delivery: The mammogram reveals a second focal lesion with an irregular border and a highly suspicious cluster of microcalcifications in the upper outer quadrant. The microcalcifications are visible in greater detail on the magnification mammogram (**c**)

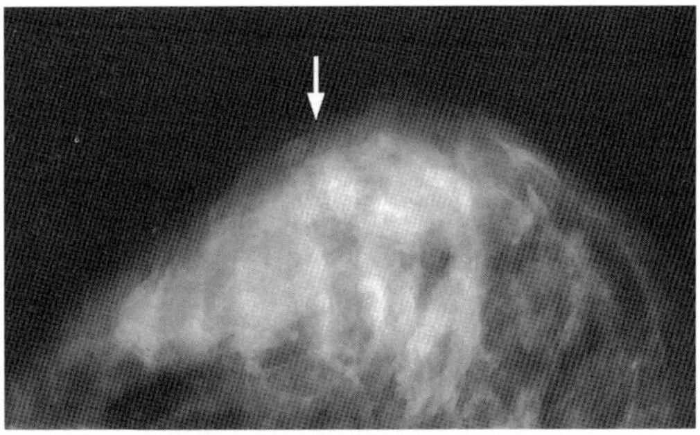

b

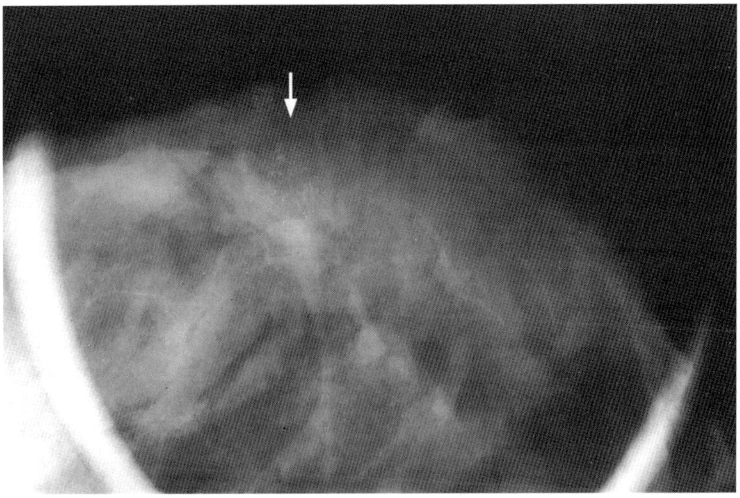

c

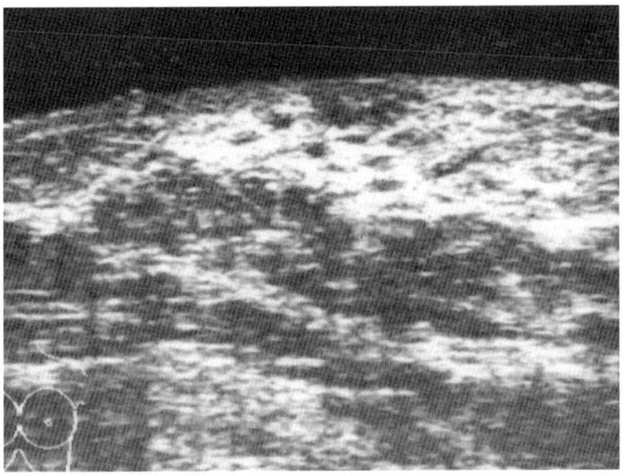

d

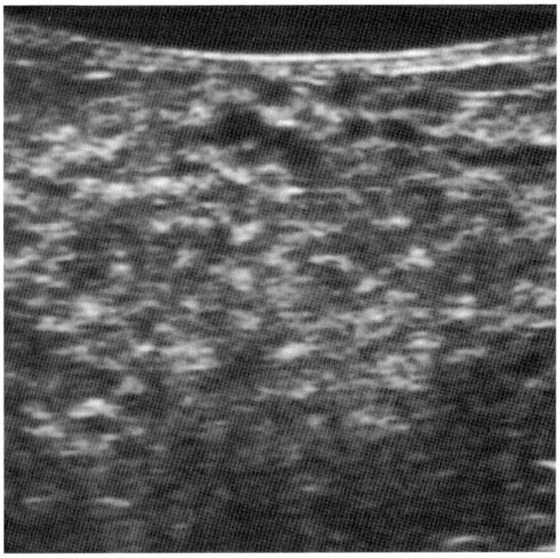

e

d Prepartum heterogeneous tissue changes in the glandular body (arrowheads) during late pregnancy (normal findings):
Whereas the peripheral glandular body appears extremely hypoechoic like fat, the tissue posterior to the nipple is primarily hyperechoic yet interspersed with hypoechoic tubular structures

e During lactation (different patient, normal findings), most of the glandular tissue shows a finely granular hypoechoic pattern. Individual expanded ducts are discernible

Sonography (Fig. 8.**10c**)

In light of the limited diagnostic value of mammography during pregnancy and lactation, ultrasound is extremely helpful in evaluating palpable findings.

Normally, the echogenicity of the breast tissue decreases somewhat during pregnancy and lactation. The echo pattern generally appears homogeneous and finely granular. Particularly in late pregnancy and lactation, the distended lactiferous ducts are discernible as tubular, extremely hypoechoic or anechoic structures (Fig. 8.**10d** and **e**).

Magnetic Resonance Imaging

MRI is not indicated during pregnancy and lactation since strong generalized contrast enhancement is expected in the engorged breast tissue and therefore identification of malignant processes would be difficult.

Breast Response with Hormone Replacement Therapy

The number of women receiving hormone replacement therapy, either for relief of menopausal symptoms or as prophylaxis against osteoporosis and arteriosclerosis, has increased within the past few years. Due to the hormonal proliferation stimulus, breast size increases in some of these women, occasionally accompanied by a sensation of fullness and breast pain.

Hormone replacement has an impact on the *diagnostic capability of mammography* for several reasons:

- A generalized increase in the extent and density of partially involuted parenchyma is possible.
- In older women, single or multiple cysts, fibroadenomas, and other benign breast changes can develop in one or both breasts.
- Cysts and fibroadenomas can enlarge and simulate a malignant process.
- After breast-conserving treatment of a mammary carcinoma, the extent and density of the parenchyma of the healthy breast can increase unilaterally since the irradiated fibrosed breast tissue generally does not respond to hormones.[7, 8, 9, 10, 11]

Discontinuing hormone replacement therapy generally leads to involution of the proliferative parenchymal effects.

Mammography (Fig. 8.**11a** and **b**)

Where previous mammograms are available for comparison, the examiner will observe a unilateral or bilateral increase in the extent and density of the parenchyma due to hormone replacement therapy. This increase can be diffuse or patchy. Generally, the specific architecture will still be discernible.

The increase in density can be so profound that mammographic interpretation is impaired. Under hormone replacement therapy, new cysts and fibroadenomas can develop or existing ones can increase in size, representing an exception to the rule that any new occurrence or increase in size of a focal lesion in a postmenopausal patient represents a sign of malignancy. Thus, particular care is necessary in further diagnostic workup of increasing densities. Multiple or single cysts or fibroadenomas can develop bilaterally or unilaterally.

Sonography

Sonography is an important diagnostic procedure in assessing mammographically dense parenchyma and as an adjunct in diagnosing probably benign focal findings detected mammographically, especially those that have recently developed or increased in size. The glandular tissue under hormone stimulation will generally appear homogeneous and moderately hyperechoic. However, variations such as those seen in breast dysplasia are possible.

If a simple cyst is diagnosed sonographically, no further workup will be required. Upon consultation with the patient, solid focal lesions that are not definitely benign mammographically and sonographically usually require biopsy to assess for malignancy. If they are suspected to represent a process due to hormonal stimulation, the patient may be given the option of discontinuing hormones for 2 or 3 months, then reimaging the breast to determine if the lesion has regressed.

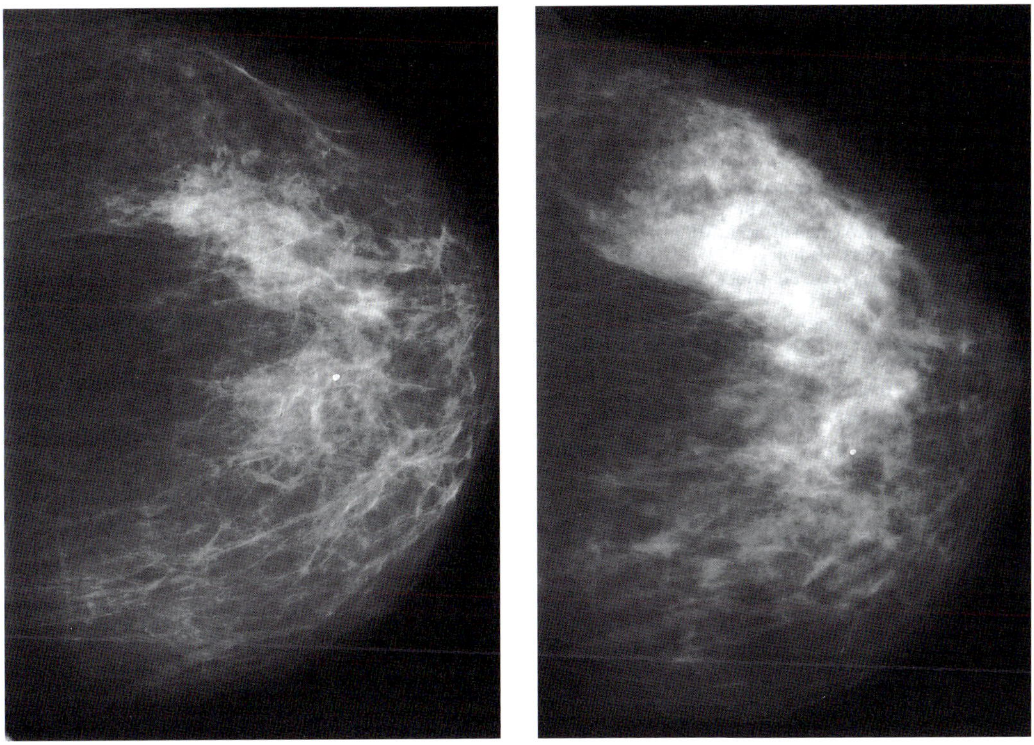

a b

Fig. 8.**11 a** and **b** Changes under hormone replacement therapy
a Normal, partially involuted breast in a 59-year-old patient
b After 12 months of hormone replacement, the patient complained of a sensation of fullness and breast enlargement. Mammography reveals extensive generalized nodular proliferation of glandular tissue. Mammographic evaluation is impaired under hormone replacement therapy compared to before

Magnetic Resonance Imaging

MRI is not indicated for diagnosing changes occuring under hormone replacement therapy. The resulting proliferative changes can be expected to enhance with MR contrast agents, impairing both detection and exclusion of malignancy.

Percutaneous Biopsy

This method can be used to diagnose uncertain focal findings developing during hormone placement therapy.

Summary

Knowledge of hormone replacement therapy is extremely important for interpreting diagnostic imaging studies. This underscores the value of taking a thorough history.

Hormone replacement therapy can produce significant parenchymal changes which can include an increase in the amount and density of parenchymal tissue, and a new occurrence or an increase in the size of focal densities. Mammographic evaluation is limited instead of improved with increasing patient age and breast involution. The additional information from sonography may be helpful in older women undergoing hormone replacement therapy. Percutaneous or excisional biopsy may be indicated for further workup of focal findings during hormone replacement therapy.

Cysts

The breasts can form *microcysts* measuring 1–2 mm diameter and *macrocysts* (which may be simple or multiloculated cysts), as well as multiple and solitary cysts. The contents of the cyst can be clear, yellowish, or milky. They can also be greenish blue (blue-domed cysts), brownish, or black as a result of previous bleeding.

Adenosis

This term refers to parallel arrangements of bundle-shaped nonneoplastic proliferations of terminal ductal segments. The most frequent forms include:

Blunt duct adenosis: Small cystic expansions of ductules containing secretion, lined with a flattened or slightly hyperplastic epithelium are typical of this frequent form of adenosis. The clustered arrangement of the ductules is suggestive of adenosis originating in the glandular lobules as opposed to the ductal segments.

Sclerosing adenosis: Sclerosing adenosis refers to focal, generalized, and tumor-like proliferations (i. e., adenosis tumor) of the epithelium and myoepithelium that originate in the glandular lobules and are accompanied by desmoplasia. Sclerosing adenosis is frequently, but not always, associated with other benign breast disorders. It can also occur in the stromal tissue of fibroadenomas, papillomas, or ductal adenomas. It can be associated with atypical lobular hyperplasia or a lobular carcinoma in situ. The relative risk of malignancy is increased by a factor of 1.5–2.

Microglandular adenosis: This rare benign form of adenosis is characterized by densely packed, isomorphic, small-diameter tubules that grow into the connective and fatty tissue either resembling a tumor or occasionally as a generalized process.

Radial scar: This term refers to single or multiple occurrences of nonneoplastic focal tubular proliferative adenosis developing around a fibrous elastoid center that radiate outward and are associated with areas of intraductal epithelial hyperplasia.

The radial scar is particularly significant as its spiculated form simulates an invasive carcinoma both macroscopically and in diagnostic imaging studies. Areas of atypical hyperplasia, and tubular, ductal, or lobular carcinomas can develop within radial scars.

Focal Fibrosis

Focal fibrosis is a proliferation of mammary stromal tissue in younger women (age from 25 to 40 years) that is associated with focal parenchymal atrophy and leads to induration. The mean focus size measures 1–3 cm in diameter. Mammography shows increased density without microcalcifications.

Forms of Epithelial Hyperplasia

- **Ductal hyperplasia (epitheliosis):** By definition, benign intraductal proliferations of the epithelium are seen in widespread or focal areas whose pattern and extent can vary. Particularly in American medical literature, the term papillomatosis is used in the same sense as epitheliosis. In Europe the term papillomatosis is used to describe particular villous epithelial textures oriented along septa of connective tissue.
- **Lobular hyperplasia:** It is characterized by an enlargement of the lobule due to extensive acinar hyperplasia in the sense of adenosis but also due to hyperplasia of the epithelium similar to epitheliosis of the extralobular ducts.
- **Atypical hyperplasia (atypia):** Ductal atypical hyperplasia occurs in ducts, and lobular atypical hyperplasia in the lobules in approximately 3.6% of all biopsies. Histopathologically, these areas show some but not all of the histologic characteristics of carcinoma in situ. Histologic and cytologic assessment of these lesions is difficult even for experienced pathologists in comparative studies, and these lesions represent a gray area in diagnosis. The relative risk of degeneration into carcinoma is from 4 to 5 times higher than in the normal population and increases with age. The absolute risk with atypical hyperplasia is 8–10% in 10 years; with a history of cancer in the family, it will increase to about 25% in 10 years. Forms of atypical hyperplasia include:
  - *Atypical ductal hyperplasia* is primarily observed in postmenopausal patients and corresponds to a lesion with some but not all of the characteristics of ductal carcinoma in situ.

- *Atypical lobular hyperplasia*, likewise, has some but not all of the characteristics of lobular carcinoma in situ. Here, the size of the lobule (in contrast to a fully developed carcinoma in situ) is not measurably enlarged.

To assess the risk of malignancy of benign breast disorders, the results of long-term studies of Prechtel[1,2] and of studies by Dupont and Page[3,4] have proven valuable. With the similar goals, a consensus meeting of American pathologists[5] recommended a slightly modified classification system:

1. *Mild epithelial hyperplasia (ductal or lobular hyperplasia)* is defined as a proliferation of a layer 2–4 cells thick. There is no increased risk of malignancy. The disorder can occur as adenosis, cystic disease, or duct ectasia corresponding to Prechtel's Grade I benign disorder. Frequency is about 70%. It may also occur in fibroadenomas, adenomas, and in mastitis.
2. *Florid epithelial hyperplasia* is defined as hyperplasia exceeding 4 layers of cells without atypia. The risk of malignancy is slightly increased to 1.5–2. It occurs as solid or papillary hyperplasia (epitheliosis), corresponding to Prechtel's Grade II benign disorder. Frequency is about 25–30%, also as papilloma with a stromal component.
3. *Atypical epithelial hyperplasia (ductal and lobular hyperplasia)* is defined as cellular atypia with disturbance of regular epithelial layering, where the myoepithelial layer and basal membrane remain intact, corresponding to Prechtel's Grade III benign disorder. The relative risk of malignancy is increased by a factor of 4 or 5. Frequency is about 4%.

The risk of malignancy for Grade I and Grade II disorders clearly differs from that of Grade III. In light of this, the overriding clinical consideration is: does the benign disorder involve atypical hyperplasia or nonatypical hyperplasia, and is there a history of cancer in the family?

Clinical Findings

- Benign breast disorders can be completely *asymptomatic*.
- They can cause pain *(mastodynia)*.
  - Breast pain due to a benign disorder will typically be more pronounced in the premenstrual phase (i. e., premenstrual tension or sensitivity to touch).
  - The pain usually is bilateral.
  - Most often it will occur as generalized pain in the upper outer quadrants. Localized pain that is not due to a cyst is not typical of benign breast disease (see also p. 228).
- In some cases, *discharge* may accompany benign breast disease. This will usually occur *bilaterally* and involve several excretory ducts. The color of the discharge is usually clear or amber-colored, occasionally yellowish green or greenish black.
- The palpable findings in the presence of a benign breast disorder can vary greatly from patient to patient.

Typical findings in the presence of a benign breast disease include:

- The tissue has a *firmer consistency*.
- Palpation reveals *finely to coarsely nodular* changes.
- The firmer consistency and nodular transformation are most often *symmetrical* and particularly pronounced in the upper outer quadrants.
- *Cysts* are usually palpable as round, elastic lumps. Deeper-lying cysts or cysts that are not completely filled may not be palpable.

Some benign breast disorders can also be associated with *unilaterally firmer consistency* or *formation of focal lumps*. With focal findings, it can be difficult or even impossible to distinguish the disorder from a malignant process. Further diagnostic workup (diagnostic imaging, percutaneous biopsy, or perhaps excisional biopsy) is indicated.

Diagnostic Strategy and Objectives

Benign breast disorders can only be classified histologically. Palpation, mammography (structural changes, radiodensity, microcalcifications), or sonography (hyperechoic glandular tissue with or without cysts or dilated ductal structures) can be suggestive of a benign breast disease, but cannot prove it.

Since there is insufficient correlation among mammographic, sonographic, or MRI findings and cellular proliferations or the degree of cellular atypia present, it is *not possible to assess the risk of carcinoma based on diagnostic imaging studies*. However, it is a general rule that the *majority of benign breast disorders* (70–80%) are *associated with no risk or only a slight risk of carcinoma*.

The increased radiodensity and firmer nodular consistency associated with typical cases of benign breast disorders *limit diagnostic accuracy* in comparison to a fatty breast. Mammographic and clinical examination can, therefore, be more difficult in these women. Annual mammography is strongly recommended to improve detection of small carcinomas, which are more difficult to discern in dense tissue.

Additional diagnostic methods are *not indicated* in the presence of typical findings of benign breast disease without an increased risk or without mammographically or clinically suggestive findings. Where *clinical examination reveals suspicious findings* (i. e., palpable findings, uncertain palpable asymmetry, or atypical discharge), *mammography* is indicated as the first step in additional workup.

Mammography can detect a carcinoma at the site of the palpable findings, or at another unexpected location, by revealing a typical density or typical microcalcifications. *The absence of microcalcifications or densities typical of malignancy* in radiodense tissue *does not exclude* a malignancy *suspected on the basis of clinical findings.*

Therefore in the presence of clinically suggestive findings or suspected cysts in radiodense tissue, *sonography* is indicated as an adjunctive modality to mammography. Ultrasound is particularly helpful when it can identify a simple cyst as the cause of uncertain palpable findings, uncertain mammographic densities, or asymmetry. Aside from this, most palpable carcinomas in radiodense tissue are also discernible as hypoechoic mases. For this reason, sonography is also used to confirm suspected malignant findings.

Some small carcinomas, and particularly carcinomas in situ, cannot be reliably identified by sonography. *Therefore the absence of ultrasound findings does not exclude a malignancy suspected on the basis of clinical or mammographic evidence.*

Percutaneous biopsy is the next most important diagnostic step and most valuable alternative to open biopsy in the diagnosis of probably benign palpable findings or changes detected at mammography.

Open biopsy is indicated as a diagnostic and therapeutic method when a malignancy is suspected, and as the diagnostic method if the finding is not readily accessible (i. e., a small deep lesion), if core biopsy yielded a borderline lesion (atypical hyperplasia), or if results of the existing diagnostic studies or of imaging versus percutaneous biopsy are contradictory.

Mammography

The mammographic appearance of benign breast disease (Figs. 9.**1 a–i**) is characterized by the following features:

- Structural changes and/or increased density in the parenchyma
- Calcifications
- Cysts

These changes can occur individually or in combination.

Structural Changes and/or Increased Density

These changes include:

- Coarsened structure.
- Finely to coarsely nodular densities, usually relatively uniform, often found along the tree-shaped structure of the mammary gland.
- Areas of increased density or generalized increased density.
- In some cases, the structures appear indistinct and not readily discernible. This is probably due to increased water retention.
- Fibrosis and/or secondary inflammatory processes can produce random and irregular densities.

Structural changes or densities are suggestive of a benign breast disorder, although they are not conclusive.

Benign changes are *typically generalized and symmetrical.* When this is the case, the findings are characteristic of benign breast disorders and cannot usually be confused with changes typical of malignancy. However, in the presence of generalized and symmetrical benign changes, detection or exclusion of carcinomas without microcalcifications is more difficult because they may easily be obscured by the surrounding dense tissue. Diagnostic problems occur with increased density, architectural distortion, or even a smooth or irregular mass:

- *Asymmetrically*, or
- *As a focal lesion* (Figs. 8.**8 a–d**, 9.**1** and 9.**3 a–h**).

Nodular, irregular, or spiculated masses can occur in certain benign breast diseases and characteristically also in the rare tumorous form of sclerosing adenosis.

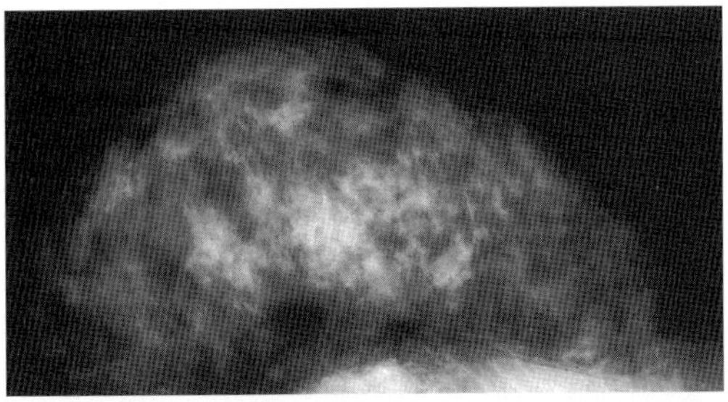
a

Fig. 9.1 a–i
a Relatively uniform, finely nodular benign breast parenchyma of increased density
b Nodular parenchymal pattern with multiple disseminated calcifications appearing as round or linear structures
c Coarsely nodular radiodense parenchymal structure compatible with benign breast disorder. There are multiple disseminated calcifications appearing as round and linear structures and isolated sedimentation phenomena or "teacups" (arrow) due to milk of calcium

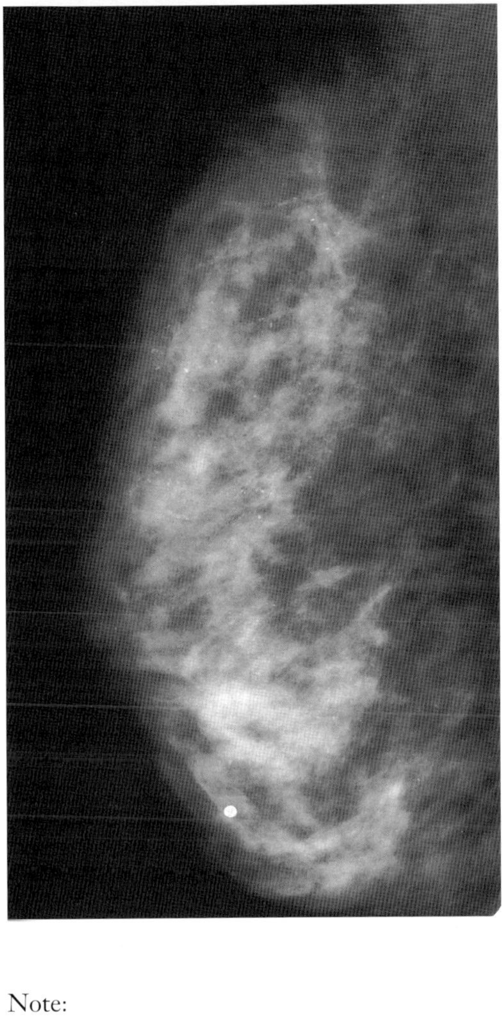
b

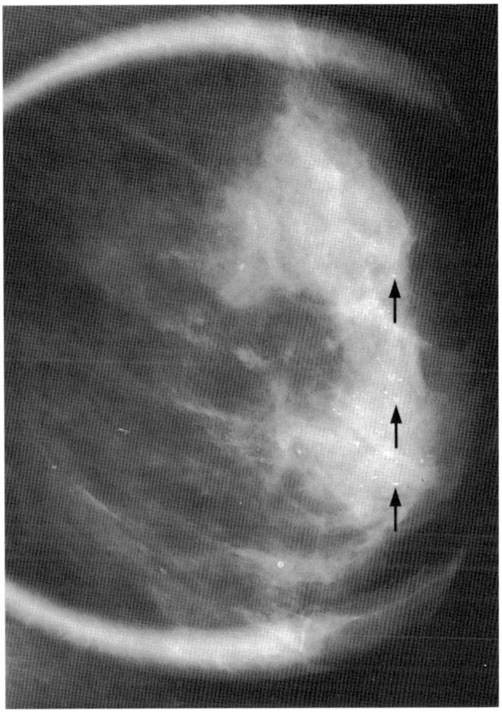
c

Note:

- Irregular foci of benign breast disease and radial scars will often produce palpable findings smaller and less pronounced than the findings expected with a carcinoma of comparable size
- A radial scar is often centrally radiolucent

These characteristics can only be regarded as suggestive of a benign process and not as conclusive evidence.[6, 7, 8] Since carcinomas can have a similar appearance, biopsy should be considered in the presence of these changes.

Significance of Changes in Structure and Density

Whereas focal and asymmetrical densities or structural changes can simulate a carcinoma at mammography and clinical examination, gener-

Fig. 9.**1 d** and **e** Circumscribed nodular mass in the left inferior medial breast. The margin is partially smooth and partially indistinct. *Histology:* Nodular adenosis 10 mm in diameter

f Mammary parenchyma has a coarsely nodular benign structure. There are multiple, uniformly distributed, relatively round, monomorphic and punctate microcalcifications. Histologic examination (performed because of a planned liver transplant) revealed simple fibrocystic benign breast disease with psammomatous calcifications

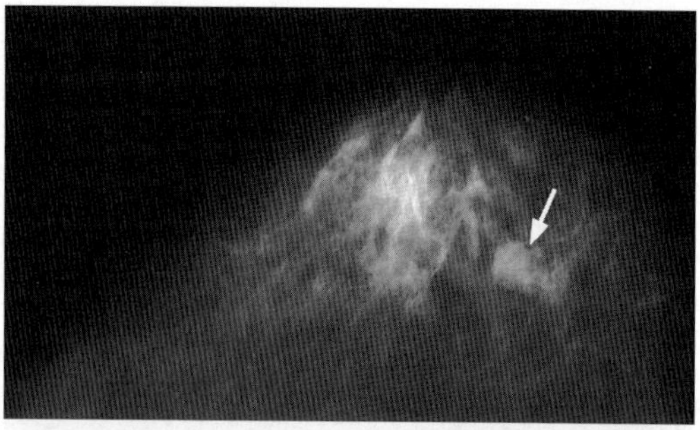

e

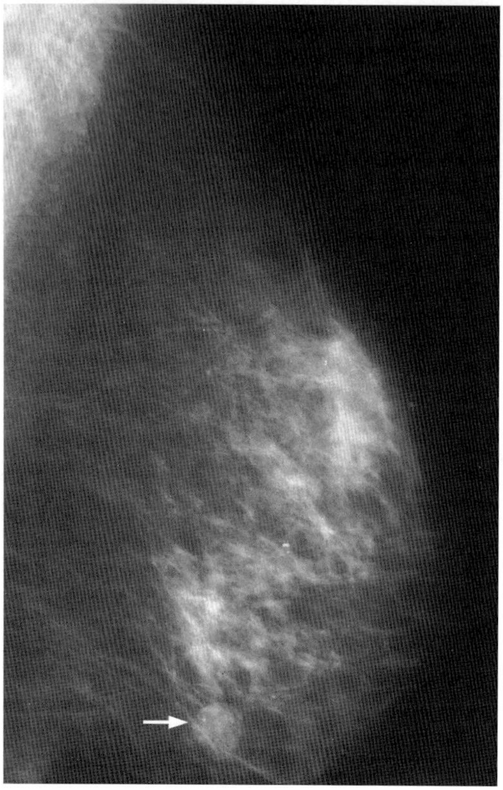

d

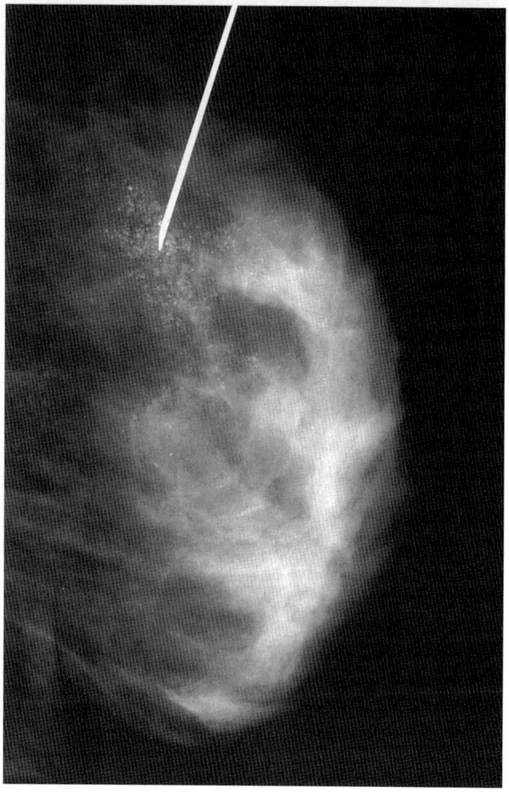

f

Abb. 9.**1 g–i** ▷

alized changes can make detection of malignant processes difficult as a result of generally increased radiodensity.

There is no correlation between the extent of structural changes or increased radiodensity and the degree of cellular proliferation or atypia. As a result, it is *not possible to correlate mammographically detected structural changes and changes in density with the possible risk of carcinoma.*

■ Calcifications

Microcalcifications frequently occur in benign breast disorders. They exhibit a broad range of variation with respect to their morphology and pattern of distribution. They can be the result of calcified secretions. Necrotic cells shed into intraductal or intralobular spaces can calcify, and calcifications can occur in the stroma. Accordingly, they may be found diffusely disseminated,

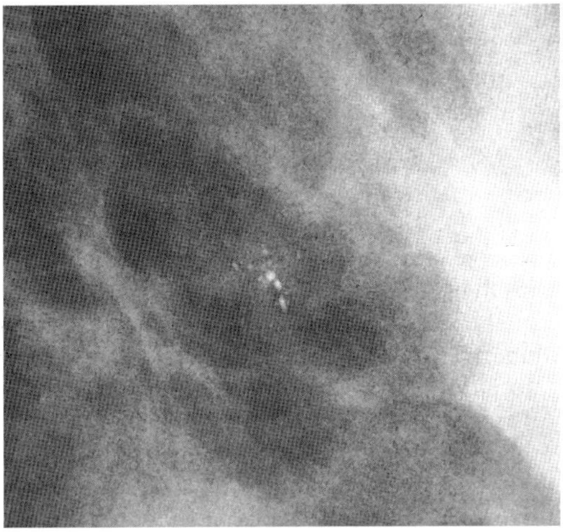
g

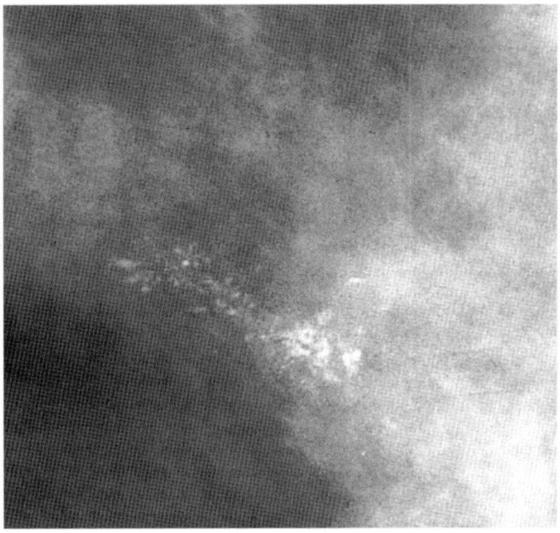
h

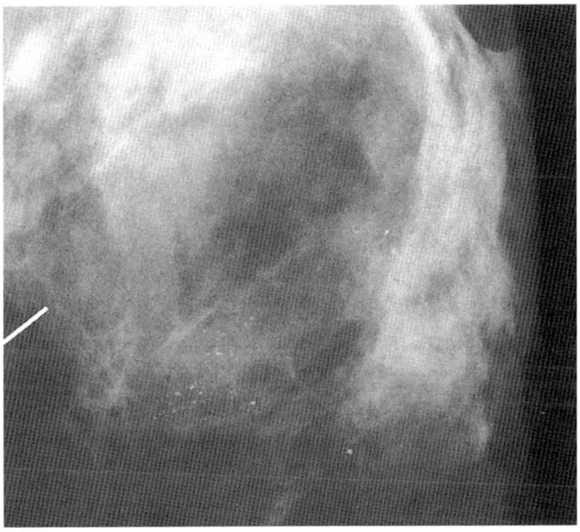
i

Fig. 9.**1 g** Magnification mammography reveals a tiny cluster of round microcalcifications arranged in a linear pattern. *Histology:* focal fibrous breast disease
h Magnification mammography shows a long cluster of round, linear, and polymorphic microcalcifications. *Histology:* focal fibrous breast disease
i Specimen radiography: One large and two adjacent smaller clusters of polymorphic microcalcifications. Fibrocystic benign breast disorder with focal sclerosing adenosis and intraductal papillomatosis

arranged in a lobular pattern, or without any clear pattern of distribution.

Spectrometry has revealed these structures to consist primarily of calcium phosphates in addition to compounds involving other elements[9].

The following forms are *typical of benign breast disorders*[10, 11, 12, 13]:

- *Isolated*, generally round *calcifications.*
- *Scattered punctate microcalcifications*, generally occurring *symmetrically.* These occur in many benign breast disorders and particularly often with sclerosing adenosis.
- *Milk of calcium in microcysts.* These correspond to the typical teacup-shaped calcifications described by Lanyi. They represent small "lakes" of milk of calcium in cystic distended lobules. The milk of calcium contains extremely fine suspended particles of calcium not resolved on the mammogramm. This accumulation of calcified milk in distended microcystic structure appears as a one "calcification."
  In the craniocaudal view, these individual "calcifications" appear as lakes of calcified milk, generally round, sometimes faceted, and frequently of different size. Their margins are often indistinct or amorphous. They are nonspecific and can vary in density. The lobular arrangement of these deposits can only be assessed when some of these calcifications lie close together in small flower-like or rosette-like clusters.
  In the mediolateral 90° view, the characteristic sedimentation of extremely fine particles in the calcified milk produces a characteristic sign: The inferior border of the small lake

that appears to be a calcification is arc-shaped and shows a horizontal surface produced by sedimentation. This surface corresponds to the fluid–fluid level of sedimented milk of calcium.
Intense compression can cause the calcium salt precipitates to well up so that the fluid–fluid level appears to form a superior dome. These so-called teacups generally occur bilaterally, but can also be observed unilaterally or asymmetrically. The typical teacup sign can usually only be demonstrated in some of the calcifications.
Where the *typical teacup sign can be demonstrated* and other changes typical of malignancy (casting or pleomorphic microcalcifications, or suggestive densities) are absent, the examiner can diagnose a *benign breast disorder.*

- *Clusters of microcalcifications following a lobular pattern.* These may be isolated or multifocal. The calcifications lie *closely clustered together* in a small area corresponding to the size of a normal or hypertrophic lobule (1–5 mm). At mammography, this will appear like a *morula or rosette.* Several lobules may be involved. Despite certain variations in the size of the individual calcifications, the individual calcifications within a cluster appear round and monomorphic. Such clusters occur primarily in the presence of *cystic and sclerosing adenosis.*

Unfortunately, aside from these typical benign calcifications, benign breast disorders can also involve *uncharacteristic and, occasionally, even suspicious calcifications.*

Uncharacteristic microcalcifications that can occur in benign breast disorders include the following forms [10, 12, 13]:

- Ill-defined and amorphous calcifications with slight to pronounced polymorphism
- Microcalcifications appearing in an isolated area that are asymmetrical with the contralateral side and not clearly benign
- Clusters of microcalcifications that are not clearly arranged in a monomorphic lobular pattern.

Suspicious calcifications may rarely also occur in benign breast disorders. These appear as:

- Casting, rod-like, V-shaped, or Y-shaped
- Coarsely granular and pleomorphic
- They may even be arranged in a segmental configuration, and/or follow the ductal structures, indistinguishable from microcalcifications associated with malignancy and therefore always necessitating biopsy

Uncharacteristic calcifications and, rarely, suspicious calcifications may be associated with benign breast disease as well. This is just an expression of the fact that benign transformation can affect both the lobules and the ductal system. Calcifications can occur in a typically benign "lobular" configuration but also in a ductal configuration simulating a malignant process, albeit less frequently. In sclerosing adenosis, myothelial and connective-tissue proliferation can lead to deformity of the lobules. This can explain the greater polymorphism of the individual calcifications detected in sclerosing adenosis as well as individual rod-like microcalcifications.

Importance of Microcalcifications in Benign Breast Disorders

On the whole, uncharacteristic and suspicious *microcalcifications occur more frequently in benign proliferative disorders* than in nonproliferative breast disorders. Microcalcifications associated with benign breast disorder nevertheless *do not permit an assessment of the risk of malignancy of the underlying breast disease* in a specific case.

In the presence of *calcifications typical of benign breast disorders,* routine follow-up is all that is needed. Biopsy should not be performed. The examiner should verify that these benign calcifications are not accompanied by additional microcalcifications or calcification clusters typical of malignancy.

Suspected microcalcifications require biopsy for histologic examination. Where *nonspecific microcalcifications* are present, the physician may elect follow-up imaging studies or further workup (i. e., needle core biopsy or excisional biopsy). This decision should be made on the basis of the analysis of the microcalcification, clinical examination, and patient history data (see also Chapter 20).

Isolated or multiple cysts can also occur frequently in benign breast disorders.

Cysts

Cysts can produce sharply defined round shadows, semicircular discernible shadows, or poorly discernible densities (when obscured by superimposition). They may merely contribute to a nonspecific increase in density, or they may not be visible at all.

Diagnosing cysts and differentiating cysts from solid masses is a task for sonography (see also p. 82 and Chapter 10).

Sonography

At sonography (Figs. 9.2 **a–e**), *benign breast disorders* are typically characterized by the following features[14, 15, 16]:

- *Mammary gland is homogeneously hyperechoic* (a frequent finding).
- *Cysts* are frequently encountered. They may appear in various sizes and can be diagnosed beginning from a size of about 2 mm in diameter.
- *Ectatic ducts* (occasionally present).
- *Extremely regular hypoechoic structures (generally tubular, less frequently nodular)* extending throughout the mammary gland. These hypoechoic structures that follow the ductal system most likely correspond to periductal fibrosis or to foci of adenosis. Where such a regular overall structure is present, there is a high probability that these changes are benign.
- *Mammary gland* is partially or entirely homogeneously *hypoechoic.* This finding is rare. Differentiation between hypoechoic areas of breast disease and fat is significantly more difficult here, and the capability to discern hypoechoic tumors is greatly reduced.

The following *focal changes* may also be due to just benign breast disorders [15]:

- *Hypoechoic foci* (Fig. 9.2 **c**). These are generally irregular, less frequently round, and circumscribed. They can appear as isolated foci, in which case they are usually suspicious. They can also occur as multiple foci. Histologically, they may correspond to foci of adenosis, foci of benign proliferative disorders, or areas of focal fibrosis (this usually is accompanied by an acoustic shadow). The tumorous form of sclerosing adenosis can also appear as hypoechoic focus.
- *Acoustic shadows with or without hypoechoic focal findings* (Figs. 9.2 **d** and **e**). Shadows can occur at multiple locations or in an isolated area. These changes may occur in the presence of diffusely proliferative fibrosis or focal fibrosis. Often, tumorous sclerosing adenosis or radial scar will appear as a hypoechoic focus with an acoustic shadow or as an isolated acoustic shadow.

Hypoechoic foci resulting from benign breast disorders usually do not show a typical hyperechoic halo and have a less pronounced acoustic shadow than "classic" carcinomas. However, carcinomas (and small carcinomas in particular) can vary considerably, and *a reliable differentiation of benign and malignant hypoechoic foci or acoustic shadows is not generally possible.*

Purpose

Identifying cysts as the cause of uncertain palpable findings or mammographically uncharacteristic densities allows sonography to *reduce the number of unnecessary biopsies.*

A malignant process in homogeneously hyperechoic benign tissue is improbable.[17] Since carcinomas are generally hypoechoic and are easily discernible in such tissue, sonography is often helpful as an adjunctive imaging modality in patients with homogeneously hyperechoic tissue. However, in the presence of clinical or mammographic suspicion (such as microcalcifications), *sonography alone cannot exclude malignancy* even in homogeneously hyperechoic tissue.[14, 16] This is because some carcinomas in situ and certain small carcinomas also appear hyperechoic and thus may escape detection by sonography.

The following applies in the presence of an heterogeneous or hypoechoic pattern:

- The capability of sonography to exclude a malignant process is reduced in the presence of a *hypoechoic mammary gland with a benign disorder* (rare).
- *Excluding a malignant process is not possible in the presence of sonographically heterogeneous breast tissue* (with hypoechoic foci and/or multiple acoustic shadows). Close correlation with clinical and mammographic findings is required.
- *Areas with acoustic shadows* or a *hypoechoic mass with and without acoustic shadows*—if reproducible—require further workup. Depending on the specific suspicion, mammographic findings, and clinical examination, further workup may include excisional biopsy, ultrasound-guided core needle biopsy, sonographic follow-up (in the case of benign-appearing or very small hypechoic area).

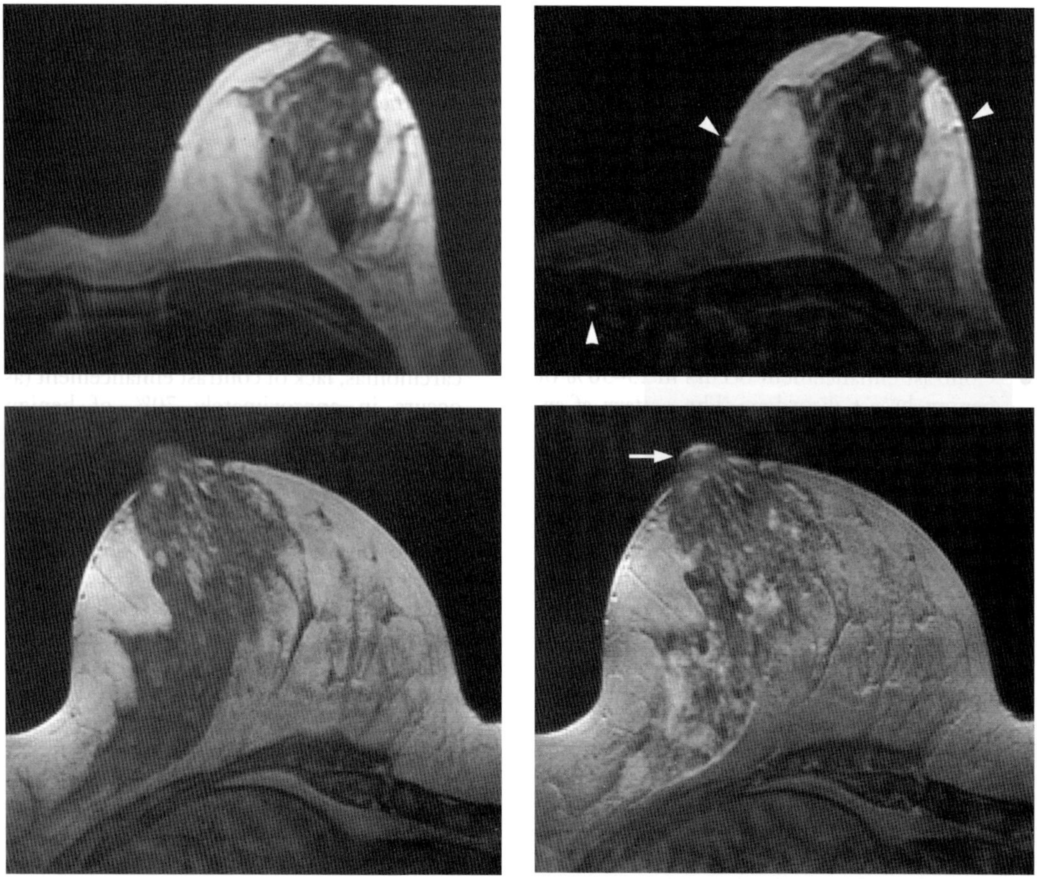

a

c

Fig. 9.3 **a–h** MRI appearance of benign breast disorders
a and **b** Most benign breast disorders (70–75%) only enhance slightly with Gd-DTPA
a Representative slice (FLASH 3D) before contrast administration
b The same slice after injection of Gd-DTPA:
Glandular tissue and fat show no significant changes in signal intensity; only vascular structures enhance (arrow). MRI examination was performed as adjunct to mammography to verify the absence of a carcinoma in radiodense tissue after a contralateral carcinoma was detected
c and **d** From 25 to 30% of all benign breast disorders demonstrate a diffuse milky to nodular pattern of enhancement (these disorders usually involve adenosis, proliferation, or atypia)
c Representative slice before injection of contrast medium. MRI was performed because of impaired mammographic assessment in the presence of radiodense breast tissue, diffusely disseminated microcalcifications, and a family history of malignancy
d The same slice after injection of Gd-DTPA. A confluent patchy pattern of gradual contrast enhancement is demonstrated in the glandular tissue. This finding is compatible with a benign breast disease, but the capability to exclude a malignant process is considerably limited.
The nipple itself (arrow) enhances in approximately 50% of all patients. In the absence of clinical suspicion this represents a normal finding

Contrast-enhanced MRI is not recommended in the following cases:

- Follow-up examination of known enhancing breast disorders (i. e., known from previous diagnostic studies).
- Differentiation between inflammatory and malignant changes. (Both enhance allowing no reliable distinction.)
- In patients undergoing hormone therapy (generally with preparations containing intermediate or high dosages of gestagen) who complain of tension (unspecific enhancement will often impair diagnostic accuracy).
- In asymptomatic patients with dense breast tissue. The majority of these patients are below the age of 40. Here frequently occult

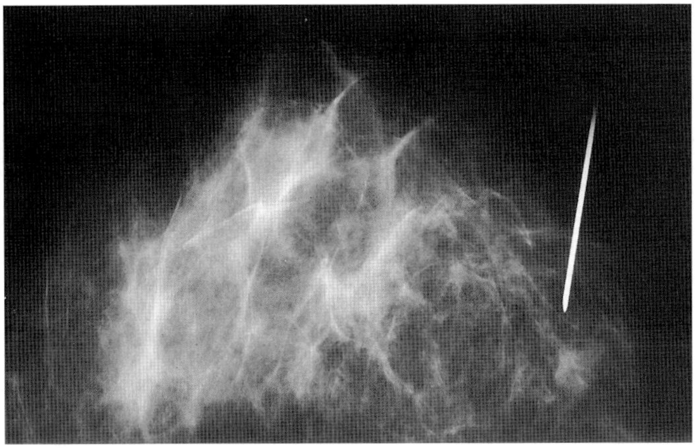

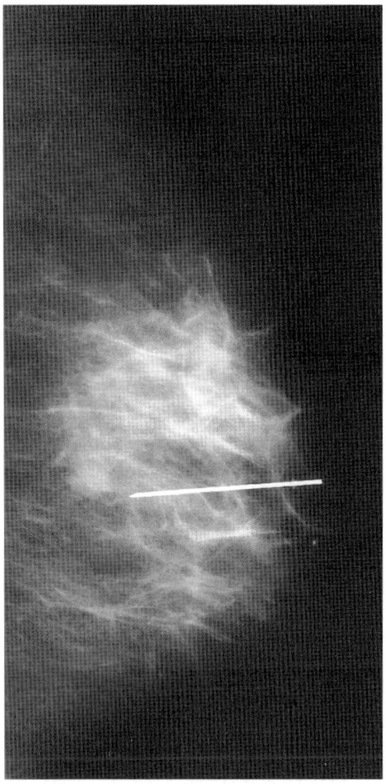

f

Fig. 9.**e–h** Occasionally, mammography and MRI (sometimes only MRI) will reveal a benign focal breast disorder. Focal fibrous breast disease will not enhance (see Figs. 8.**8 a–d**). In a benign proliferative breast disorder, the focus can enhance significantly, which represents a suggestive MRI finding
e and **f** Mammographically suspicious indistinct lesion on the craniocaudal and mediolateral preoperative localization images

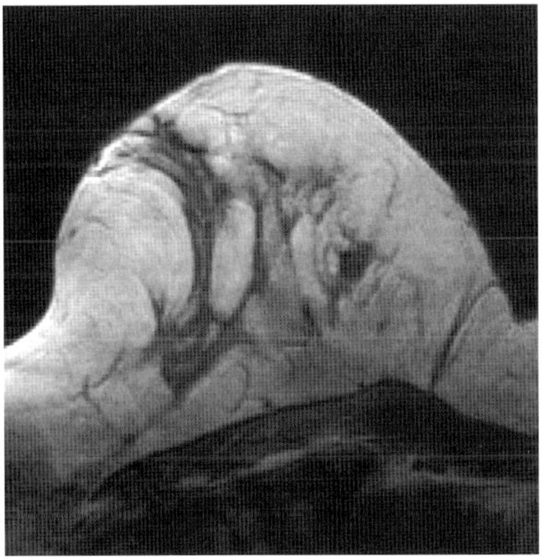

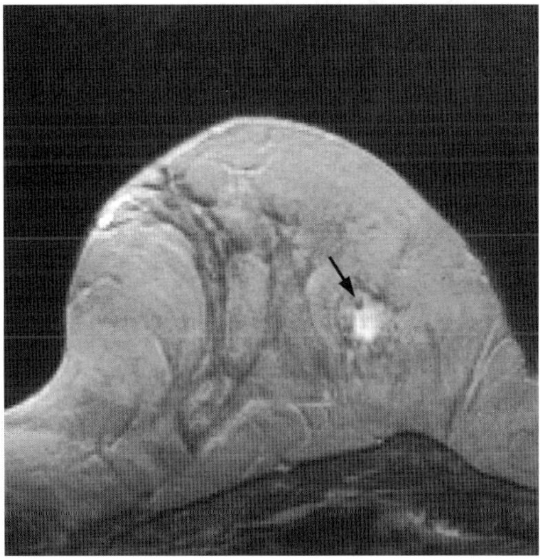

h

Fig. 9.**g** Slice through the suspicious lesion before contrast injection (MR examination was part of a study protocol)
h After injection of Gd-DTPA, the indistinct focal lesion enhances rapidly and early, behaving in the same manner as a malignant process on MRI. Histologic examination revealed mildly proliferative benign focal breast disease accompanied by a pronounced but unspecific inflammatory reaction.

fibroadenomas or areas of adenosis will be detected (unspecific enhancement may be encountered in about 1 of 5 cases) leading to expensive workup, while the chance of detecting a malignancy is low since the prevalence of malignancy (about 3 to 5 in 1000 patients or even fewer for patients below 40) is low in unselected patient populations.

Contrast-enhanced MRI, however, may be quite helpful in the following indications:

- In radiodense tissue to exclude *additional foci* or a *contralateral malignancy* where conservative treatment of a small breast carcinoma is planned.
- In radiodense tissue with a *high risk of malignancy*, such as locating a primary tumor. It has yet to be decided whether adjunctive contrast-enhanced MRI is cost-effective in monitoring high-risk patients.
- In selected cases with radiodense tissue with *uncharacteristic disturbed architecture or asymmetry, in patients with severe scarring.*
- In radiodense tissue in the presence of (multiple) *contradictory findings* (except for microcalcifications).

With these indications, the absence of enhancement during contrast MRI can help exclude a carcinoma. Focal enhancement on an MR image can provide an indication for percutaneous biopsy, and MRI can help guide the biopsy. MRI can thus aid in early detection of carcinomas or secondary foci in tissue that is difficult to assess by other imaging modalities.

Percutaneous Biopsy

There are three methods of obtaining biopsies of nonpalpable mammographic lesions for histopathologic or cytopathologic examination: excisional biopsy, fine-needle aspiration, and core needle biopsy. In an effort to minimize the number of excisional biopsies, percutaneous fine-needle aspirations for cytologic smears and core needle biopsies have become increasingly common practices.

Diagnostic accuracy correlates with the size and homogeneity of the focus, the amount of tissue obtained, and the examiner's experience.[20, 21, 22, 23]

The pathologist and cytologist require representative tissue specimens in sufficient quantity for examination. Such specimens cannot always be obtained.

Heterogeneous changes in benign breast disorders and the occasional presence of atypical focal hyperplasia can limit the diagnostic accuracy of fine-needle aspiration or core needle biopsy. For these reasons diagnostic open biopsy is recommended in the following cases:

- In the presence of ductal atypia or radial scar, or where findings are insufficient for examination
- If there is a discrepancy between mammographic changes and cytopathologic findings

In the case of a malignancy proven by percutaneous biopsy, open surgery will be necessary for treatment.

Summary

Histologically, benign breast disorders encompass a broad spectrum of tissue changes. We differentiate the following types according to their prognosis:

- Benign nonproliferative breast disorders (70% of all benign disorders) without an increased risk of carcinoma
- Benign proliferative breast disorders without cellular atypia (approximately 25% of all benign disorders) with a slightly increased risk of carcinoma (by a factor of 1.5–2)
- Benign proliferative breast disorders with cellular atypia (4–5% of all benign disorders) with an increased risk of carcinoma (by a factor of 5)

Diagnostic imaging studies do not permit reliable assessment of risk. *Above all, diagnostic imaging studies cannot reliably identify the benign breast disorders that entail a genuinely increased risk* (by a factor of 5). *Clinical signs* of benign breast disorders can include pain, palpable findings, and, rarely, discharge.

The primary *mammographic signs* are increased density and microcalcifications.

Sonography may reveal hyperechoic tissue texture. Often cysts can be identified. Hypoechoic structures or acoustic shadows may also be found.

On MRI examination, nonproliferative disorders usually enhance only slightly, while contrast enhancement can vary greatly in adenosis and proliferative benign disorders (up-

take can vary equally in proliferative changes with and without atypia).
Depending on the extent of the benign changes, findings in all modalities will *overlap* with changes associated with preinvasive and early invasive carcinomas.

Diffuse benign changes are usually recognizable as such but can often *limit visualization of malignancy. Focal changes* usually differ qualitatively and quantitatively from surrounding benign tissue. Such changes require particularly careful workup. Mostly diagnostic imaging studies are unable to reliably distinguish these changes from malignant processes. Therefore focal changes frequently lead to *false positive findings* and necessitate percutaneous or open biopsy of benign changes.
Clinical examination and mammography are the methods of choice for assessing benign breast disorders detected by *screening*, and they are fully adequate for this purpose. In the presence of *questionable or suggestive mammographic or clinical findings, adjunctive procedures* are indicated for the following reasons:

- To minimize the number of excisional biopsies of benign findings
- To improve early detection of malignancy where the risk of malignancy is high and visualization is limited

In the presence of uncharacteristic focal findings, adjunctive sonography is recommended as a first step of the workup. Biopsy should follow in all cases where carcinoma is not excluded with reasonable certainty.
Contrast-enhanced MRI may be helpful in selected cases with breast tissue that is difficult to assess by other methods (e. g., due to severe scarring or pronounced asymmetry), if a high risk of malignancy exists.
Open biopsy remains the most reliable method for assessing borderline lesions (e. g., benign breast changes with atypias), or contradictory findings. In the case of malignancy, it will constitute the first therapeutic measure as well.

References

1 Prechtel K. Mastopathie. Histologische Formen und Langzeitbeobachtungen. Zentralbl Pathol. 1991; 137:210
2 Prechtel K, Gehm O, Geiger G, Prechtel P. Die Histologie der Mastopathie und die kumulative ipsilaterale Mammakarzinomsequenz. Pathologe. 1994;15:158
3 Dupont WD, Page DL. Risk factors for breast cancer in women with proliferative disease. N Engl J Med. 1985;312:146
4 Dupont WD, Page DL. Relative risk of breast cancer varies with the time since diagnosis of atypical hyperplasia. Hum Pathol. 1989;20:723
5 Consensus Meeting: Is fibrocystic disease of the breast pre-cancerous? Arch Pathol Lab Med. 1986;110:171
6 Adler DO, Helvie MA, Obermann HA. Radial sclerosing lesion of the breast: mammographic features. Radiology. 1990;176:737
7 Mitnick J, Vazquez M, Harris M, Roses D. Differentiation of radial scar from scirrhous carcinoma of the breast: mammographic pathologic correlation. Radiology. 1989;173:697
8 Orel SG, Evers K, Yeh IT, Troupin RH. Radial scar with microcalcifications: radiologic–pathologic correlation. Radiology. 1992;183:479
9 Bässler R, Schnürch HG. Standards der pathologischen Aufarbeitung des Mammakarzinoms. Ein Beitrag zur Qualitätssicherung in Pathologie und Klinik. Gynekologe. 1994;27:23
10 American College of Radiology. Breast imaging reporting and data system. 1993
11 Lanyi M. Diagnostik und Differentialdiagnostik der Mammaverkalkung. Berlin: Springer; 1986
12 Linden SS, Sickles EA. Sedimented calcium in benign breast cysts: the full spectrum of mammographic presentations. AJR. 1989;152:967
13 Tabar L, Dean PB. Teaching Atlas of Mammography. New York: Thieme; 1985
14 Bassett LW, Kimme-Smith C. Breast sonography. AJR. 1991;156:449
15 Jackson VP, Hendrick RE, Feig FA. Imaging of the radiographically dense breast. Radiology. 1993;188:297
16 Pamilo M, Soiva M, Anttinen I et al. Ultrasonography of breast lesions detected in mammography screening. Acta Radiol. 1991;32:220
17 Stavros AT, Thickman D, Rapp CL et al. Soled breast nodules: use of sonography to distinguish between benign and malignant lesions. Radiology 1995;196:123–134
18 Beck R, Heywang-Köbrunner SH, Untch M. Contrast-enhancement of proliferative dysplasia in MRI of the breast due to the menstruation cycle. ECR '93 Book of abstracts. 1993:151
19 Kuhl C et al. Fokale und diffuse KM-anreichernde Läsionen in der MR-Mammographie bei gesunden Probandinnen: Bandbreite des Normalverhaltens und Zyklusphasenabhängigkeit. Radiologe. 1995;35(4):86
20 Jackman RJ, Nowels KW, Shepard MJ et al. Stereotaxic large core needle biopsy of 450 nonpalpable breast lesions with surgical correlation in lesions with cancer or atypical hyperplasia. Radiology. 1994;193:91
21 Jackson VP. The status of mammographically guided fine needle apsiration biopsy of nonpalpable breast lesions. Radiol Clin North Am. 1992;30:155
22 Schöndorf H, Schöndorf N. Die Aspirationszytologie als diagnostische Methode beim Mammakarzinom. Gynekologe. 1994;27:17
23 Brenner RJ, Fajarto L, Fisher PR, Dershaw DD et al. Percutaneous core biopsy of the breast: effect of operation experience and number of samples or diagnostic accuracy. AJR. 1996;166:341–6

Suggested Reading

Heywang-Köbrunner SH. Contrast-enhanced MRI of the Breast. Munich: Karger;1990

10. Cysts

Cysts are by far the most common mass in the female breast. Approximately half of all women 30 to 40 years and up develop fibrocystic changes in the breast that manifest themselves in single or multiple cysts of varying sizes. Larger cysts occur in 20–25% of all women.[1,2] Simple cysts, characterized by all hollow fluid-filled space lined with epithelium, are benign lesions.

Cysts become clinically important when the patient presents with pain, or when palpable findings require further diagnostic studies to determine if they are benign or malignant. Asymptomatic cysts may also be initially detected by mammography or sonography.

Cysts can simulate tumors and conceal malignancy.

■ Histology

Cysts are locally distended peripheral ductal segments filled with fluid. They usually occur in the terminal ductal lobular units and are associated with fibrocystic changes in the breast. While simple cysts are always benign, "complicated cysts" can sometimes harbour malignancy.

■ Definition

Simple cysts consist of two layers of cells, an inner layer of epithelial cells and an outer layer of myoepithelial cells. They are benign processes that are not associated with an increased risk of cancer.

The term "complicated cysts" refers collectively to cysts or conglomerate cysts detected in imaging studies or by clinical examination that are "complicated" by inflammation or bleeding or contain neoplastic tissue changes in their wall or lumen. In the widest sense of the term, these include cavities containing hemorrhage and necrotic carcinomas.

Simple cysts are usually lined with linear epithelium surrounded by a layer of compressed connective tissue. Like the surrounding fibrocystic disease, the cyst wall can exhibit various forms of epithelial hyperplasia, sometimes even atypia. The risk of malignant degeneration only depends on the cellular changes of the underlying fibrocystic alterations. Simple cysts themselves are not premalignant lesions.

Complicated cysts have a heterogeneous origin, occuring in either preformed cavities (lactiferous ducts or cysts) or in cavities resulting from necrosis or bleeding.[3,4]

Inflammatory changes in cysts occur in retention cysts or in the presence of chronic mastitis. Cystic cavities can also develop in centrally necrotic tumors, or they can occur as a result of secretion and recurrent bleeding, as in intraductal papillomas and papillary carcinomas.

■ Medical History and Clinical Findings

Cysts can be totally asymptomatic. As they become larger, they manifest themselves as palpable findings, sometimes associated with breast pain.

Cysts are typically seen to develop acutely. They may wax and wane. However, based on the history, it is mostly impossible to distinguish a suddenly developed cyst from a slowly developed lesion (e.g., carcinoma) that has just been noticed by the patient.

Generally, cysts will first appear after the age of 30 or 40, occurring with peak frequency in premenopausal and perimenopausal women between the ages of 40 and 45.

In women under 40 and especially under 30, fibroadenomas tend to occur more frequently than cysts; after 40, the opposite is true. Since the risk of cancer is also higher in this age group, special care should be taken to exclude the possibility of breast cancer in these patients.

Breast Examination

Cysts are generally palpable as smooth-contoured, mobile masses. Most frequently, they are firm and somewhat compressible. However, they can also manifest themselves as hard masses. Particularly in the presence of conglomerate cysts and surrounding inflammation, distinguishing a cyst from a malignant growth can be difficult.[3, 4] Since some malignancies are relatively smooth-contoured and mobile, further diagnostic studies are always indicated in the presence of a clinical diagnosis of suspected breast cysts.

Objectives of Diagnostic Studies

1. To differentiate between simple cysts and noncystic changes, such as benign tumors or breast cancer (most frequent diagnosis to be excluded).
2. To distinguish simple cysts from other cystic masses. These include complicated cysts accompanied by inflammation, papilloma, or proliferative changes as well as cystic carcinomas (mural cancer growing into a cyst and carcinomas with central necrosis that can have the appearance of a cystic mass) (see also Fig. 10.**3**).

If a simple cyst is confirmed, further diagnostic studies will not be necessary. In the presence of complicated cysts or solid masses, further studies are essential, and if necessary the mass should be biopsied.

Diagnostic Strategy

Sonography is the method of choice for diagnosing cysts.[5, 6, 7]

In women under 35, sonography should be the initial imaging study in the workup of a palpable lump. If it confirms that the mass is a cyst, the workup is completed. If the cyst is painful, aspiration may be performed for symptomatic relief.

In women over 35 years of age and in particular in women over 40, both mammography and sonography must be performed due to the increasing risk of carcinoma. Mammography may, for example, reveal a carcinoma close to (or even remote from) the cyst, which—when small or preinvasive—may go undetected sonographically. Therefore mammography should be used liberally.

If the diagnosis of a cyst is equivocal sonographically, aspiration should be attempted (which, in addition, can be complemented by pneumocystography, see p. 161). In patients with frequently recurring masses, a repeat mammogramm is not necessary if a recent mammogram exists and the new lump is proven to be a cyst based on the sonogram.

When mammographic and sonographic findings are consistent with a cyst, and malignancy is excluded in the remaining breast tissue as well, the workup is done. If the lesion is solid, the diagnostic workup of solid masses is followed (see p. 339). If the diagnosis of a cyst is equivocal and aspiration is attempted, the further workup will depend on the result of aspiration (see pp. 160–161).

Sonography

Unit Settings/Examination Technique

Optimum unit settings are particularly important in diagnosing cysts. If the gain is set too low, solid hypoechoic processes can appear anechoic, which can lead to serious diagnostic errors.

In case of doubt, the following simple technique can be helpful (Figs. 10.**1 e–g**). Gradually increase the gain on the unit until the echoes in the lesion begin to appear:

- Typically, cysts will fill with echoes from the periphery, whereas echoes in solid structures will simultaneously increase at different places within the mass.
- Occasioinally, reverberation echoes will also be visible in cysts. They are more prominent in the upper part of the cyst adjacent to its leading wall and are parallel to the transducer. (Reverberation echoes are artifacts and do not represent tissue in the cyst.)

Turning and tilting the transducer can visualize the entire length of septa, making it possible to distinguish them from intracystic processes (Fig. 10.**1 h**). Changing the patient's position and repeating the examination can be helpful in identifying sedimentation, which layers in the dependent portion of the cyst appears as hypoechoic material on its floor.

Typical Appearance (Fig. 10.**1 a–k**)

The simple cyst is characterized by its smooth thin wall, absence of internal echoes, and distal

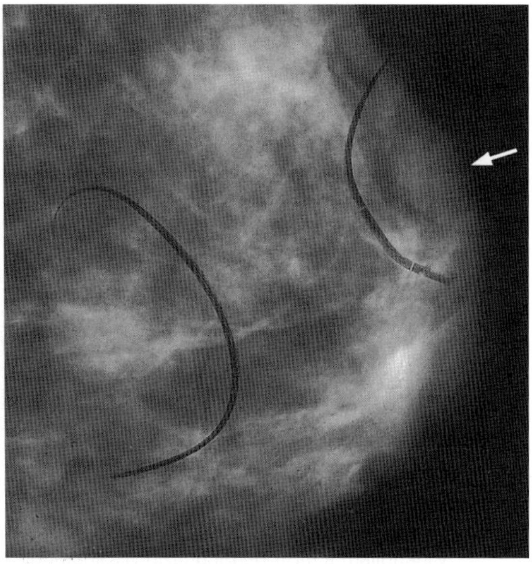

a

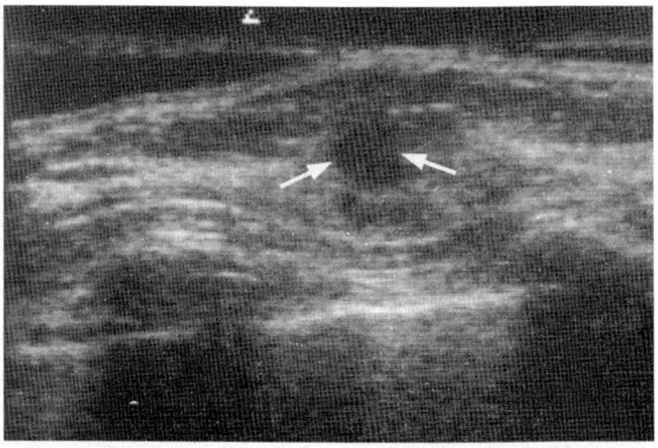

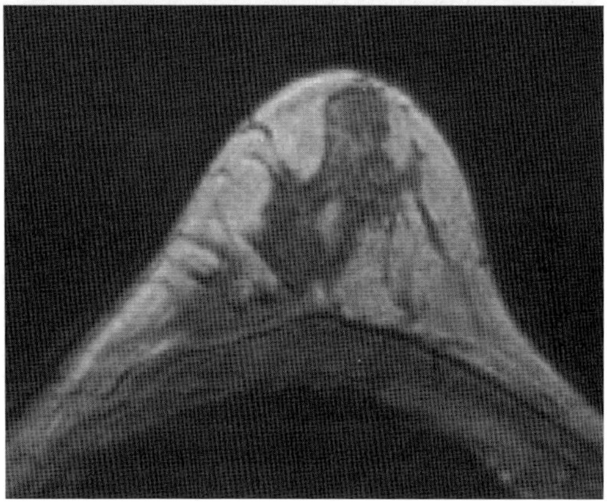

c

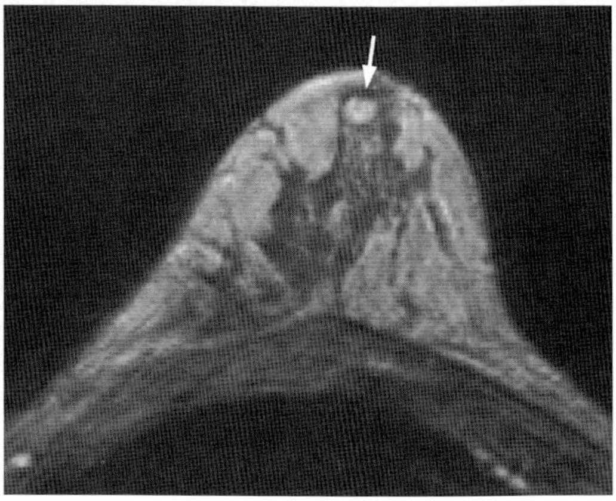

Fig. 11.**6a–d** Imaging of the nonfibrosed fibroadenoma. Since most nonfibrosed fibroadenomas show definite contrast enhancement and are consequently not distinguishable from a smoothly outlined fibroadenoma, core biopsy should be preferred rather than MRI as the most cost-effective method to evaluate a suspected fibroadenoma (young woman, soft to palpation and sonographically without acoustic shadowing)
a A palpable moveable tumor that is mammographically smoothly outlined anteriorly and not quite smoothly outlined posteriorly, located about 8 mm behind the nipple (as well as an additional lesion located centrally)
b Sonographically noncystic round hypoechoic lesion (arrow) with moderate sound transmission, not quite smoothly outlined
c and **d** MRI before (**c**) and after (**d**) intravenous injection of contrast medium. The nodule exhibits—as typical, but not diagnostic, of a "young" fibroadenoma—a smoot outline and intense enhancement. *Histology:* nonfibrosed intracanalicular fibroadenoma

- If the lesion is also visualized with other methods (mammography, sonography, physical examination) and not clearly classified as benign, it needs further evaluation by *percutaneous or excisional biopsy.*
- If the lesion is only detected by MRI in an asymptomatic patient, it should be *followed by MRI* (e.g., repeat MRI after 4 and 12 months, or after 6 and 18 months).

It should be pointed out that a ring-like enhancement or an early washout of contrast agent, if present, would speak against a fibroadenoma. This finding should lead to further workup (biopsy).

Accuracy

Because of the recognized high sensitivity of MRI in detecting malignancies, and the resultant high reliability of negative MRI findings in sclerosed fibroadenomas (contrast-enhanced MRI combined with a T2-weighted pulse sequence), MRI appears to the suitable for the diagnosis of the sclerosed fibroadenoma. The high sensitivity of MRI in the detection of young enhancing fibroadenomas and the inadequate specificity in differentiating them from circumscribed malignancies is problematic.

Therefore percutaneous biopsy is most appropriate for evaluating the suspected fibroadenomas.

For the evaluation of suspected fibrous fibroadenomas (older woman, mammographically detected contour irregularity without direct signs of malignancy, sonographically diminished elasticity, moderate sound transmission or even attenuation), MRI appears appropriate. It appears to be particularly advantageous if the lesions are small, deep, and multiple.

Diagnostic Goals

The most important role of imaging in the diagnosis of fibroadenoma consists of differentiating it from well-circumscribed malignancies with similar findings. In addition to the well-circumscribed ductal carcinoma, this includes medullary and papillary carcinomas, lymphomas, sarcomas, and metastases. The phyllodes tumors can also have a similar pattern. All these tumors can occasionally be completely well circumscribed, even surrounded by a mammographically detectable halo (see p. 169 for significance of the halo).

An excision of all circumscribed or round lesions, performed as a safety measure to find all rare circumscribed malignancy, does not appear in the best interest of the patient and cannot be justified for economic reasons. Even if only lesions deemed benign with a probability of benignity lower than 98% were all biopsied, a biopsy rate of over 1:10, or worse, would result. (This means that less than 1 carcinoma will be found in 10 recommended biopsies). It is for this reason that imaging methods should be used as much as possible to avoid unnecessary biopsies.

Overview of the Diagnostic Strategy

- The typically calcified fibroadenoma is mammographically pathognomonic. Additional evaluation or follow-up examinations are not necessary.
- Mammographically well-circumscribed solid masses (definition see p. 169), which are primarily fibroadenomas, are benign in 98% of the cases. In this situation follow-up mammography at intervals of 6, 12, 24, and 36 months is appropriate.
- The remaining solitary, circumscribed nonpalpable, and most likely benign lesions that do not entirely fulfill the above-mentioned criteria may be subjected to percutaneous or excisional biopsy.
  Because of the characteristic doubling rates of breast carcinomas and the rather slow growth rates of some circumscribed malignancies, the intervals of follow-up examinations should not be less than 6 months. The follow-up period should not be less than 3 years, and the current examination should be compared with the initial and not with the most recent examination.
- When masses do not contain calcifications, sonography should be used to differentiate between cyst and solid tumor, as well as to characterize palpable lesions that are hidden by mammographically dense tissue.
- Sonography cannot achieve a definitive differentiation of mammographically indeterminate noncystic masses from malignancy.
- A lesion seen only sonographically and exhibiting the typical features of a fibroadenoma (p. 173) may be followed at regular intervals or undergo a percutaneous biopsy if neither the patient's history nor clinical and mammographic findings reveal evidence of malignancy.
- For further evaluation of a suspected fibroadenoma that has been newly discovered and appears clinically and mammographically benign but does not fulfil all criteria of a benign lesion, percutaneous biopsy is appropriate. If percutaneous biopsy reveals a fibroadenoma, an excisional biopsy is not necessary.
- If a small sclerosed fibroadenoma not amenable to percutaneous needle biopsy because of its small size or location, or if the le-

sions are multiple, MRI (contrast-enhanced MRI combined with T2-weighted pulse sequence) can be obtained.

- Increasing size of a circumscribed tumor or suspected malignancy (irregular contour, suspected calcifications) is an indication for biopsy.

Summary

The most important role of the diagnostic methods in diagnosing a fibroadenoma is the definitive differentiation, if possible, from the rare circumscribed malignancies and the avoidance of high rates of excisional biopsies exclusively performed for diagnostic purposes.

The mammographically pathognomonic finding of a calcified fibroadenoma unfortunately only makes up for a small proportion of the fibroadenomas. The typical mammographic finding is the well-circumscribed nodule (see definition, p. 169), with or without halo. Its risk of malignancy is less than 2%.

Sonography serves to separate fibroadenomas from cysts and to diagnose fibroadenomas that are mammographically obscured by dense tissue, but not to characterize unclear mammographic findings. If the sonographic lesion corresponds to a newly detected finding, confirmation of the presumed diagnosis by percutaneous biopsy is recommended.

Exceptions and variations of the typical mammographic and sonographic findings are common. They require further evaluation, which can be achieved by follow-up examinations, percutaneous biopsy, MRI, or excision. Percutaneous biopsy should be done first because of its cost-effectiveness. MRI should be considered for fibrosed fibroadenomas (very small lesions, multiple lesions, unfavorable location).

When a lesion is being followed, the follow-up examinations should be done initially at 6 months and then at intervals of 12 months for at least 3 years. If any suspicion arises, e.g., if the lesion increases in size, excisional biopsy should be considered.

Papilloma

The papilloma is a benign fibroepithelial tumor of the breast. It represents 1–1.5% of the breast tumors. Even relatively small papillomas can become symptomatic by causing a clear or bloody nipple discharge. The role of clinical evaluation and diagnostic imaging (including galactography, see p. 69) consists of determining the localization and extent of the papilloma or papillomas. Occasionally a papilloma can be detected as a palpable finding or mammographic density and is then to be differentiated from other nodular-shaped masses.

It is important to know that certain types of papilloma can be associated with an increased risk of malignancy, depending on presentation (singular or multiple) and localization (subareolar versus peripheral).

Because of the difficult differentiation among papilloma, papillary carcinoma, or other nodular lesions, excision of papillomas is often diagnostically and therapeutically desirable.

Histopathology

They are classified as:[2, 14, 15, 16, 17]

1. *Intraductal, subareolar, solitary papilloma:* It generally extends over a length of 0.5 to 3.5 cm and is subject to involutional changes. These tumors are benign. Related to the occasional coexistance of atypical hyperplasia or foci of in situ carcinoma, they are followed by papillary or other carcinomas after excision in 4%.
2. *Small peripheral intraductal papillomas:* They are situated in the peripheral ductal segments and generally are coexistent finding of proliferative changes seen in fibrocystic breasts. They are associated with an increased recurrence rate and cancer incidence of 12%.
3. *Papillary adenoma of the nipple:* It is a benign tumor, frequently leading to erosions and occurring unilaterally and bilaterally. In 12% of the cases, concurrent or subsequent ipsilateral and contralateral carcinomas are found.
4. *Juvenile papillomatosis:* It is a disease of puberty and adolescence, featuring atypical papillary duct hyperplasia, which has been observed in families with an increased incidence of cancer. An increased risk of breast

cancer has not jet been found in these patients.

Properties

Papillomas usually show evidence of secretory activity (watery to yellowish discharge). They are very friable and bleed easily (brownish or bloody discharge). Papillomas have the tendency to infarct. Old papillomas can become completely fibrosed and can contain calcifications.

Because of their intraductal location and high vulnerability, they can

- Lead to watery to bloody discharge
- Distend ducts
- Distend cysts
- Be surrounded by a blood-containing cavity

Differentiation

The histologic differentiation from a papillary carcinoma is not always easy. Singular or multiple papillomas must be differentiated from papillomatosis. In contrast to singular and multiple papillomas, which are spatially separate tumors, papillomatosis manifests itself as regional epithelial hyperplasia and can be part of proliferative changes in fibrocystic breasts. In papillomatosis the risk of malignancy is increased—as in other proliferative changes—depending on degree and extent of cellular atypia.

Clinical Findings

Discharge can be found in 80% of the papillomas and can be watery, yellowish, brownish, or bloody, whereby a bloody discharge strongly suggests a papilloma. Carcinomas can also cause a bloody discharge (in up to 25% of the cases) and rarely a watery discharge, occurring in only 2–3% of carcinomas with discharge. A thorough diagnostic evaluation is therefore indicated.

Not infrequently, the localization of one or multiple papillomas can be suspected clinically if nipple discharge can be elicited by pressure on the so-called *trigger points.*

Only a few papillomas are primarily detected by palpation, mammography, or sonography. These papillomas are usually large, superficial, or have caused a retention cyst or "hemorrhagic cyst" through ductal obstruction.

Cytology of Nipple Discharge

The cytologic evaluation of nipple discharge can be easily performed and does not put any demand on the patient. A positive finding (cords of papillary cells, suspected cells, blood) should be an indication for further evaluation.

Cytology of the nipple discharge, which is based on the necrotic changes of the shed cells found in the discharge, is only of moderate sensitivity. A negative finding does not exclude a carcinoma. Furthermore, a reliable differentiation between carcinoma and papilloma cannot be expected from the cytologic assessment of the nipple discharge.

Diagnostic Strategy and Goals

Since most papillomas are detected by their secretory activity, the diagnostic questions to be answered are:

- *Confirmation of a papillary lesion.* In addition to papillary tumors, there are other causes of nipple discharge (as to the differential diagnosis of pathologic nipple discharge, see Chapter 20)
- *Localization* (search for the point of origin of the secretion)
- *Extent* (one papilloma or multiple papillomas)

Initially, noninvasive methods like mammography, sonography, and a careful clinical examination are utilized.

Clinical examination (trigger point) as well as *mammography* (for large papillomas in a fatty breast) can point to the correct localization in some cases. The full extent is rarely appreciated mammographically or clinically.

In selected cases (intracystic or large papillomas, very rare small papillomas located in the subareolar ducts), a papilloma can be detected *sonographically*.

In many instances, localization and extent cannot be adequately evaluated with noninvasive methods. Above all, this applies to small papillomas surrounded by nonfatty tissue. In these cases, galactography is indicated as a supplemental examination. By showing filling defects or, less frequently, truncated ducts, it can detect papillomas and allows an assessment of their extent. Absence of any filling defects or truncated ducts—together with cytologic absence of suspected cells or cords of papillary cells—excludes

ity and enlargement of the parenchymal lobules as found in LCIS.

Clinical Presentation and History

Clinically, there is no characteristic finding.

Some lesions of LCIS are diagnosed in excisional biopsies performed because of a worrisome palpable finding or asymmetry. Others are incidental histologic discoveries in biopsies performed for fibroadenomas or adjacent microcalcifications.

Mammography

There are also no mammographic findings characteristic of LCIS. This implies that LCIS generally cannot be distinguished from benign changes or normal breast parenchyma. Rarely is an asymmetry found mammographically. Microcalcifications—which are generally uncharacteristic in morphology and distribution—are only found in a few cases of LCIS.

Sonography

Sonographically, LCIS is not recognizable.

Magnetic Resonance Imaging

Only limited experience is available so far. In the few examined cases, a mostly moderately diffuse enhancement was observed, and in our own patients, a focal enhancement was seen twice, similar to the enhancement found in proliferative benign changes.

Percutaneous Biopsy

Percutaneous biopsies are not suitable for the detection and exclusion of LCIS, since the diagnosis of LCIS from small samples or even single cells is difficult and diagnostically unreliable.

Therapeutic Decisions after Documented LCIS, Goals and Value of Diagnostic Methods

Utilizing diagnostic methods with the goal of disclosing or excluding LCIS is at the present infeasible because of absence of characteristic features. Therefore utilizing diagnostic methods is restricted to the possible early detection of an invasive carcinoma. Presently, mammographic and clinical follow-up, supplemented by sonography in case of indeterminate findings, is recommended.

Whether other modalities, such as MRI and percutaneous biopsy, can be cost-effectively applied to the early detection of an invasive carcinoma in these patients at risk needs to be confirmed by well-designed clinical trials.

Because of the uncertain clinical significance and prognosis of LCIS, therapeutic recommendations vary. As part of a large multicenter study conducted in the USA (NSABP-B 17), all cases with LCIS are recorded and followed to get a better understanding of this tumor entity.

The current therapy consists of simple excision and regular clinical and mammographic follow-up examinations, for early diagnosis of an invasive carcinoma, should one develop.

Ductal Carcinoma in Situ (DCIS) (Intraductal Carcinoma)

Definition

Histopathologically, as well as clinically and prognostically, DCIS comprises a heterogenous group of carcinomas. As a result of mammography and screening, the incidence of DCIS detected in biopsies has increased from 2–4% to 10–29%.

According to the definition of these tumors, malignant cells are exclusively found within the lactiferous ductal system, i.e., intraductal, without destruction of the basement membrane.

They extend contiguously or noncontiguously through the ductal system, explaining the frequent multifocal and multicentric tumor manifestations found on average in 30% of all DCIS and in over 60% of the DCIS of large extent.

Incidence

The peack incidence of DCIS occurs between the ages of 40 and 60 years. Since most cases of

DCIS contain microcalcifications, and consequently are mammographically detectable, the detection rate has markedly increased with the expanding use of mammography. While the proportion of DCIS of all discovered carcinomas in patients with clinical findings is only 3–5%, it has now reached 20–30% in the screening group.[2, 3, 4, 5, 6] In particular, mammographic detection of those subtypes of DCIS that are associated in a high percentage with the (subsequent) development of an invasive carcinoma (see below) can indeed be considered an early one.

Furthermore, some noncalcified DCIS are incidentally discovered histologically in biopsies performed for other reasons.

Histology

Histologically, five types found at different frequencies are distinguished. These are lesions not only of different histologic pattern, but also of diverse clinical and prognostic properties, dominated by the comedo DCIS in distinction to the remaining tumors that are grouped together as non-comedo DCIS (Table 13.**1**).

The variation of the numerical values is attributable to the so-called mixed types with two or more components encountered in 30–50% of cases, particularly in large lesions.

Comedo DCIS

This subtype of DCIS is characterized by a dominant solid intraductal tumor component with the formation of areas of central necrosis that form calcifications and can occupy 50% or more of the ductal diameter.

In comparison to the other subtypes, the comedo carcinoma is of an increased malignant potential, characterized by an increased proliferation rate of the tumor cells with a high nuclear grading leading to the formation of pleomorphic hyperchromatic cell nuclei. It is histologically more anaplastic appearing than other subtypes of DCIS.

There is a relationship between tumor size and likelihood of microinvasion[7] as well as between tumor size and likelihood of ipsilateral residual tumor.[8] The foci of microinvasion are the origin of the axillary nodal metastases found in 1–3% of the cases.[9, 10, 4, 8]

Prognostically important are the cytomorphologic criteria and the marked overexpression of the c-erb-B-2 oncogene encountered primarily in comedo DCIS.

Table 13.**1** Subclassification and incidence of intraductale carcinomas related to all intraductal carcinomas

Comedo carcinoma	30–50%
Solid carcinoma	9–22%
Cribriform carcinoma	20–28%
Micropapillary carcinoma	8–14%
Papillary carcinoma	4–7%

Non-comedo Carcinoma

The *solid subtype* and the *cribriform carcinoma* are predominantly confined to one quadrant and express a higher degree of differentiation. *Micropapillary carcinomas* generally extend in several quadrants and exhibit a high percentage of multicentric growth. The *papillary carcinoma in situ* is divided into the typical DCIS confined to the duct and the intracystic papillary DCIS.

Importance

Based on current knowledge, there seem to be important prognostic differences between the subgroups of DCIS. While up to 50% of comedo carcinomas can be expected to progress to invasive ductal carcinoma, the noncomedo carcinoma seem to have a lower progression rate.[11, 7, 12, 13, 14, 15, 16, 17, 18]

New Classification

Though the traditional histopathological classification is generally accepted, there have been discordances, above all of the clinical and prognostic criteria, and new classifications have been proposed. They part from evaluating histopathologic patterns and entities in favor of evaluating cytonuclear differentiation (nuclear grading), architecture, and the presence or absence of various forms of necrosis.

1. The **Van Nuys classification**[19, 20] combines nuclear grading and necrosis as the determining criteria. This classification divides:
- **High-grade DCIS with comedo-type necrosis,** corresponding to the classic comedo carcinoma

- **Non-high-grade DCIS without comedo-type necrosis** (non-comedo carcinoma), encompassing solid, cribriform, papillary and micropapillary subtypes, and
- **Non-high-grade DCIS** with comedo-type necrosis, representing an intermediate type with a favorable prognosis and resembling the second type

2. The **classification** proposed by **Holland and coworkers**[16] completely abolishes the conventional terminology and replaces it with cytonuclear and architectural criteria. The authors define specific proliferation patterns with cellular polarization and three categories of cytonuclear differentiation, associated with characteristic calcifications:
   - **Poorly differentiated DCIS** with amorphous calcifications
   - **Intermediately differentiated DCIS** with an amorphous, laminated, coarse and fine-granular calcifications, and
   - **Well-differentiated DCIS** with laminated, psammomatous, and fine-granular calcifications

Therapeutic Decisions

In view of the remaining questions as to the exact prognostic classification of the subtypes of DCIS and because of the still outstanding exact comparison of the efficiency of the available therapies, a standard treatment for DCIS does not exist. In most cases, DCIS is treated today with a simple mastectomy without axillary dissection. Only if the findings are extensive is sampling of the axillary lymph nodes recommended. Mastectomy is associated with a cure rate approaching 100%.

At the present time, several studies are in progress to evaluate whether DCIS with minimal extension can be successfully treated by breast-conserving surgical intervention and whether or not radiotherapy is necessary.

There is a connection between the extent at the time of the primary diagnosis and therapy and the likelihood of locally recurrent disease. Comparing patients having DCIS <25 mm with patients having DCIS >25 mm, Lagios et al.[7] found an increase in multicentricity from 14% to 46%, in occult invasion from 0% to 46% and in axillary nodal involvement from 0% to 4%.

Clinical Findings and History

In population screening, only 10% of DCIS lesions are clinically apparent. The clinical findings mostly present as a palpable abnormality, rarely as a pathologic secretion or Paget disease of the nipple. DCIS very rarely becomes symptomatic through localized (unilateral and usually not related to the menstrual cycle) pain.

Diagnostic Methods: Value and Goals

Mammography alone, above all by demonstrating microcalcifications, makes it possible to detect DCIS even in asymptomatic patients. But this is associated with problems since:

- DCIS is a true indicator of a subsequent invasive carcinoma only in part of the lesions. If mastectomy is recommended as the therapy of choice, perhaps 50% of patients with comedo DCIS and 75% with non-comedo DCIS are overtreated.
- The microcalcifications found in DCIS (primarily microcalcifications in comedo DCIS) show a relatively characteristic pattern in some lesions and are only then reliably distinguishable from the frequent calcifications found in benign conditions. Surgical removal of all calcifications that might represent DCIS (including the non-comedo type) could increase the sensitivity of detecting DCIS but would result in an unacceptable high biopsy rate (more than 10 excisions of benign findings for each detected DCIS).

On the basis of current knowledge, good sensitivity and acceptable specificity may only be achieved by:

- Thorough analysis of the mammographic calcifications.
- One should proceed to supplemental methods only after thorough analysis of microcalcifications, guided by critical appraisal of the limitations of the supplemental methods (see p. 218).

Currently, sonography and MRI do not play an important role in the detection and diagnosis of DCIS. Even with percutaneous biopsies, the diagnostic accuracy of the carcinoma is situ is less than that of the invasive carcinoma.[21]

Mammography

Microcalcifications are the *cardinal finding* of DCIS, but *microcalcifications* can be *absent* in

DCIS. DCIS can mammographically appear as a density or an asymmetry, can become clinically symptomatic, or can be incidentally diagnosed histologically (in excisional biopsies performed for an unrelated reason).

■ Image Presentation

Mammographically, DCIS can become visible:

- Through microcalcifications. They are the only finding in about 80–85% of DCIS lesions detected by mammography, rarely surrounded by soft tissue density. (The surrounding soft tissue density, encountered in some of the DCIS without invasion, can be explained as reactive periductal fibrosis.)
- As a spiculated mass often without central density (10% of DCIS lesions).
- As an irregularly outlined or uncharacteristic mass (about 5–10% of DCIS lesions).
- As well-circumscribed nodular mass (<1% of DCIS lesions).

Importance of Microcalcifications

Mammographic microcalcifications are the most *important characterizing feature* of DCIS, but their presence should *by no means be equated with the presence of DCIS.*

Actually, up to 80% of excised microcalcifications—depending on the technical quality of the mammographic films and experience of the examiner—turn out to be benign. Therefore, it represents an important diagnostic challenge to analyze the microcalcifications and above all to differentiate malignant calcifications from calcifications occurring in context with benign conditions (mostly in mastopathy).

Image Presentation of Microcalcifications in DCIS

The following calcifications can be found in DCIS:

1. *In the comedo type,* the central cells undergoing necrosis calcify. These necrotic cylinders can be extruded under pressure from the macroscopic specimen like common cutaneous comedos, as implied in the name given in analogy with this condition. Since this necrotic cellular materials is always within the lactiferous ductal system, it leads to:

- Typical segmental arrangement of the so-called ductal calcifications following the ductal system (Figs. 13.**1a–c**). Depending on the location within the breast, a linear, branching arrangement, with or without segmental or triangular distribution with the apex oriented toward the nipple can be observed. Rectangular, club-shaped and butterfly-shaped formations, depending on the projection, may occur as well.
- Typical microcalcifications, so-called rod-like casting of the small lactiferous ducts with branching configurations (Y-shaped, V-shaped), linear and/or comma-shaped calcifications (Fig. 13.**2**).
- Typical, markedly polymorphous, coarse granular microcalcifications up to 2 mm in diameter (Fig. 13.**3**).

These calcifications are considered characteristic since—depending on their number and size—they indicate the presence of DCIS, usually the comedo type, with a high degree of specificity (in about 80% of the cases). It should be pointed out that comedo-DCIS does not always calcify and that about 20–25% of the cases of calcified comedo-DCIS fail to exhibit this characteristic pattern.

2. *In the cribriform and micropapillary subtype of the non-comedo carcinoma* (Fig. 13.**4a–h**), the very tiny, often round cavities that are part of the typical histomorphologic architecture of these DCIS fill with secretion and calcify. Therefore, calcific manifestation of the non-comedo DCIS is:

- Frequently very delicate
- Occasionally fine granular, irregular to bizarre
- But sometimes also fine granular, relatively monomorphic

This means that the rod-like casts characteristic of comedo-DCIS are often absent.

- As for comedo-DCIS, the *arrangement* of the calcifications may often be segmental

Such microcalcifications are considered less characteristic—in particular, if a segmental arrangement is not definitely recognizable—since they are very frequently encountered in benign changes as well and are indicative of a malignancy in only 5–20% of the lesions.

In addition to these uncharacteristic calcifications, less frequently non-comedo DCIS may

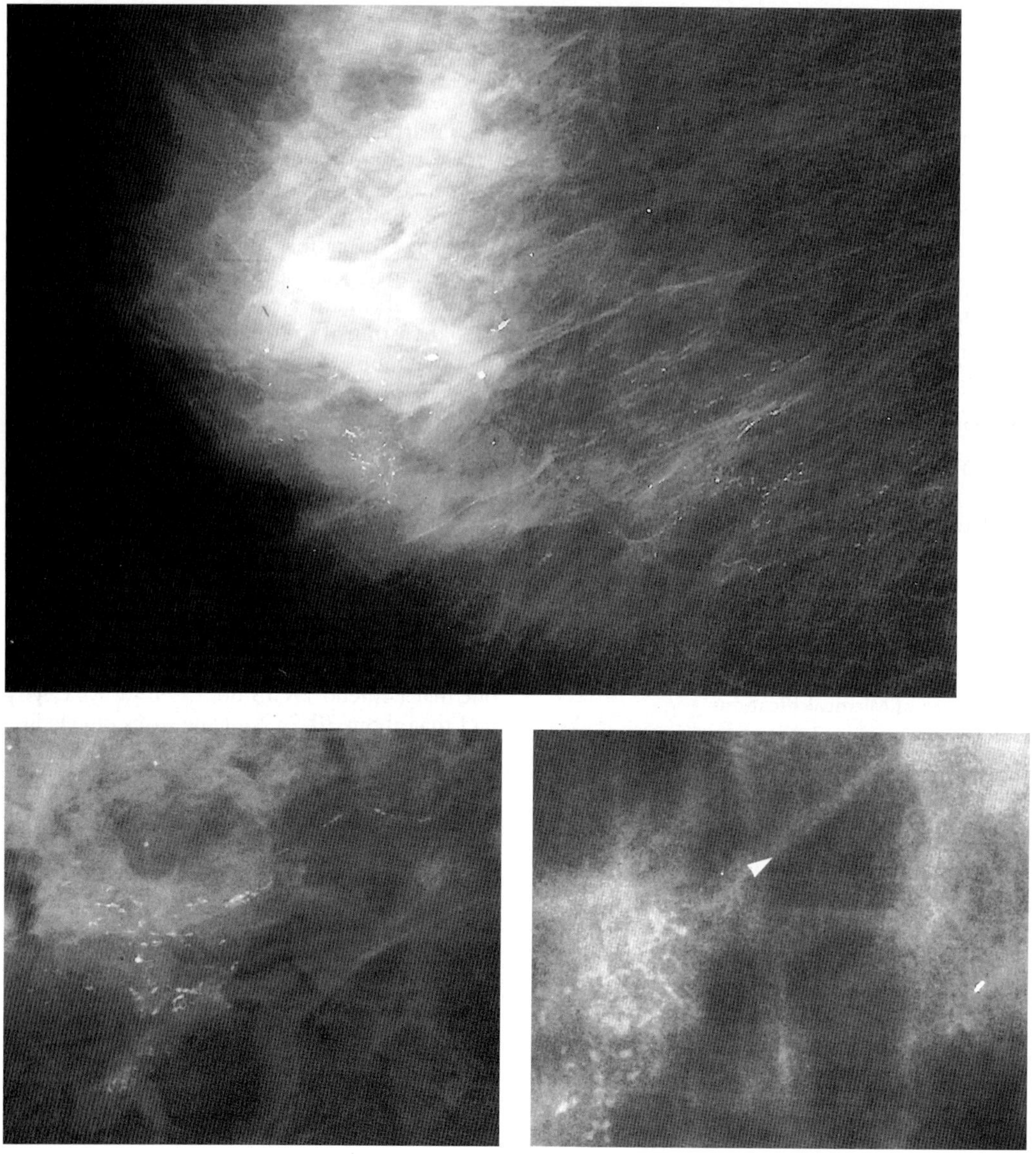

a b c

Fig. 13.**1 a–c**
a Typical segmental arrangement of microcalcifications, extending from the prepectoral region to the nipple: DCIS, comedo type
b The specimen radiograph (magnification) shows the elongated casts of individual calcifications and their branching pattern to better advantage
c Characteristic triangular group formation, with the apex of the triangle pointing toward the nipple. *Histology:* comedo DCIS

develop comedo-type calcifications, facilitating early detection and differentiation from benign changes.

Altogether, exact mammographic assignment to a certain histologic subtype only succeeds in some cases. The list presented above should be seen as a basis for a better understanding of the microcalcific formations, but by no means as a substitute for histology. Moreover, a subtype rarely manifests itself, alone. More often, the various subtypes are mixed and occur together. Therefore, the radiologist should not attempt to predict the histology of DCIS on the basis of the mammographic pattern of calcifications.

In a prospective study, the comedo subtype was more likely accompanied by linear calcifications (78%)[5] than the non-comedo subtypes, which was more likely associated with fine-granular calcifications (53%).

Methodical Prerequisites for the Analysis of Microcalcifications

The comprehensive evaluation of microcalcifications requires mammography in at least two projections. High image quality concerning optimized contrast, correct exposure of the area in question, good contrast, and acceptable noise level are absolute prerequisites.

For demonstrating the teacup appearance of benign microcalcifications, one mediolateral view, perhaps as an added view, should be obtained in a 90° lateral projection, usually with magnification.

Magnification mammography is of utmost importance for improving the analysis of the morphology of the individual calcifications.

■ Accurary of Mammography for the Detection and Differential Diagnosis

Mammography alone has made it possible to detect carcinomas in situ on a large scale. It is therefore the decisive method for detecting and diagnosing carcinomas in situ. Since carcinomas in situ not visible mammographically are generally clinically asymptomatic, the true sensitivity is unknown.

DCIS presenting as "characteristic calcifications" or spiculate density is mammographically detectable with a very high sensitivity and good specificity. DCIS with less characteristic calcifications that are aggregated in groups too small for analysis as well as DCIS presenting as an uncharacteristic or a smoothly outlined density may not always be diagnosable by imaging. Since these changes are too uncharacteristic, they cannot all be pursued by immediate biopsy in order to maintain an acceptable specificity.

It is well known that part of the DCIS may not be visible mammographically and may only be discovered as an incidental histologic finding. Prevalence as well as significance of mammographically invisible DCIS cannot be assessed at the present time.

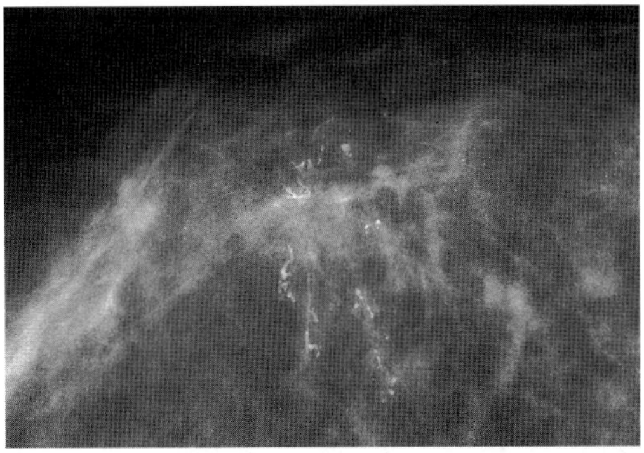

Fig. 13.**2** Magnification mammography with typical irregular, linear calcifications and branching pattern: comedo DCIS

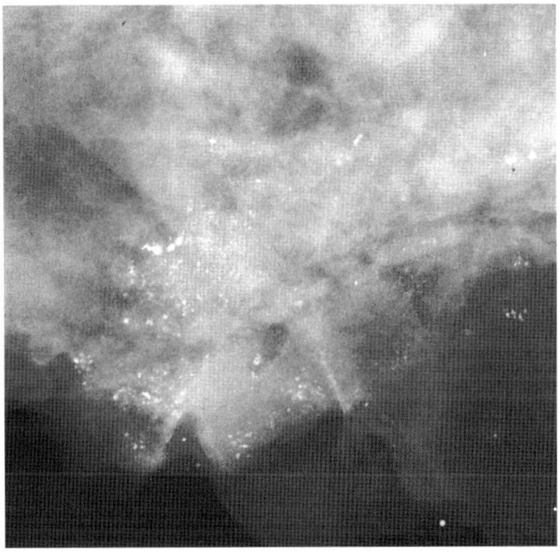

Fig. 13.**3** Predominantly larger granular, pleomorphic microcalcifications next to a few elongated casts. Specimen radiography: peripheral location of the calcifications

■ Additional Roles of Mammography for DCIS

In addition to detecting DCIS (usually on the basis of microcalcifications), mammography is given the important role of providing information concerning its extent (as feasible through microcalcifications) as accurately as possible. This is necessary since a complete removal of DCIS is of great therapeutic significance and since DCIS generally is neither palpable nor macroscopically demarcated.

The mammographic assessment of size, however, is only a crude estimate, since noncalcified components of the DCIS are usually mammographically not apparent. This means

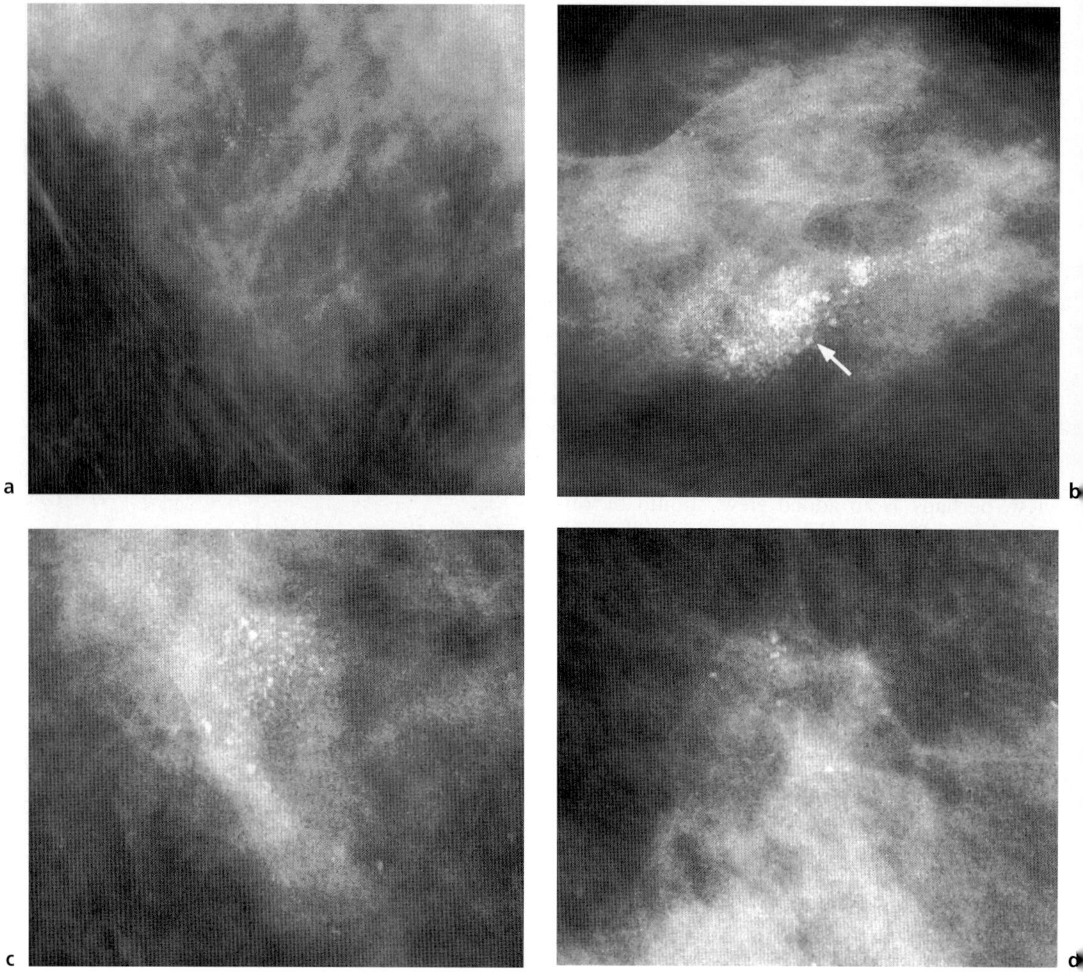

Fig. 13.**4 a–h** Magnification × 4
a Magnification mammography shows two groups of fine granular calcifications
b The specimen radiograph clearly depicts the individual fine granular configuration as well as the ductal distribution. *Histology:* micropapillary cribriform DCIS
c Fine granular pleomorphic microcalcifications, in clusters, which, however, contain casting shapes as well: cribriform DCIS
d Faint spiculated mass with several fine granular calcifications: cribriform–papillary DCIS

that *the extent of intraductal carcinomas is often mammographically underestimated.* To assess the extent as best as possible:

- *Preoperative mammography* must be performed using optimal technique (magnification).
- *Specimen radiography* should be used routinely and with optimal technique, i.e., as standard and magnification views.
- All *microcalcific foci* (especially those close to the cut surface) are *to be marked* on the specimen for the pathologist.
- Postoperative mammography of the surgical site should be performed if breast-preserving surgery is planned, including standard and magnification views. This is important in order to detect any remaining calcifications that might necessitate a second resection or mastectomy, and to document residual benign calcifications for future mammograms obtained as part of the follow-up care.[22]

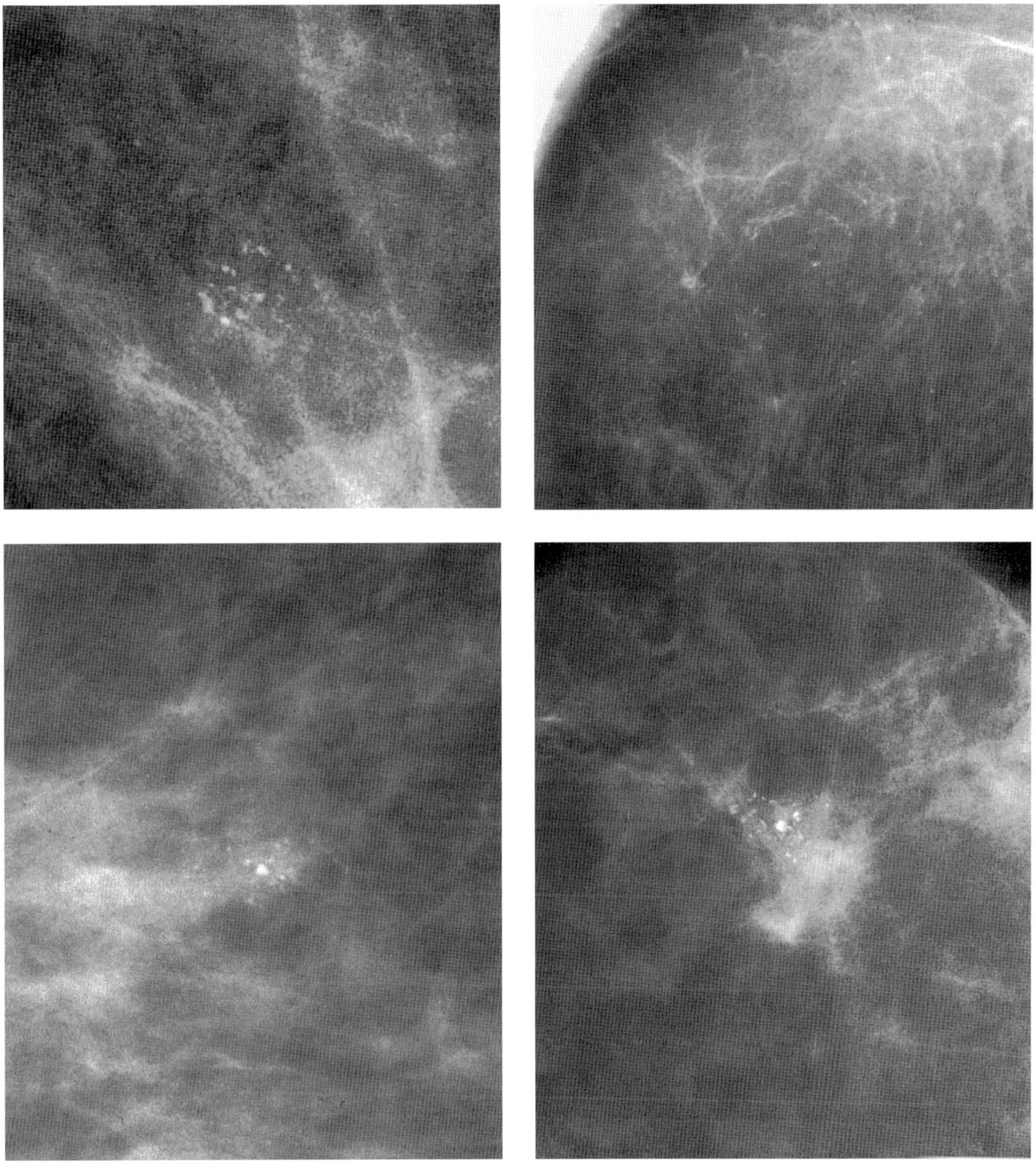

e f g h

Fig. 13.**4 e** Small cluster of fine granular microcalcifications: DCIS, papillary type
f Even magnification mammography shows very small, partially punctated, partially elongated microcalcifications arranged in a branching, ductal distribution: DCIS with micropapillary and solid subtypes
g Small group of predominantly fine granular microcalcifications within a focal mass with delicate spiculation: small-cell DCIS, 5 mm in size, with desmoplastic reaction
h Magnification specimen radiography

Sonography

Image Presentation

Most carcinomas in situ have no characteristic sonographic presentation, i.e., they cannot be distinguished sonographically from normal parenchyma. Only in a few carcinomas in situ—in particular, if a high resolution transducer is used—larger microcalcifications may be visualized or suspected by relatively strong echoes, or dilated hypoechoic ductal structures be interpreted as evidence of DCIS. However, numerous other causes exist for dilated ducts.

Accuracy

All evidence considered, sonography does not afford a reliable diagnosis of DCIS.

Importance

Consequently, sonography does *not* contribute to the detection, exclusion, or differential diagnosis of DCIS.

Magnetic Resonance Imaging

The experience with MRI concerning DCIS is still rather limited.

Image Presentation

Preliminary results suggest that most *comedo DCIS lesions* show relatively intense and early enhancement, following the pattern of invasive carcinomas. However, some comedo DCIS exhibit delayed, occasionally diffuse enhancement (as in benign proliferative breast disease). There is as yet not sufficient knowledge on whether and how often comedo DCIS has minimal enhancement. Based on preliminary results, *non-comedo DCIS lesions* generally enhance slowly and moderately. In some lesions, even minimal enhancement can be expected. Consequently, a reliable differentiation from enhancing benign breast conditions is generally not possible.

Accuracy

Comprehensive data as to the accuracy of MRI for DCIS are still unavailable. With good technique and cautious interpretation (considering any type of enhancement as a possible indicator), the sensitivity of MRI should be about 80%. The specificity (especially the demarcation of the non-comedo DCIS from benign breast conditions), however, is low.

Significance

Because of unanswered questions as to sensitivity and specificity, MRI currently is not to be recommended for diagnosing or evaluating presumed DCIS. In particular, MRI is not indicated for the differentiation of indeterminate microcalcifications.

Larger clinical studies are needed to explore whether *contrast-enhanced MRI* can be meaningfully employed for preoperative assessment of the extent of the lesion and for the detection of additional foci without microcalcifications in patients suspected of having a comedo carcinoma in situ, and whether it can play a role as supplemental examination for early detection of invasive foci in the long-term follow-up of patients with known DCIS.

Percutaneous Biopsy

The data of the accuracy of percutaneous biopsy methods are also limited. They primarily refer to the accurate assessment of mammographic microcalcifications. In a recently published multicenter study, 167 cases of DCIS were found histologically in the needle aspiration biopsy performed on 1637 cases of microcalcifications. All needle aspirations were obtained with the patient supine, lying on a special examination table. Up to 10 tissue cores measuring 2 mm in diameter and 20 mm in length were retrieved. The specificity was stated as 99%. In addition to the examination technique used, the short follow-up periods, which were as short as 6 months, should be noted. However, for carcinomas in situ in particular, mammographic changes may only be visible after a period much longer than 6 months. False negative results of percutaneous biopsies have so far been documented more frequently with microcalcifications than with masses. Whether the above results obtained with special examination tables can be transferred to biopsies with stereotactic needle placement performed with add-on equipment is uncertain. It is currently necessary that groups of microcalcifications that are very suggestive undergo an excisional biopsy, even if percutaneous biopsy (with conventional needles) is negative. With new needles that work with a vacuum, it may be possible to remove areas of microcalcifications and their surroundings completely and thus achieve optimum accuracy.

Summary

LCIS cannot be diagnosed clinically or mammographically. It is often discovered incidentally through excisional biopsies performed because of questionable abnormal palpation or indeterminate mammographic findings. The therapeutic consequence consists of categorizing a patient with histologically proven LCIS as a patient at risk, i.e., to subject her to annual clinical and mammographic examinations for the early detection of a developing invasive carcinoma.

The term DCIS encompasses a group of histologically and prognostically heterogeneous noninvasive carcinomas. Its discovery has risen with the increasing use of mammography. Microcalcifications are the cardinal finding in DCIS. Therefore mammography is the primary imaging method since it alone permits the detection and analysis of microcalcifications.

While the comedo subtype produces a mammographically characteristic (ductal) pattern of individual forms and distribution, the noncomedo subtypes are more difficult to differentiate from the numerous microcalcifications that are associated with benign breast conditions. The rigorous use of magnification mammography adds significantly to increasing the accuracy.

Sonography plays no role in the detection, exclusion, or differential diagnosis of DCIS. The experience with contrast-enhanced MRI is limited at the present time and MRI does not contribute to the differential diagnosis of microcalcifications.

At present, further investigations and data are necessary to determine whether and under which conditions percutaneous biopsy methods (aspiration cytology, core needle biopsy) might eventually be able to replace excisional biopsy for evaluating microcalcifications. Presently, the limitations of percutaneous biopsy must be critically taken into account, particularly when suspected microcalcifications are to be evaluated.

References

1. Stegner HE. Histopathologie der Mammatumoren. Licht- und elektronenmikroskopischer Atlas. Stuttgart: Enke; 1986
2. Schnitt SJ, Silen W, Sadowsky NL, Connolly JL, Harris JR. Ductal carcinoma in situ (intraductal carcinoma of the breast). N Engl J Med. 1988;318:898–903
3. v. Dongen JA, Harris JR, Petersen JL, Fentiman IS, Holland R, Salvadori E, Stewart HJ. In situ breast cancer: The EORTC consensus meeting. Lancet. 1989;25–7
4. Holland R, Hendriks JHCL, Verbeek ALM, Schuurmans Stekhoven JH. Extent, distribution and mammographic/histological correlations of the breast ductal carcinoma in situ. Lancet. 1990;335:519–22
5. Stomper PC, Conolly JL. Ductal carcinoma in situ of the breast: correlation between mammographic calcification and tumor subtype. AJR. 1992;159:483–5
6. Dershaw DD, Abramson A, Kinne DW. Ductal carcinoma in situ: mammographic findings and clinical implications. Radiology. 1989;170:411–15
7. Lagios MD, Margolin FR, Westdahl PR, Rose MR. Mammographically detected duct carcinoma in situ: frequency of local recurrence following tylectomy and prognostic effect of nuclear grade on local recurrence. Cancer. 1989;63:618–24
8. Silverstein MJ. Intraductal breast carcinoma (DCIS). Clinical factors influencing treatment choice. Abstract: 7th International Congress on Senology, Island of Rhodes. 1992
9. Lagios MD, Westdahl PR, Margolin FR, Rose MR. Duct carcinoma in situ: relationship of extent of noninvasive disease to the frequency of occult invasion, multicentricity, lymph node metastases and short-term treatment failures. Cancer. 1982;50:1309–14
10. Ashikari R, Huvos AG, Snyder RE. Prospective study of non-infiltrating carcinoma of the breast. Cancer. 1977;39:435–9
11. Millis RR, Thynne GSJ. In situ intraduct carcinoma of the breast: a long term follow-up study. Br J Surg. 1975;62:975–62
12. Eusebi V, Foschini MP, Cook MG, Berrino F, Azzopardi JG. Long-term follow-up of in situ carcinoma of the breast with special emphasis on clinging carcinoma. Semin Diagn Pathol. 1989;6:165–73
13. Solin LJ, Yeh IT, Kurtz J et al. Ductal carcinoma in situ (intraductal carcinoma) of the breast treated with breast-conserving surgery and definitive irradiation. Correlation of pathologic surgery and definitive irradiation. Correlation of pathologic parameters with outcome of treatment. Cancer. 1993;71:2532–42
14. Bellamy COC, McDonald C, Salter DM, Chetty U, Anderson J. Noninvasive ductal carcinoma of the breast: the relevance of histologic categorization. Hum Pathol. 1993;24:16–23
15. Holland R, Petersen JL, Millis RR et al. Ductal carcinoma in situ: a proposal for a new classification. Semin Diagn Pathol. 1994;11:167
16. Holland R, Hendriks JHCL. Microcalcifications associated with ductual carcinoma in situ: mammographic-pathologic correlation. Semin Diagn Pathol. 1994;11:181–92
17. Silverstein MJ, Lagios MD, Craig PH et al. A prognostic index for ductal carcinoma in situ of the breast. Cancer. 1996;77/11:2267–74
18. Schwartz GF, Finkel G, Garcia JC, Patchefsky AS. Subclinical ductal carcinoma in situ of the breast. Treatment by local excision and surveillance alone. Cancer. 1992;70:2468–74

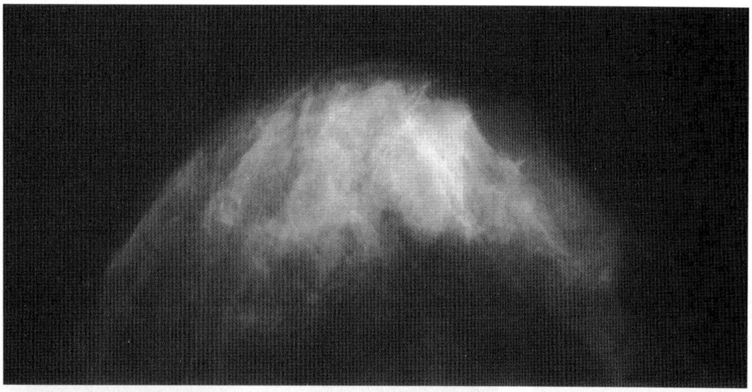

a

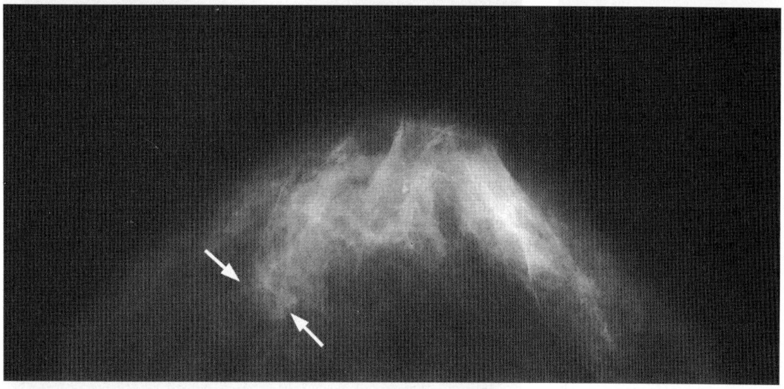

b

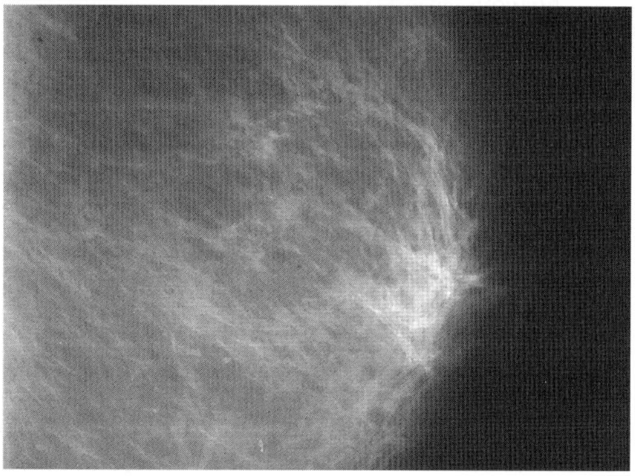

c

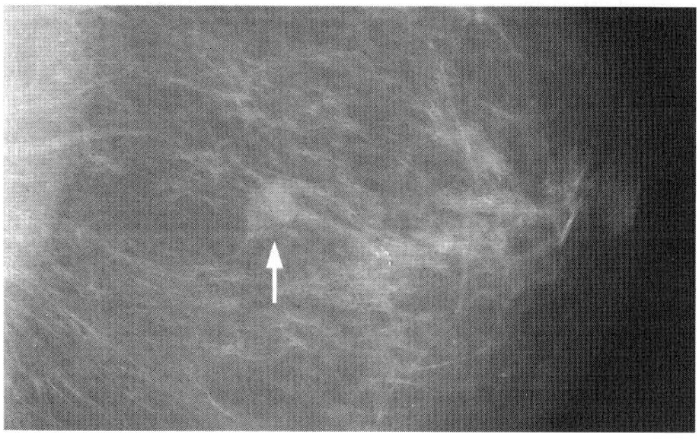

d

Fig. 14.7 **a–h** Follow-up mammography
a and **b** Current CC view (**b**) and previous CC view (**a**) obtained 3 years earlier. In comparison with the previous view, the current a new density equal to the density in the remaining parenchyma (arrows). Since it is new or has increased in size, it must be considered suspect despite its radiodensity equal to that of the parenchyma. Retrospectively, a subtle structural alteration can already be appreciated in the same area 3 years ago, i.e., the parenchyma in this area is not oriented toward the nipple. *Histology:* ductal carcinoma, multifocal

Fig. 14.7 **c** and **d** A round structure measuring a few millimeters is shown here. It could represent a small cyst, a very small fibroadenoma, or a papilloma in the parenchyma. The next follow-up examination revealed an increase in size, rendering this structure (arrow)—in particular, since it does not correspond to a cyst sonographically—very suspicious for malignancy (close-up of an oblique view). *Histology:* intraductal carcinoma with minimal invasion (pT1a)

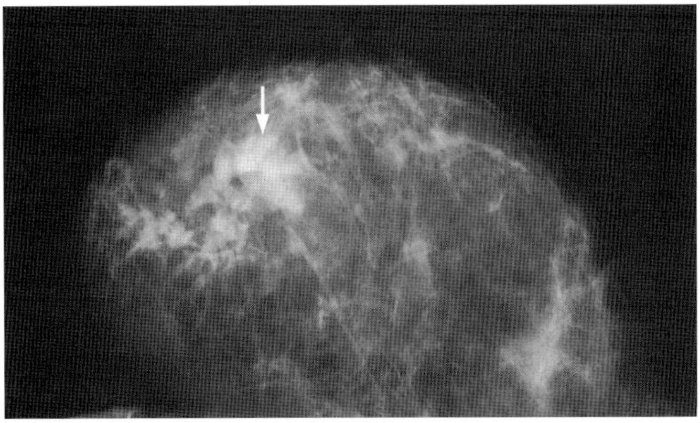

e

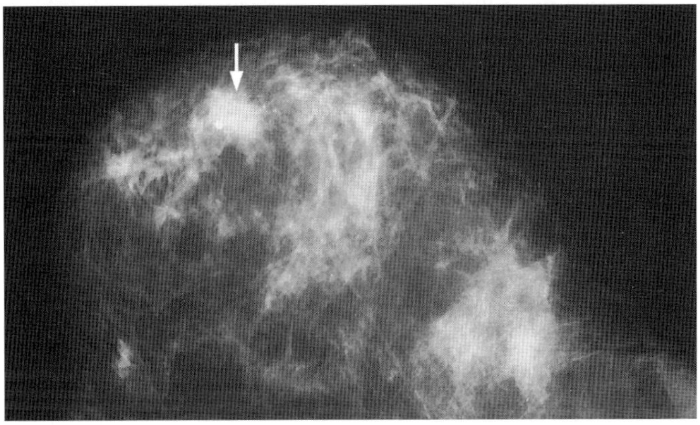

f

Fig. 14.7**e** This mammogram of a 46-year-old patient reveals asymmetric densities with distorted architecture and slightly increased density medially, which were not mentioned as suspicious by the interpreting radiologist
f Three years later, the density of the mass has increased, and its margins are now spiculated. (The density of the entire parenchyma appears increased since a high-contrast film was used.) Decrease in size is certainly not a sign of benignity and can be explained by retraction due to fibrosis. Another small mass has appeared adjacent to the thoracic wall. *Histology:* well-differentiated, slowly growing tubular carcinoma

g

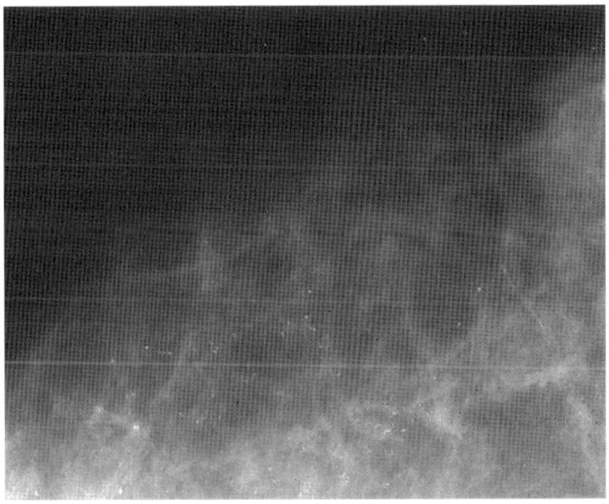

h

Fig. 14.7**g** Mammography with unequivocally suspicious calcifications (elongated individual forms), confined to the upper inner quadrant—not categorized as suspicious by the initially interpreting radiologist
h Six years later, the microcalcifications are essentially unchanged. The surrounding soft tissues have even decreased in density due to postmenopausal involution. Because of the suspicious appearance of the individual calcifications and despite the lack of any interval change, excisional biopsy was recommended. *Histology:* extensive DCIS with microinvasion. This finding confirms that any progression seen on follow-up examination mandates prompt definitive evaluation, but that stability—as illustrated in this case—cannot be taken as assurance of benignity of an otherwise suspicious finding

The Influence of Histology on Mammographic Presentation

As already mentioned, histologic type and growth pattern of the carcinoma affect the mammographic presentation. Knowing the histologic features and the different manifestations of the various types of carcinomas is important for detecting breast carcinomas. Though the histopathologic classification cannot be deduced, it can sometimes be suspected from the particular presentation of the carcinoma.

In this context, the relationships between histology and mammographic features are recapitulated.

Invasive ductal carcinoma can have diverse manifestations, and any of the signs of malignancy listed in Table 14.**1** can be present, alone or with others (e.g., irregularly outlined mass, circumscribed mass, diffuse growth pattern, focal microcalcifications, diffusely distributed microcalcifications, or no microcalcifications).

Invasive lobular carcinoma frequently grows along established tissue planes without forming a mass and without inciting fibrosis. Therefore, it is often difficult to recognize. Occasionally a spiculated mass or other focal lesion (not infrequently similar to the density of the normal parenchyma) is observed. Very rarely even a round mass can be present. Because of its diffuse growth, lobular carcinomas have the highest percentage of mammographically overlooked carcinomas. Lobular carcinoma does not form microcalcifications.

Tubular carcinoma frequently presents as a spiculated mass with long, reactive, fibrotic strands. It can contain microcalcifications. Regardless of the individual shapes of these microcalcifications, the spiculated mass is an indication for biopsy. Microcalcifications often are the manifestation of DCIS accompanying a tubular carcinoma and can assume characteristic configuration or arrangement.

Medullary, mucinous and papillary carcinomas belong to the types of carcinoma that present as round lesions. However, the most frequent round, well-defined carcinoma histologically is the invasive ductal carcinoma, not otherwise specified (Figs. 14.**2 g–h**). Round carcinomas frequently show areas of indistinctness or subtle undulation (microlobulation) that speak against benignity (Fig. 14.**8 a**). Some of these carcinomas, however, can be smoothly outlined throughout and might even be surrounded by a halo. *Intracystic papillary carcinoma can be completely round if the papillary cancer is in situ.* Any macroscopic infiltration is detected only if the affected portion of the cyst wall is seen tangentially (Fig. 14.**8 b**), showing irregularity with extension into adjacent tissue. Carcinomas with a completely smooth outline (some with a halo sign) constitute less than 2% of the smoothly outlined solid lesions. While medullary and mucinous carcinoma only rarely show microcalcifications (usually single and atypical), some papillary carcinomas, such as papillary carcinoma in situ, can have microcalcifications.

Paget disease of the nipple becomes clinically apparent through eczema of the nipple or areola. The eczema is induced by seeding of malignant cells into the nipple or areola or both. It can arise from any carcinoma within the breast that extends to the areola through the ductal system. A direct retroareolar site of origin in the major ducts is also possible. Eczema suggestive of Paget disease of the nipple always demands a thorough evaluation of the breast to the level of the thoracic wall (mammography, magnification mammography, supplemental methods). In most cases, Paget disease of the nipple has no mammographic findings. Occasionally focal changes in the nipple–areolar complex are seen. Mammography should be obtained, however, to try to detect an underlying carcinoma within the breast.

Inflammatory carcinoma (Fig. 14.**6 c**) is characterized by diffuse thickening of the skin as well as by increased trabecular markings in the subcutaneous tissue and parenchyma, caused by carcinomatous lymphangiosis. Focal thickening as well as malignant-type microcalcifications can be present.

Breast carcinoma associated with nipple discharge. Pathologic discharge is always an indication for mammography and supplemental cytologic examination. Positive cytology confirms an underlying malignancy, but negative cytology does not exclude it. The majority of discharge-inducing breast carcinomas are mammographically detectable. Rarely can such breast carcinomas be hidden in mammographically dense tissue. To localize these carcinomas, *galactography* is indicated.

Filling defects in the ductal system and truncated ducts speak for a carcinoma (Fig. 14.**9**). A definite differentiation between papillomatosis, benign papilloma, or papillary carcinoma can

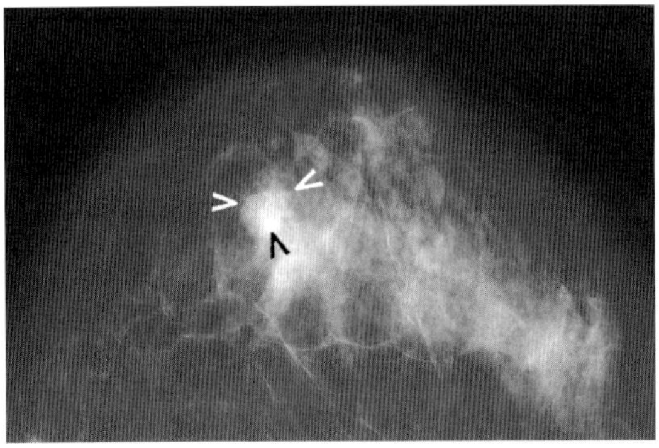

a

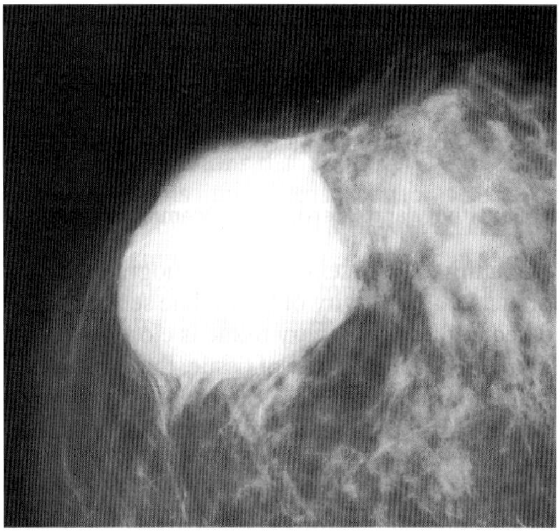

b

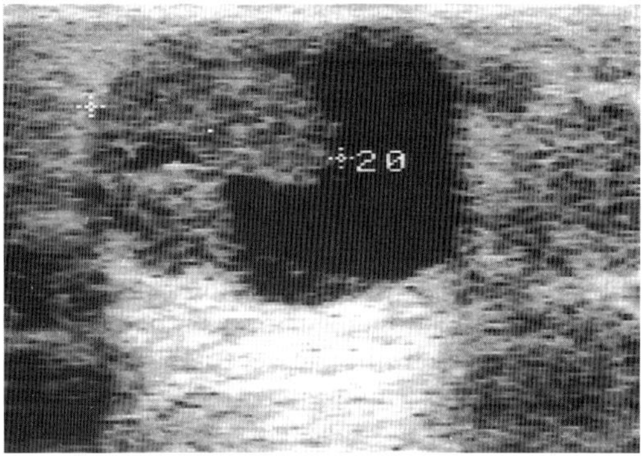

c

Fig. 14.**8 a–c** Additional specific manifestations
a Medullary carcinoma, 1 cm in size. In this case, the outline of the round carcinoma is relatively sharp, but microlobulation (arrow heads) raises the possibility of a malignancy (sonography, see Fig. 14.**11 b**)
b and **c** Mammographically smoothly outlined lesion
b Some areas of indistinctness might be explained by superimposed residual mastopathic tissue, but the pattern should raise concern about possible spiculation
c Sonography shows that the smoothly outlined lesion with good sound transmission consists of a solid and a liquid component. *Histology:* papillary carcinoma. Remark: A small focus of invasion outside the wall of the cyst is only detectable if this segment of the wall (not illustrated here) is tangentially projected on the mammographic view. Sonographically, macroscopic invasion can be noted as irregular interface with the adjacent tissue

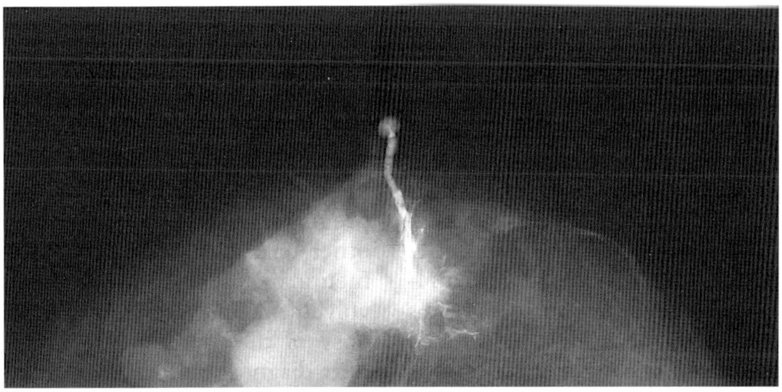

Fig. 14.**9** Galactography of a patient with pathologic nipple discharge and suspicious cytologic smear. Mammography, sonography, and palpation were unremarkable. Galactography, craniocaudad view: There are small persistent filling defects, best explained as remnants of debris. There is an appreciable change in caliber and ductal cut-off 2–3 cm behind the nipple. This region must be considered suspicous. *Histology:* extensive, partially intraductal, partially invasive, poorly differentiated ductal carcinoma

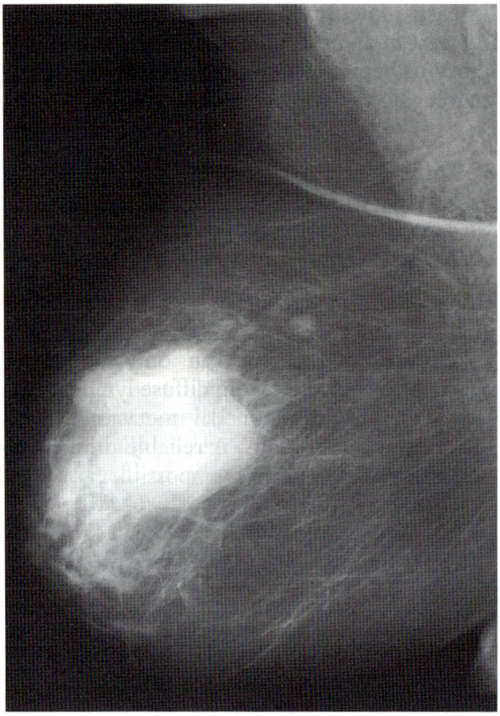
a

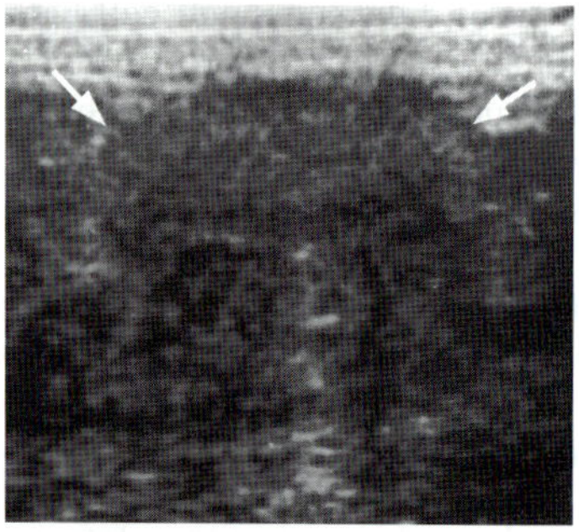
b

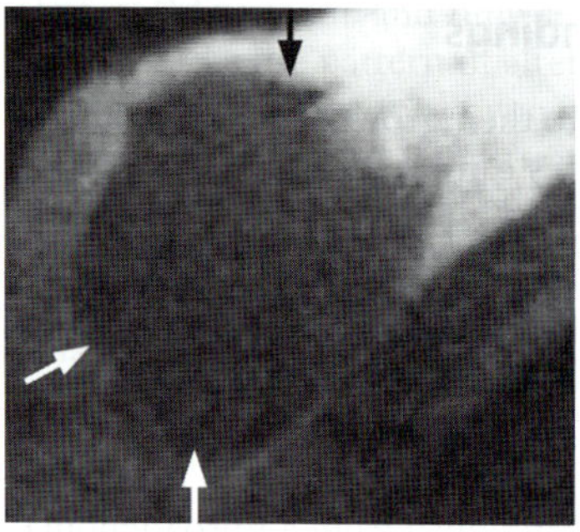
c

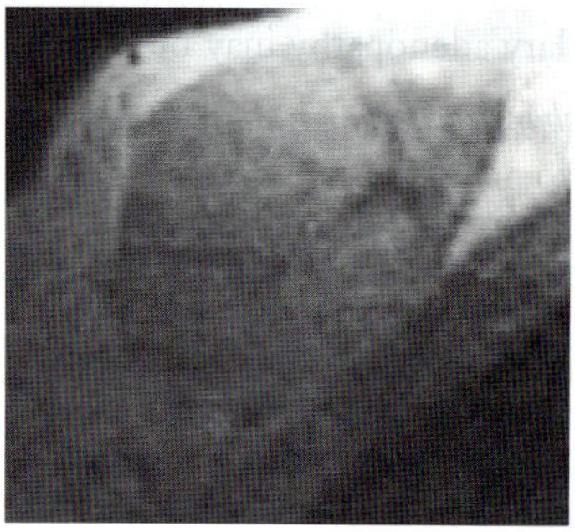
d

Fig. 15.**3 a–d** Nodular non-Hodgkin lymphoma
a Seventy-six-year-old woman with a left breast mass, that is largely well defined. *Histology:* lymphoma
b Sonographically, this lymphoma is seen as lobulated, hypoechoic lesion (arrows)
c It is low signal on the T1-weighted images (arrows)
d Lobulation is apparent on the T2-weighted images (contrast medium was not available at the time of this examination), whereby the areas of high signal-intensity corresponded histologically to lymphomatous tussie. The linear signals of low intensity turned out to be fibrous structures

Percutaneous Biopsy

The diagnosis of a lymphoma can generally be made by fine needle or core biopsy of tumorous infiltrates. Malignant lymphomas are often diagnosed by excisional biopsies. The immunohistochemical subclassification is generally based on the adequate material obtained from an excisional biopsy.

Summary

Hematologic malignancies can present as a focal lesion or as an indistinct diffuse process. There are no morphologic criteria to distuinguish the individual hemotologic malignancies, nor are there reliable differentiating criteria toward benign tumors (for well-circumscribed masses), carcinomas (for irregularly outlined lesions) or inflammatory carcinoma, lymphedema, or inflammation (for diffuse involvement). The final diagnosis and exact classification rest on the excisional biopsy.

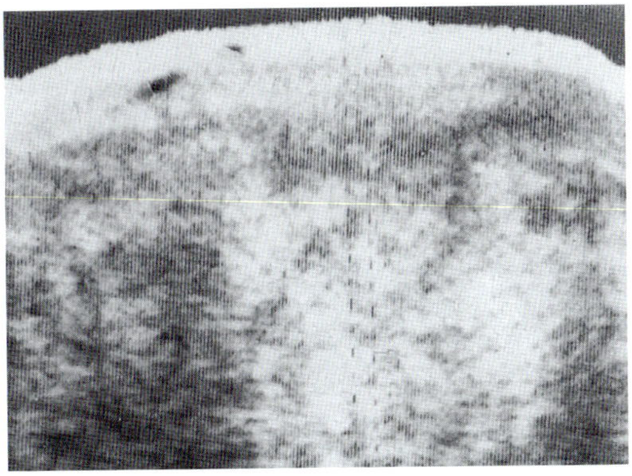

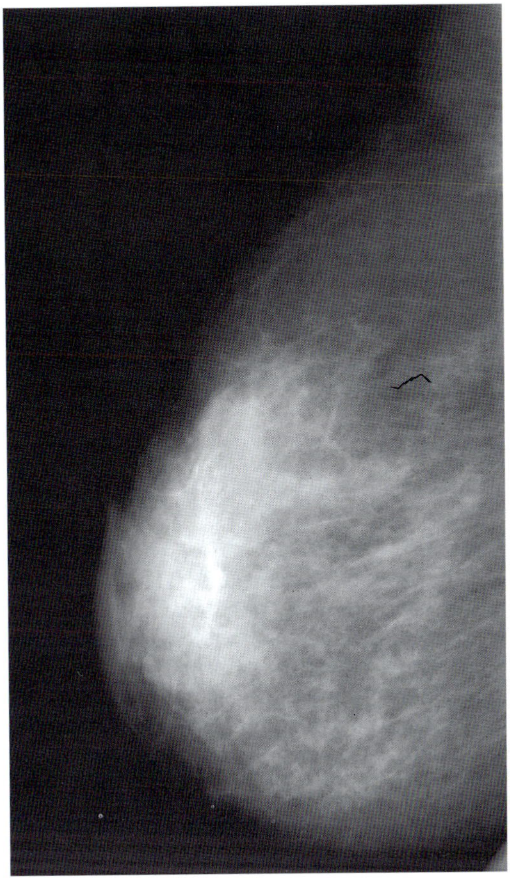

Fig. 15.**4** Diffuse non-Hodgkin lymphoma
a In addition to predominantly periareolar skin thickening, this older mediolateral mammogram shows diffuse interstitial thickening throughout the mammary tissue
b Sonographically (old examination), the diffuse lymphomatous involvement is manifested as skin thickening and increased echogenivity in the subcutaneous space and parenchyma, with resultant loss of the normal echo structure

Metastases

Metastases in the breasts are rare (about 1–5% of the malignancies). They can arise from:

1. An extramammary tumor of any origin
2. A contralateral breast carcinoma
3. A malignancy of hematologic origin (see p. 272)

Metastases should be considered in findings with multiple masses or diffuse increased breast density in cases with a history of known primary carcinoma or metastases, but a specific manifestation is not known.[29]

The therapeutic approach depends on the overall prognosis.

Histology

The most frequently observed metastases arise from the opposite breast, followed by malignant melanomas, bronchial carcinomas, ovarian carcinomas, and sarcomas. Moreover, metastases can arise from gastrointestinal carcinomas, cholangiocarcinomas, thyroid carcinomas, head and neck carcinomas, and urogenital carcinomas, including cervix carcinoma in women and prostate carcinoma in men. The metastases of most extramammary *malignancies* exhibit a *nodular* growth: rather round than oval, and sometimes lobulated.

Metastatic spread can produce *single or multiple* lesions. Metastases are usually distinct in outline and rarely somewhat indistinct. Spiculations do not occur. They are usually located in subcutaneous fat rather than in the core of the breast tissue.

Some extramammary malignancies also have metastases that show a *diffuse growth pattern.* This is most frequently observed in ovarian carcinomas, but has been occasionally described with other malignancies.

Metastases from a carcinoma of the contralateral breast can be hematogenous or lymphogenous via the lymphatics crossing the sternum.

Clinical Findings

If adequate in size and situated superficially, *focal metastases* may be palpated as:

- Smoothly outlined, round
- Usually moveable, rarely fixed
- More often firm than soft lesions (depending on the property of the primary tumor)
- The size of the palpable finding approximates the mammographic size (since reactive changes of the surrounding tissue—as found, for instance, in scirrhous carcinoma—are absent).[29]

Reliable criteria differentiating these from fibroadenomas and cysts do not exist. History of rapid growth often suggests the diagnosis.

If the *involvement is diffuse*, skin thickening and diffuse swelling are observed. Pain is infrequent.

Metastases from a carcinoma of the contralateral breast usually occur via direct extension. They are detectable through skin thickening, palpable thickening, peau d'orange, nodules, or swelling.

Diagnostic Strategy and Goals

With the appropriate history, metastases should be considered if single or multiple, new or growing lesions are found clinically or mammographically, or if diffuse changes of undetermined etiology are encountered.

If the excisional biopsy of a breast lesion—without appropriate history—suggests a metastasis, the search for a primary tumor is warranted.

Appropriate special stains and immunohistology of the excised tissue may assist in determining the origin of the metastasis.

Mammography

(Fig. 15.**5 a**)

Focal metastases are generally visualized mammographically:[24, 29, 30]

- As round, sharply outlined lesions, frequently without any significant marginal indistinctness. Particularly suggestive is the perfectly round shape.
- Single or multiple.
- They can also be partially or totally hidden in dense tissue.
- Aside from coarse calcifications involving necrotic areas, calcifications are extremely rare and, as far as we know, only described as amorphic calcifications in ovarian carcinoma.
- Multiple round lesions containing subgroups of lesions that are about equal in size—reflecting intermittent dissemination—are characteristic and considered important evidence of the presence of metastases.

Reliable criteria that distinguish individual metastases from smoothly outlined benign lesions (fibroadenomas) *do not exist.*

Elongated, polymorphic or ductally oriented microcalcifications, or spicules preclude, for all practical purposes, a metastasis.

Diffuse metastases can become manifest as:

- Skin thickening
- Thickened trabecular markings
- Diffuse, asymmetrically increased density of the parenchyma

Metastases from a carcinoma of the contralateral breast can involve the entire breast diffusely, or appear as cutaneous and subcutaneous thickening extending from the parasternal region laterally (Fig. 15.**6**).

Sonography

(Fig. 15.**5 b**)

Sonography is used to exclude a simple cyst and to verify the presence of palpable findings in mammographically dense tissue.

Sonographically localized metastases:[31]

- Usually present as sharply outlined, round, hypoechoic lesions, with homogeneous in-

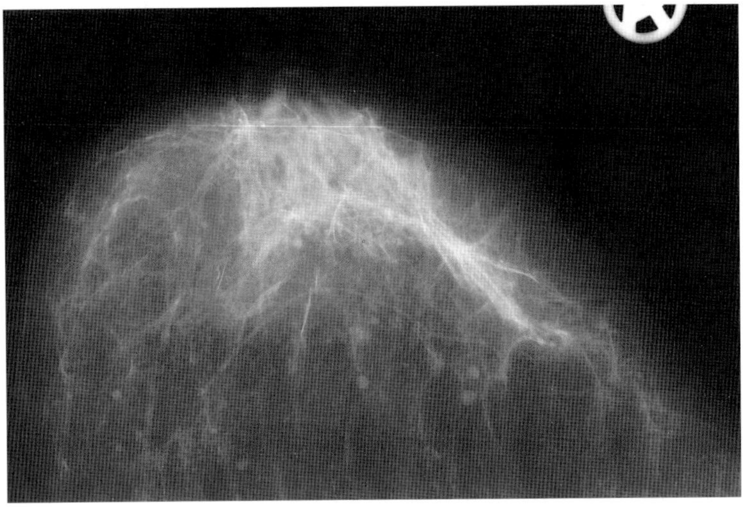

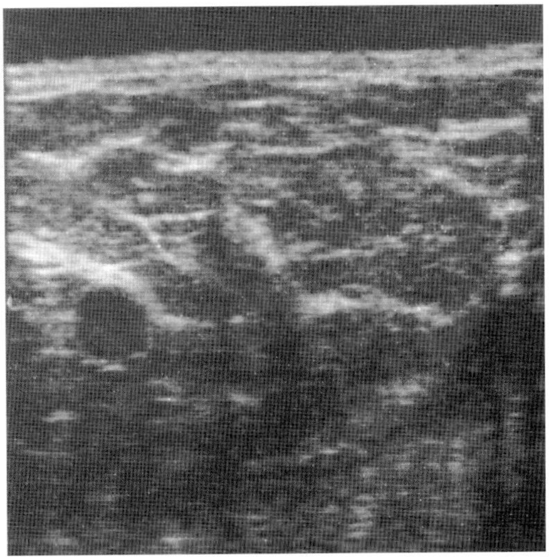

Fig. 15.5 **a** and **b** Multiple small nodular metastases in a patient with known metastatic malignant melanoma
a Craniocaudal mammogram. The multitude of nodules with several nodules equal in size suggests (even without the clinical history) a metastatic process. Despite the smooth outline, the perfectly round configuration favors metastases over benign lesions
b Sonography of a small metastasis—also exhibiting a perfectly round configuration.

ternal structure, and with no or only minimal reactive changes in the surrounding tissue
- Usually have distal acoustic enhancement, sometimes no enhancement or acoustic shadowing (in the presence of intense fibrosis) is seen
- A certain indistinctness of the outline might be appreciated
- Heterogeneity of the internal structure can develop with central necrosis
- Metastases often are easily moveable, rarely fixed
- The consistency varies from firm to soft elastic

Consequently, *sonography does not allow a reliable differentiation* from other and, in particular, from benign lesions that are sharply outlined, such as adenomas.

Diffuse metastatic spread is sonographically:

- Recognized by diffuse skin thickening and obliteration of the echogenic interface with the subcutaneous layer
- Cooper's ligaments may be thickened and appear hypoechoic, secondary to lymphatic stasis caused by tumor cells
- The changes of the parenchyma are often uncharacteristic; overall, the parenchyma appears somewhat hypoechoic

Magnetic Resonance Imaging

The experience is based on only a few individual cases, which showed the metastases as smoothly outlined, nodular, enhancing lesions.

Percutaneous Biopsy

Percutaneous biopsy is very well suited to confirm the presence of malignancy. The diagnosis of a "metastasis" is usually made by excisional biopsy. The larger tissue sample obtained with excisional biopsy may permit better histologic evaluation and immunohistologic examination, but even then the site of origin of the primary tumor cannot be determined in all cases.

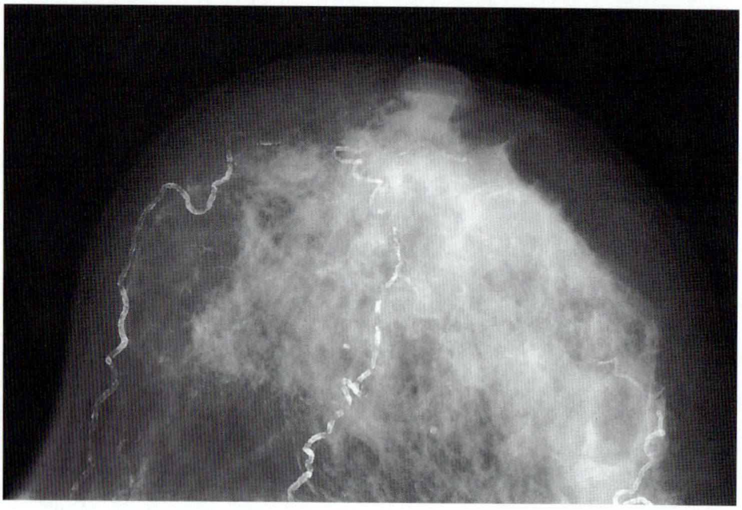

Fig. 15.**6** The medially rotated craniocaudal mammogram shows subtle skin thickening medially, and slightly accentuated interstitial markings in a locally metastasizing contralateral breast carcinoma. (Slightly rotated view for better visualization of the medial skin and subcutis)

Summary

Metastatic spread can become manifest as diffuse, ill-defined changes (skin thickening, increased consistency) or by forming single or several nodular lesions.
Reliable criteria distinguishing metastases from other nodular, usually sharply outlined lesions or from other diffuse changes (mastitits, inflammatory carcinoma) do not exist. Several round lesions, including subgroups of equal size, suggest a metastasizing process.
With the history of a known carcinoma, metastases should be considered if nodular or diffuse changes are found. Confirmation and analysis as to their site of origin rest on the histologic examination.

Other Very Rare Tumors

The following very rare tumors, classified as semimalignant tumors, are listed here:

- fibromatosis
- hemangiopericytoma
- hemangioendothelioma

Fibromatosis (= Extra-abdominal Desmoid)

The fibromatosis of the breast grows as locally invasive. Local recurrence occurs frequently following incomplete excision. It arises from the fascia and consequently is frequently fixed to the pectoral muscle. *Histologically*, it consists of proliferative fibroblasts and extensive fibrosis.[32]

Mammographically[33], it is seen as irregular thickening with fibrous strands and retractions, and cannot be distinguished from the geographic growth of a scirrhous carcinoma.

Sonographically, extensive acoustic shadowing can be expected, as found in scirrhous carcinoma.

There is no experience with MRI. Excision is recommended for diagnosis and therapy.

Hemangiopericytoma and Hemangioendothelioma

Both tumors are rare. The diagnosis is made histologically.

References

1. Bässler R, Zahner J. Über Rezidive und Metastasen des Cystosarcoma phylloides (Phylloide Tumor, WHO). Geburtshilfe Frauenheilkd. 1989;49:1
2. Cohn-Cedermark G, Rutquist LE, Rosendahl I et al. Prognostic factors in cystosarcoma phylloides: clinicopathologic study of 77 patients. Cancer. 1991;68:2017
3. Hart WR, Bauer RC, Oberman HA. Cystosarcoma phylloides: a clinicopathologic study of twenty-six hypercellular periductal stromal tumors of the breast. Am J Clin Pathol. 1978;70:211
4. Norris HJ, Taylor HB. Relationship of histologic features to behavior of cystosarcoma phylloides: analysis of ninety-four cases. Cancer. 1967;20:2090
5. Buchberger W, Strasser K, Heim K et al. Phylloides tumor, findings on mammography, sonography and aspiration in 10 cases. AJR. 1991;157:715
6. Friedrich M. Ultraschalluntersuchung der Mamma. In: Frommhold W, Dihlmann W et al. Hrsg. Bd 1/1: Schinz, Radiologische Diagnostik in Klinik und Praxis. 7. Aufl. Stuttgart: Thieme; 1987
7. Liberman L, Bonaccio E, Hamele-Bena D, Cohen MA, Abramson AF, Dershaw DD. Imaging characteristics of benign and malignant phyllodes tumors. Radiology. 1996;198:121–4
8. Cole-Beuglet C, Soriano R, Kurtz AB. Ultrasound, x-ray mammography and histopathology of cystosarcoma phylloides. Radiology. 1983;146:481
9. Grebe P, Wilhelm K, Brunier A, Mitze M. MR-Tomographie des Cystosarcoma phylloides. Ein Fallbeispiel. Akt Radiol. 1992;2:376
10. Heywang-Köbrunner SH. Contrast-enhanced MRI of the Breast. Munich: Karger; 1990
11. Gutman H, Pallock PE, Ross MJ et al. Sarcoma of the breast: implications for extent of therapy. Surgery. 1994;116:505
12. Chen KTK, Kirkegaard DD, Bocian BB. Angiosarcoma of the breast. Cancer. 1980;46:368
13. Rosen PP, Kimmel M, Ernsberger D. Mammary angiosarcoma, the prognostic significance of tumor differentiation. Cancer. 1988;62:2145
14. Sordillo PP, Chapmans R, Hajdu SI et al. Lymphangioma. Cancer. 1981;48:1674
15. Berger SM, Gershion-Cohen J. Mammography of breast sarcoma. AJR. 1962;87:62
16. Elson BC, Ikeda DM, Anderson I et al. Fibrosarcoma of the breast: mammographic findings in 5 cases. AJR. 1992;158:993
17. Hoeffken W, Lanyi M. Röntgenuntersuchung der Brust. Stuttgart: Thieme; 1973
18. Liberman L, Dershaw DD, Kaufmann R, Rosen PP. Angiosarcoma of the breast. Radiology. 1992;183:649–54
19. Grant EG, Holt RW, Chun B et al. Angiosarcoma of the breast: sonographic, xeromammographic and pathologic appearance. AJR. 1983;141:691
20. Barth V. Mammographie. Intensivkurs und Atlas für Fortgeschrittene. Stuttgart: Enke; 1994
21. Giardini R, Piccolo C, Rilke F. Primary non-Hodgkin's lymphomas of the female breast. Cancer. 1992;69:725
22. Hugh JC, Jackson FJ, Hanson J et al. Primary breast lymphoma: an immunohistologic study of 20 new cases. Cancer. 1990;66:2602
23. Kennedy BJ, Bornstein R, Brunning RD et al. Breast involvement in acute leukemia. Cancer. 1970;25:693
24. McCrea ES, Johnston C, Haney PJ. Metastases of the breast. AJR. 1983;141:685
25. Meyer JE, Kopans DB, Long JC. Mammographic appearance of malignant lymphoma of the breast. Radiology. 1980;135:623
26. Paulus DD. Lymphoma of the breast. Radiol Clin North Am. 1990;28:833
27. Liberman L, Giess CS, Dershaw DD, Deutch BM, Louise DC. Non-Hodgkin's lymphoma of the breast: imaging characteristics and correlation with histopathology. Radiology. 1994;192:157–60
28. Tohno E, Cosgrove DO, Sloane JP. Ultrasound Diagosis of Breast Diseases. Edinburgh: Churchill Livingstone; 1994
29. Bohmann LG, Bassett LW, Gold RH et al. Breast metastases from extramammary malignancies. Radiology. 1982;144:30
30. Paulus DD, Libshitz HJ. Metastases to the breast. Radiol Clin North Am. 1982;20:561
31. Derchi LF, Rizzato G, Guiseppetti GM et al. Metastatic tumors in the breast; sonographic findings. J Ultrasound Med. 1985;4:69
32. Wargotz ES, Norris HJ, Austin KM et al. Fibromatosis of the breast: a clinical and pathological study of 28 cases. Am J Surg Pathol. 1987;11:38
33. Kalisher L, Long JA, Peyster RG. Extraabdominal desmoid of the axillary tail mimicking breast carcinoma. AJR. 1976;126:903

16. Post-traumatic, Post-surgical and Post-therapeutic Changes

Post-traumatic and Post-surgical Changes

Following surgery or trauma, marked and characteristic tissue changes develop, independent of the inducing cause.

Acute changes can be separated from late changes:

1. **Acute changes:** hematoma, seroma, edema, fat necrosis (acute)
2. **Late changes:** scar formation, retraction, dystrophic calcifications, fat necrosis (chronic): oil cyst, lipophagic granuloma

■ Histology

Hematomas and seromas occupy either a surgical cavity or a traumatic tear, or spread into the surrounding parenchyma, connective tissue, and adipose tissue.

After the formation of these fluid collections, resorption takes place. Tissue necrosis is generally called "fat necrosis," even though it only in part concerns fat cells. It is caused by traumatic injury of the cell membrane. The subsequent healing process is marked by the appearance of foam cells as well as of leukocytic, round cell and histiocytic infiltrates, permeating the affected area or causing resorption and repair along the border of the cavity. Beginning along the border, granulation tissue, rich in fibroblasts, grows centripetally. Initially, this tissue is hypervascular and is later transformed into a poorly vascularized, densely packed scar fibrosis. Confluent foci of necrotic fat can liquefy centrally, producing oil cysts, which have a tendency to calcify.

■ Clinical History and Findings

Following surgery or major injury, location and time of the trauma are well known. Both hematoma and fat necrosis can, however, also occur "spontaneously." The eliciting trauma is often not remembered. Instead, the patient notices a nodule, which may or may not be painful and is caused by a hematoma or fat necrosis. Sometimes an associated subcutaneous hematoma suggests the site of the trauma or hemorrhage.

Hematomas are generally completely resolved and transformed into scar tissue, while fat necroses present as tumor-like lipophagic granulomas or oil cysts. The lipophagic granuloma presents as a clinically suggestive palpable nodule, usually of medium to firm consistency and of poor demarcation. Despite their smooth mammographic demarcation, oil cysts are also generally palpated as indistinctly demarcated fixed nodules.

■ Diagnostic Strategy and Goals

Fresh hematomas and seromas are easily diagnosed by sonography in the context of preceding surgery and corresponding clinical findings. This is, however, rarely necessary. An oval, sometimes even ill-defined mass at the surgical site may normally be present up to a year after surgery. For objective exclusion of a malignancy, mammographic evaluation of the lesion is necessary in all cases where doubts exist whether the suspected hematoma, seroma, or fat necrosis may explain all of the changes. The patient's statement of a preceding trauma may not prove a traumatic etiology, and it should be verified that findings are consistent with trauma rather than malignancy.

Old hematomas also can usually be diagnosed correctly by mammography in context with the clinical history, but a centrally necrosing malignancy must be excluded in the differential diagnosis.

Fat necroses are readily diagnosed by mammography if they present as calcifying liponecrosis or oil cysts but not as lipophagic granuloma, which requires surgical evaluation unless it can be diagnosed by its characteristic clinical course.

Most scars have characteristic mammographic features and generally are positively diagnosed by correlation with the clinical findings, possibly aided by marking of the skin. On occasion it may be difficult, however, to exclude a malignant lesion without further workup.

Selected cases with palpable nodules or increased consistency on clinical examination can pose a problem as to the exclusion of residual or newly evolving malignancy, with mammographically increased density and architectural distortion, atypical dense center of the scar, or uncharacteristic calcifications. MRI might supplement mammography, in particular in the presence of extensive scar formation, and biopsy of suspicious findings my be necessary.

Dystrophic calcifications are usually clearly identified by mammography on the basis of their form, size, and location within or along scars. When these calcifications are first forming, differential diagnostic problems can be encountered.

Mammography

Acute Changes

Fresh hematomas/seromas are seen as an ill-defined mass (Figs. 16.**1 a–c**), sometimes only appreciated as a difference between both sides. Hematomas, which occupy a surgical cavity, usually present as round to oval masses with some contour irregularity. Air–fluid levels can be found in the acute postoperative period (Fig. 16.**2 a–d**).

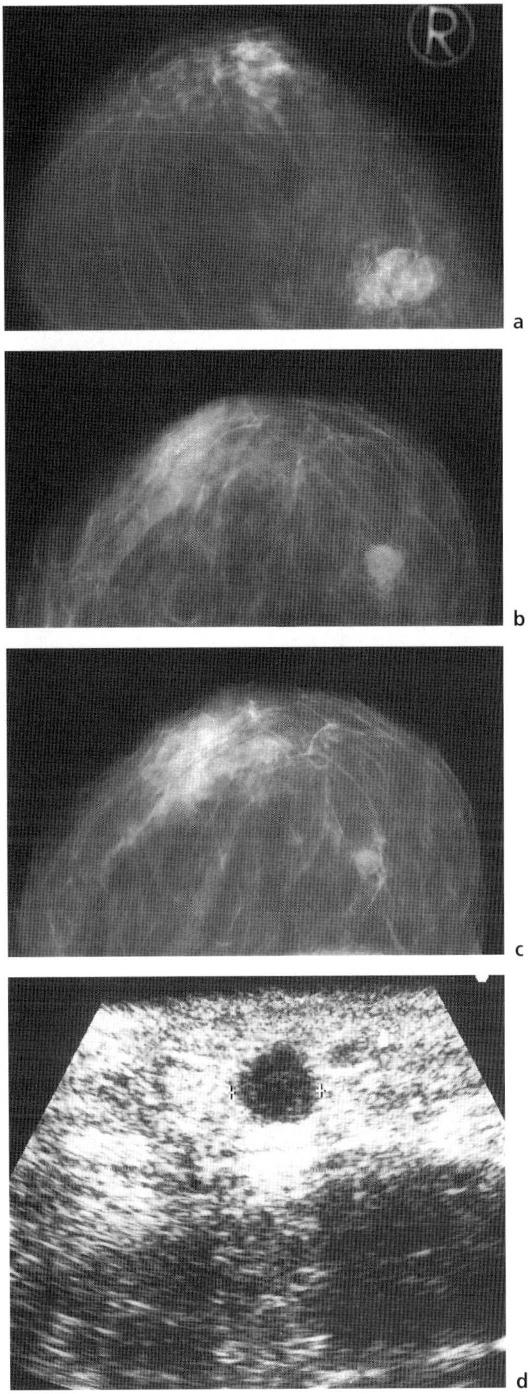

Fig. 16.**1 a–d**
a Patient after trauma. A soft, circumscribed resistance is palpated beneath a cutaneous hematoma, corresponding mammographically to a lobulated, indistinctly outlined soft-tissue density: hematoma
b and **c** Trauma while working in the garden. Irregularly outlined focal lesion in the medial half of the breast (**b**), 9 days later (**c**) markedly resolved
d Sonography (13 MHz). Round hypoechoic area, measuring 6.5 mm in diameter, with distal acoustic enhancement

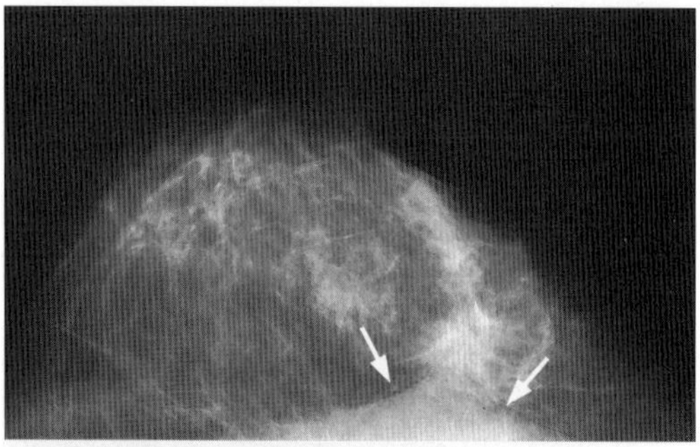
a

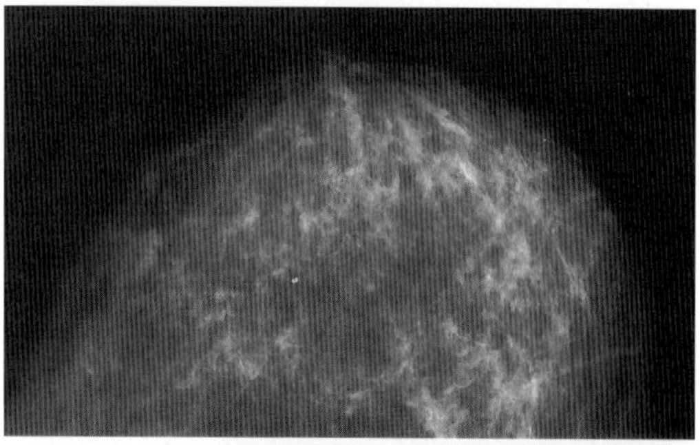
c

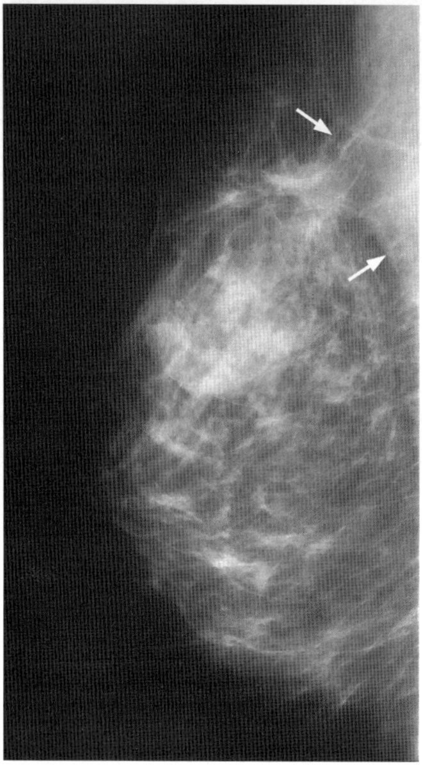
b

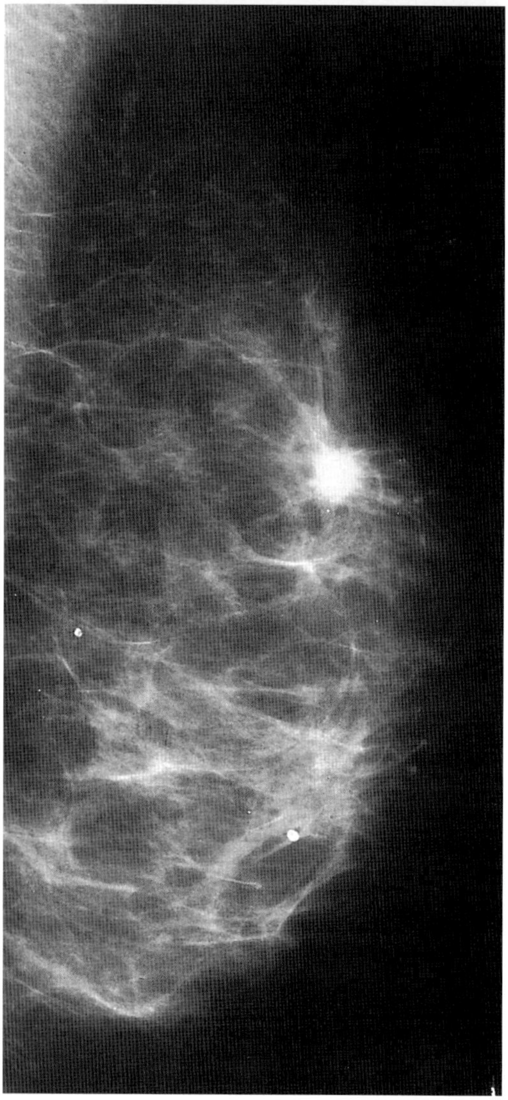
d

Fig. 16.**3 a–d**
a and **b** Scar formation in the upper outer quadrant with skin retraction and thickening, architectural distortion as well as retraction of the pectoral muscle (arrows). The craniocaudad view reveals a localized mass with a central density, which is not visible in the mediolateral view (scar). Different appearance on different views is typical for scarring
c Delicate spiculation without a central mass is seen in the medial half of the breast: small cellular solid carcinoma, measuring 13 mm in diameter, with lobular infiltration
d Granuloma: in the upper half of the breast, a 7 mm focal finding with relatively thick spicules (ML view)

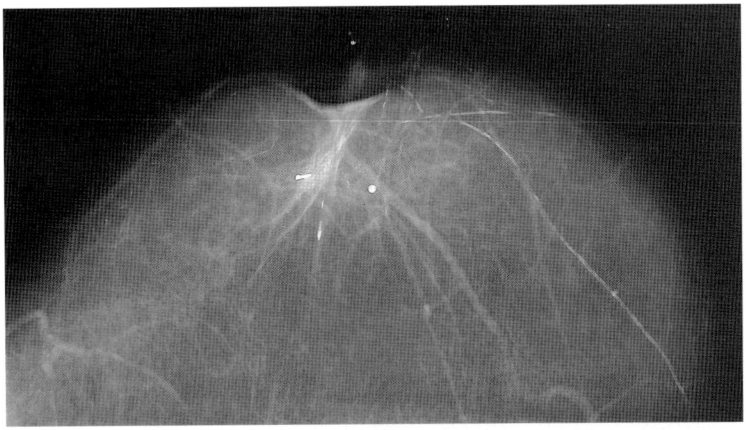
a

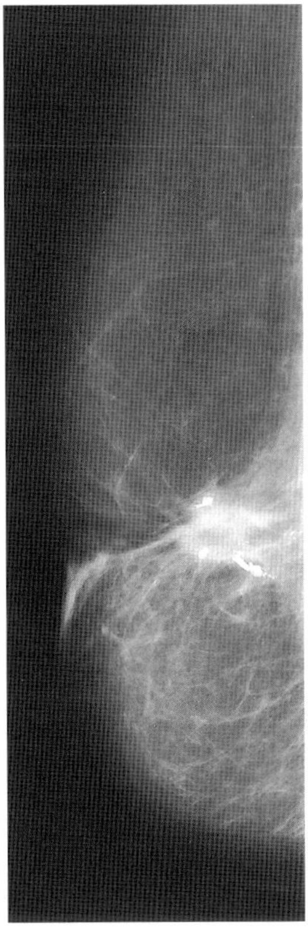
b

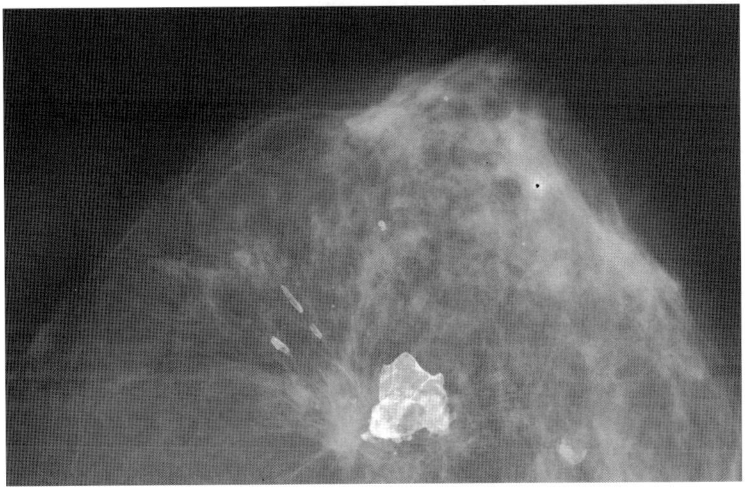
c

Fig. 16.**4 a–i** Calcifications after breast-conserving therapy
a–f Calcifications seen in scarring
a Cicatricial periareolar skin thickening and retraction, linear scarring causing thickened parenchymal structures and elongated coarse stromal calcification with adjacent calcifying liponecrosis. Extensive vascular calcifications (CC view)
b At the periphery of the architectural distortion, coarse amorphous stromal calcifications. Areolar retraction (ML view)
c Coarse calcifications adjacent to a spiculated mass are due to fat necrosis following lumpectomy and breast conservation

microcalcifications can evolve that are not always distinguishable from ductal calcifications (Fig. 16.**4 f**).

Calcifying liponecrosis and oil cysts are definitively diagnosed by mammography and do not require further evaluation. Evolving microcalcifications in fat necrosis, however, can appear rather pleomorphic as well as clustered (Fig. 16.**4 f**). Magnification mammography can improve the morphologic evaluation by better visualizing any evolving round and ring-like configurations as signs of benignity. Furthermore, demonstrating the relationship to a typically round or oval radiolucent area (Fig. 16.**4 f**) can be helpful. If uncertainty remains, biopsy is indicated.

Calcified suture material is identified as elongated string-like structures, sometimes with knots. Their double contour resembles periductal calcifications and chronic galactophoritis ("plasma cell mastitis").

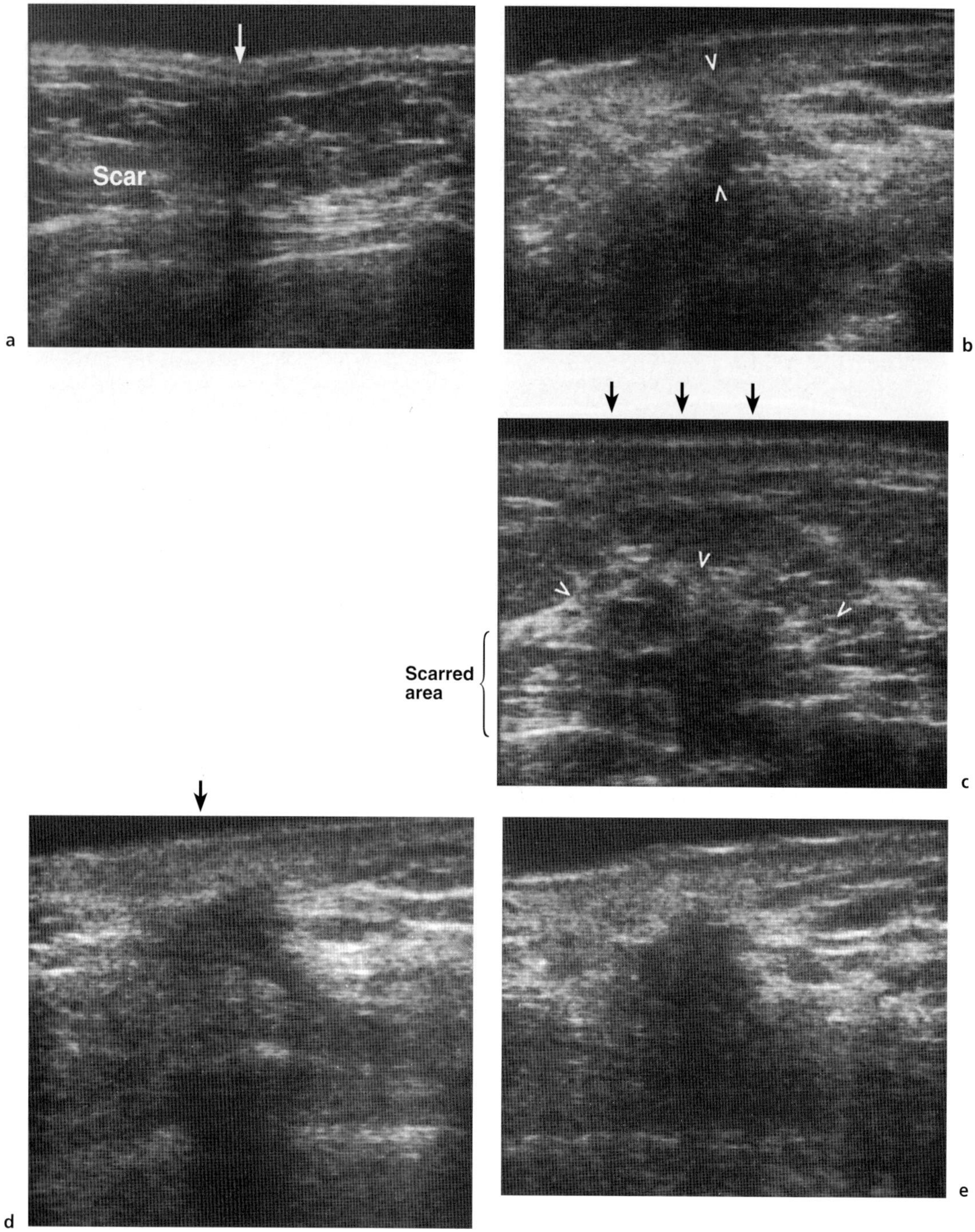

Fig. 16.**7 a–e** Sonographic manifestations of scars
a Typical scar with acoustic shadowing (arrow) starting at the skin level and interrupting all tissue layers
b Scar-related architectural distortion (arrowheads)
c Extensive distortion of the architecture with hypoechoic areas (arrowheads)
d Scar-related hypoechoic area that appears as a hypoechoic mass
e Hypoechoic, irregularly outlined scar with acoustic shadowing

- Discrete to marked architectural distortion with occasional hypoechoic structures in the subcutaneous space, acoustic shadowing, interruptions, or distortion of the parenchyma
- Occasionally one or more hypoechoic, indistinctly outlined areas with or without distal acoustic shadowing
- Areas with marked acoustic attenuation

Above all, the sonographic exclusion or detection of a malignancy can be considerably impaired or even impossible in the presence of hypoechoic areas and marked acoustic shadowing. Well-documented serial sonographic studies, if available, can be helpful.

Magnetic Resonance Imaging

Acute Changes

Hemorrhage can—depending on its age—have a variable signal intensity on precontrast T1-weighted images. Following injection of Gd-DTPA, minimal to moderate, usually somewhat delayed enhancement can be observed. Early or intense enhancement or both may occur infrequently.

Hematomas and seromas are visualized as a cavity of low to high signal-intensity, depending on their age and fluid composition. Following injection of contrast medium, the signal intensity of the nonenhancing content of the seroma or hematoma remains unchanged. The capsule—as far as it is developed—and the traumatized surrounding tissue usually show minimal to moderate enhancement, which generally is delayed.

Utility. Other imaging modalities are less expensive and more readily available to follow the uncomplicated resolution of hemorrhage, seromas, or hematomas, and MRI is not justified. The mostly diffuse and moderate enhancement in fresh scar tissue makes it impossible to exclude malignancy by MRI.

Since most (about 85%) malignancies have more rapid and intense enhancement than scar tissue, contrast-enhanced MRI may provide pertinent information, even early after surgery, if residual tumor or additional foci are suspected. In particular, for irregularly outlined scars or very dense tissue that defy adequate mammographic evaluation, MRI can detect focally enhancing residual tumor early, which is of special importance if the tumor does not contain any microcalcifications. MRI is therefore meaningful—even after a recent surgical intervention, e.g., before radiation therapy—when doubt remains concerning completeness of excision or whether the finding was excised at all.

Late Changes

While fresh scar tissue generally shows minimal to moderate enhancement, old scar tissue after complete fibrosis no longer exhibits relevant enhancement.

This usually is the case after the 3rd to 6th postoperative month, and thereafter MRI allows a reliable differentiation between scar tissue and malignancy.

Utility. As a supplemental method, contrast-enhanced MRI offers new information relevant for the detection or exclusion of malignancy whenever evaluation is difficult or diagnostic uncertainty persists.

Mammography remains the method of choice to detect and to assess microcalcifications.

Percutaneous Biopsy

Scar tissue can compromise percutaneous biopsy because of needle deviation and the difficulty of retrieving an adequate specimen from fibrotic tissue. This is most important for aspiration cytology. Whenever a definite mass exists clinically, mammographically, sonographically, or on MRI, evaluation by core biopsy may be useful.

muscle, despite the known retractive changes, by using all technical resources (coned-down views, tilting of the X-ray tube, oblique projections tailored to the individual situation).
- Generous use of magnification technique.

If breast density limits adequate penetration after radiation, the choice of target or filter, or both, by which the energy of the X-ray beam can be optimized, can influence image quality.

Post-therapeutic Changes

The following changes are usually seen:

1. Diffuse changes including trabecular coarsening, skin thickening, and diffusely increased breast-density secondary to irradiation and axillary dissection
2. Localized parenchymal changes of the skin and breast tissue due to the surgical scar
3. Localized parenchymal changes secondary to fat necrosis manifested as liponecrosis, oil cysts, or a lipophagic granuloma
4. Calcifications caused by any of the above mentioned reasons

These various changes are only partially separable, and together they determine the mammographic pattern. For didactic reasons, these changes are treated separately.

Diffuse Changes of the Parenchymal Structure

(Figs. 16.**8 a–c**)

Hyperemia with increased transudation as well as edema secondary to axillary dissection and radiotherapy cause mammographically:

- Diffusely increased parenchymal density
- Diffusely increased trabecular markings
- Thickening of the skin and areola

These acute changes can resolve slowly during the first 2 years after therapy. Chronic edema can resolve or undergo fibrotic transformation, which produces a similar mammographic pattern to that seen with edema.

The slow transformation of a chronic persistent edema into fibrosis (Figs. 16.**9 a–c**) can be recognized mammographically by

- Slight resolution of the diffusely increased parenchymal density corresponding to the replacement of fluids with connective tissue and partial resorption of the edema
- Thinner and sharper demarcation of the increased trabecular markings
- Some resolution of the initial thickening of the skin and areola
- Calcifications that can develop owing to cell necrosis

If the described resolution and transformation is reversed by a renewed increase in the diffuse changes, or if the diffuse changes remain un-

a

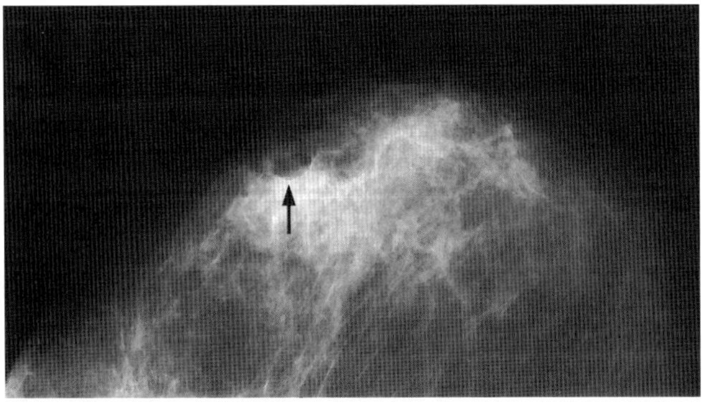

Fig. 16.**8 a–c** Diffuse acute structural changes of the parenchyma
a Status post segmentectomy (tylectomy): 5 days after surgery, diffuse infiltrative density in the lateral half of the breast with air pocket (arrow) and skin thickening

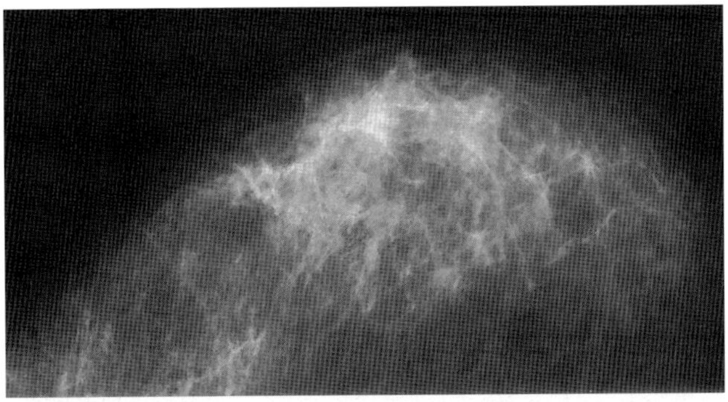

b

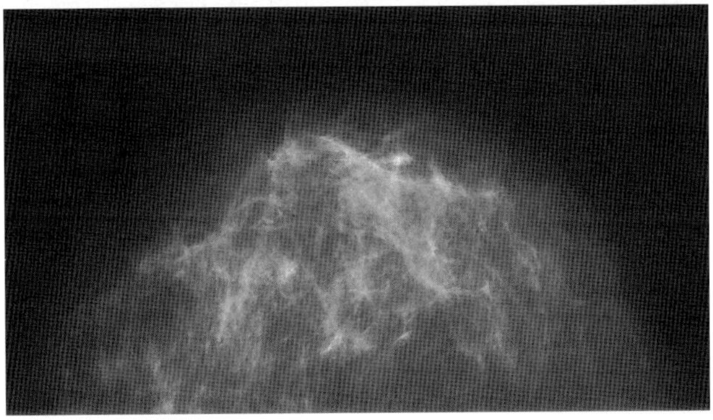

c

Fig. 16.**8 b** Three weeks after completion of radiation therapy: thickening of the skin and areola, diffusely increased reticular markings, and delicate cicatricial radial structural transformation at the site of the excision
c Four years after completion of radiation therapy, almost complete resolution, with skin thickening confined to the region of the scar and underlying radial structural transformation

changed without recognizable resolution, the following conditions have to be considered in the differential diagnosis:

- Secondary mastitis
- Venous stasis (heart failure, mediastinal or axillary space occupying lesion)
- Carcinomatous lymphangiosis

Localized Changes of the Cutaneous and Parenchymal Structures

They may occur with:

- Scar formation following surgery
- Fat necrosis that can transform into *oil cysts*, calcifications, or a *lipophagic granuloma* secondary to radiation-compromised microcirculation and subsequent development of necrosis, (partial) resorption, or formation of granulation tissue.

Scar formation is characterized by:

- Parenchymal asymmetry
- Associated architectural distortion and spiculations that can have extensions to the skin, the pectoral muscle or chest wall (Fig. 16.**10**)
- Masses caused by delayed resorption of large hematomas or seromas (Fig. 16.**11 a–d**), by dense fibrosis, or by lipophagic granulomas (Fig. 16.**12**)
- Calcifications (see p. 289)

Evaluating the course of these changes is of great importance for their correct interpretation.

The postoperative mammogram is obtained before the initiation of radiation therapy. It is only needed in women whose cancer contained microcalcifications and is done to check for if residual calcifications that may signify residual tumor, requiring reexcision. These studies may show hematomas or seromas. Large hematomas may not resolve completely, resulting in a persistent mass of variable extent. Characteristically, follow-up examinations will document decrease in size and increase in scar formation with spiculation.

A parenchymal scar seen as a spiculated structure without central density can be recog-

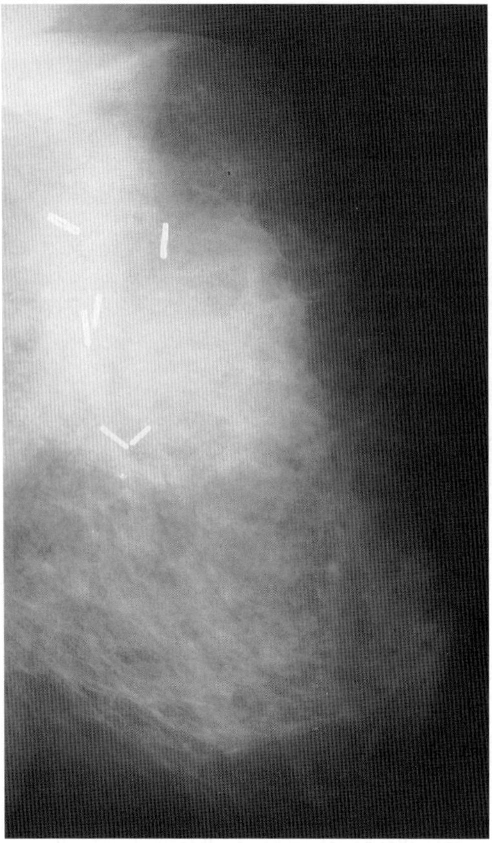
a

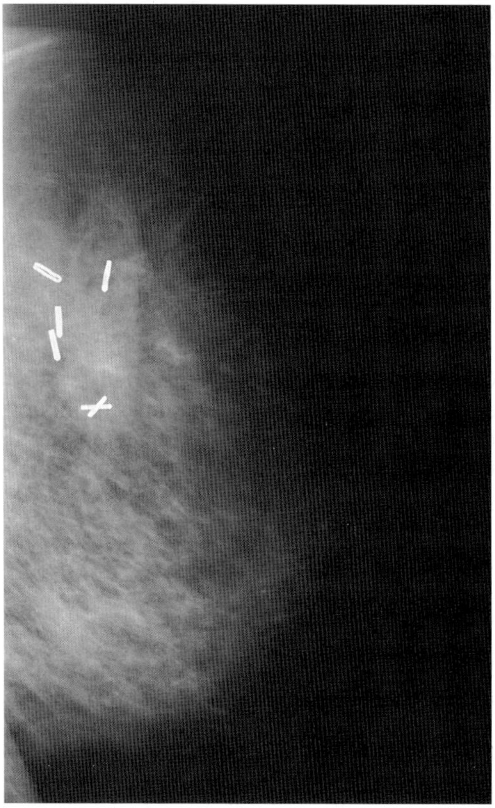
b

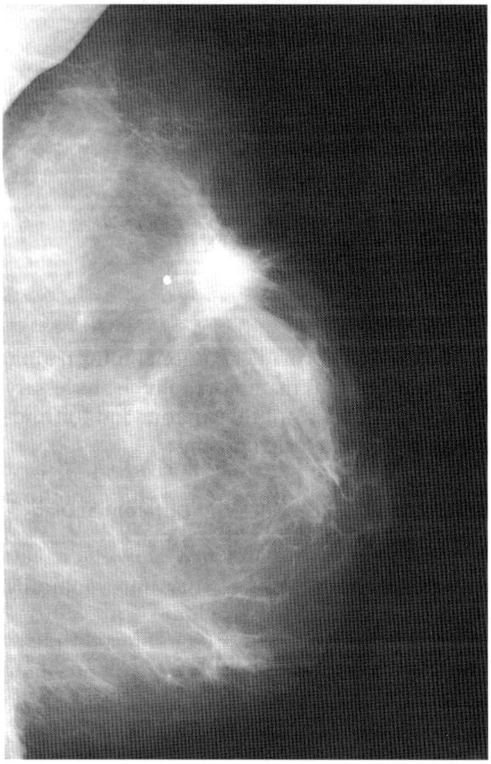
c

Fig. 16.**11 a–d** Focal changes after limited surgery and irradiation
a, b Case 1: mammograms done 6 and 12 months after breast conservation show an ill-defined hematoma with adjacent surgical clips on the initial study (**a**) that has resolved on the later examination (**b**). Diffusely increased breast density with diffusely coarsened trabecular markings are present on both studies
c, d Case 2: a spiculated scar at a lumpectomy site shows considerable reduction in its size from a study done 1 year (**c**) after treatment to another done 2 years (**d**) after therapy

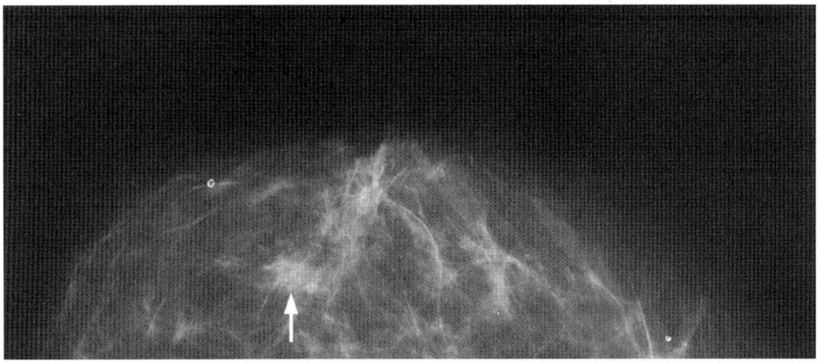
a

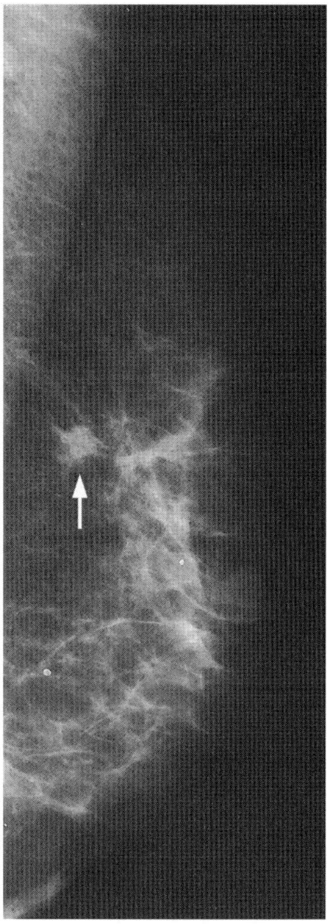
b

Fig. 16.**12 a–d** Lipophagic granuloma mimicking a malignancy. This patient had a mammogram 18 months after biopsy of a suspicious finding that turned out to be a proliferative mastopathy. A previous postoperative mammogram was not obtained.
This mammogram again shows a suspicious density in the region of the scar (arrow)
a Mammography, craniocaudal view
b Mammography, mediolateral view
c and **d** Because of the suspicious finding, an excisional biopsy was recommended. A supplemental contrast-enhanced MRI was obtained as part of a trial designed for preoperative patients

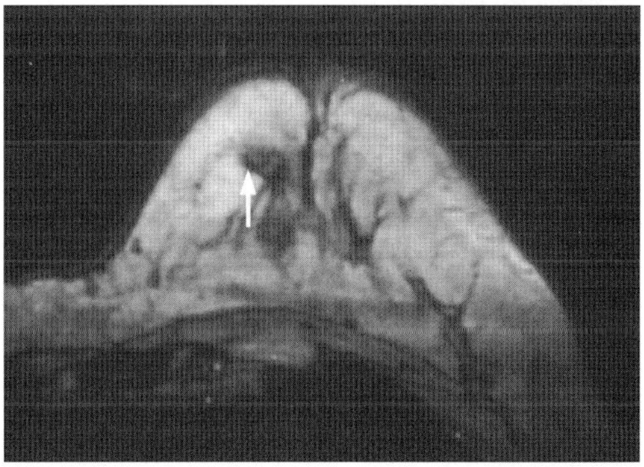
c

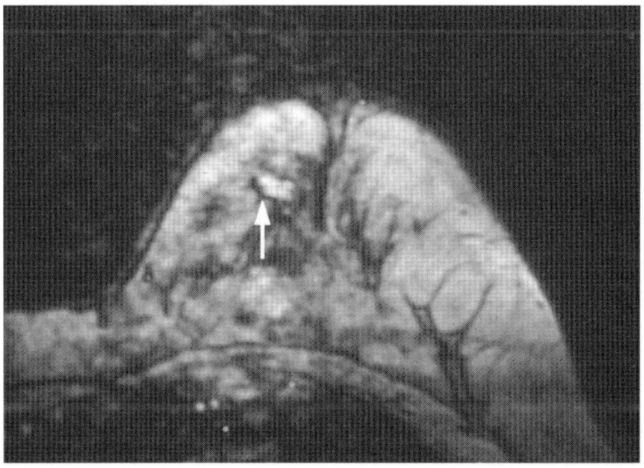
d

Fig. 16.**12 c** Representative section through the lesion before i.v. administration of contrast medium
d Same section as in **c** after injection of the contrast medium Gd-DTPA. The lesion shows a rapid intense enhancement with irregular margin to be considered as definitely suspect. *Histology:* Lipophagic granuloma (from Heywang-Köbrunner SH[1])

- Enlarging scar
- microcalcifications
- Diffusely increased density (diffusely growing recurrence)

Focally Growing Recurrence

(Figs. 16.**13 a** and **b**)

About 70% of intramammary recurrences develop in the vicinity of the scar, and early treatment failures tend to be at the biopsy site. The most important feature of focal recurrences and also the best criterion for distinguishing them from post-therapeutic changes is the temporal evolution:

1. Newly occuring mass and/or tumor calcifications
2. Enlarging mass or scar
3. Increasing radiodensity
4. Increasing architectural distortion

These changes can be very discrete and can be underestimated or overlooked with variations in technique (different exposures) (see Technical Difficulties, p. 293).

Newly occurring mass and suggestive calcifications in quadrants other than the one harboring the primary tumor are generally easily recognized. Apart from recurrence, the differential diagnosis also includes benign changes, such as cysts or fibroadenomas. Cysts should be excluded sonographically. A new lipophagic granuloma occurring after therapy cannot be distinguished from recurrent disease by any imaging method and therefore usually requires biopsy.

Microcalcifications as Evidence of Recurrence

Mammography is necessary to detect microcalcifications that can be an early sign of recurrence. Since microcalcifications can develop after radiation, thorough analysis of their individual configuration and their distribution is of great importance (Figs. 16.**13 c** and **d**).

The criteria for the analysis of microcalcifi-

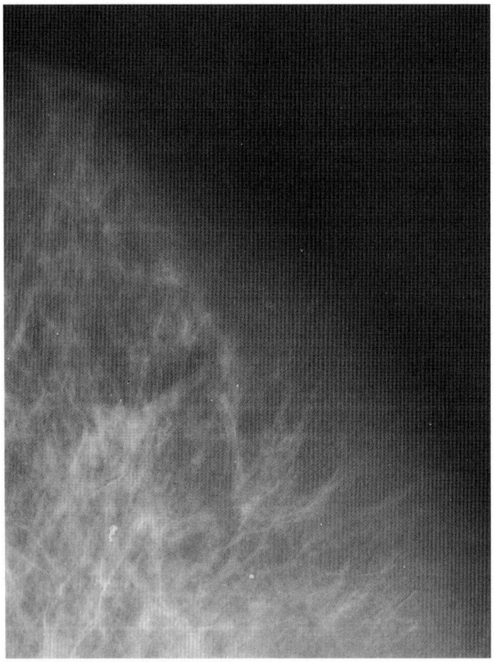

a

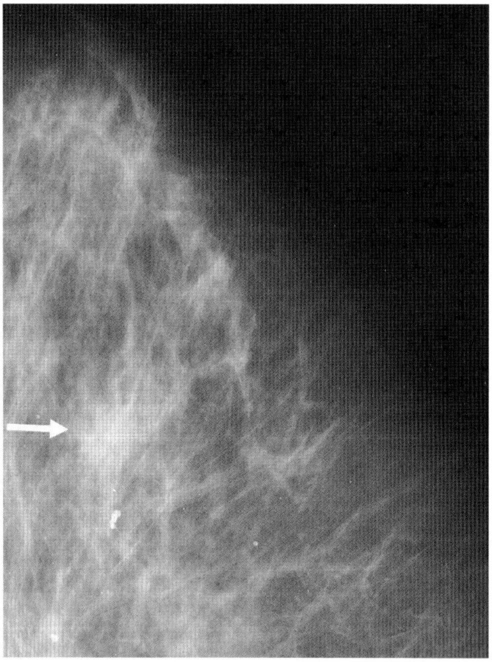

b

Fig. 16.**13 a–f** Mammographic presentations of recurrences

a Four years after breast conservation, a few coarse calcifications are present at the surgical site due to fat necrosis

b Three years later, a new mass (arrow) has developed at the scar due to a 1 cm recurrent infiltrating ductal carcinoma cations are also applicable to recognizing recurrent disease (see Chapter 20). Calcifications associated with recurrent breast cancer have a pattern identical to those found with de novo breast cancers.

It is important to consider the *time of the appearance* in the differential diagnostic consideration.

If the entire tumor was removed, documented by specimen radiography, histopathologic examination, and postoperative mammogram, a recurrence within 12–18 months after irradiation would be unusual. Instead, dystrophic calcifications tend to evolve during this time span.

Diffusely Increased Density as Evidence of Recurrence

Diffusely growing recurrences are most difficult to diagnose. They can be multicentric, present as carcinomatous lymphangiomatosis, or they can even be manifested by the growth of dispersed small-cell malignancies. They can be diagnosed as recurring or increasing diffuse density and structural coarsening, and as areas of increasing parenchymal density, together with a clinical increased consistency and possibly with a reduction in size and retraction of the breast (Figs. 16.**13 e** and **f**). In our experience, more than half of diffusely growing recurrent tumors were early recurrences with unusually rapid tumor growth, primarily affecting young women.[2]

Sonography

Diffuse Structural Changes

Early changes. Radiation induces varying degrees of skin thickening. In the acute stage, the edema-related echogenicity increases in the subcutaneous space and decreases in the parenchyma, leading to a loss of the normal echo pattern (Figs. 16.**14 a** and **c**).

Resolution. Over a period of 1–2 years, skin thickening and other early changes slowly regress. Some skin thickening may persist. Increased fibrosis found in the irradiated tissue frequently causes diffusely increased echogenicity.

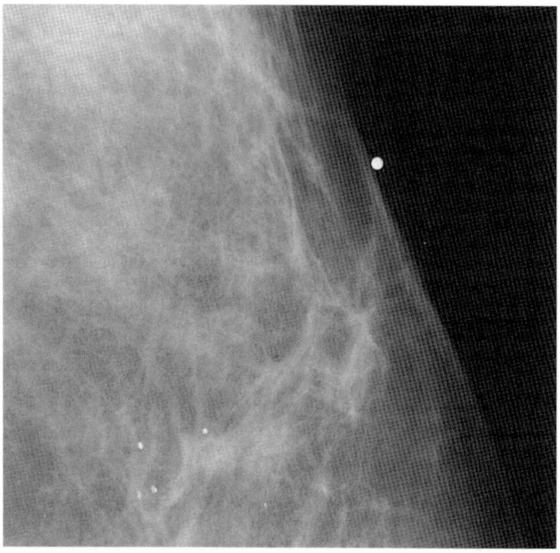

c

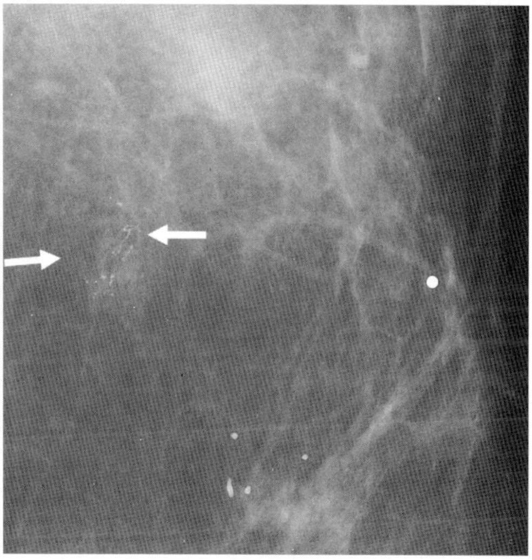

d

Fig. 16.**13 c** Two years after breast conservation, some deformity is noted in the lateral aspect of the breast. A skin marker localizes the scar
d A year later, new pleomorphic linear calcifications (arrows) have developed. These were due to new DCIS

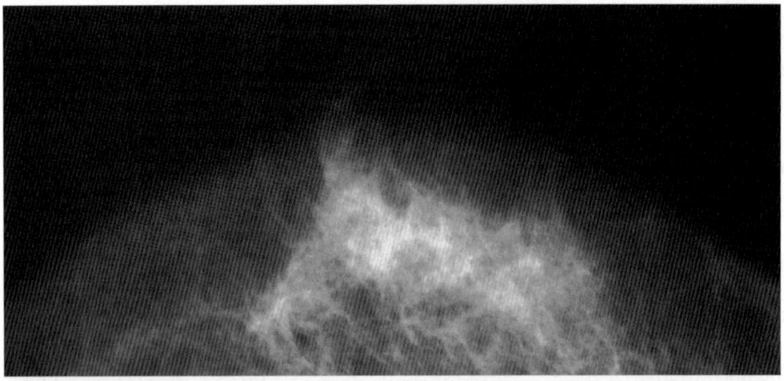

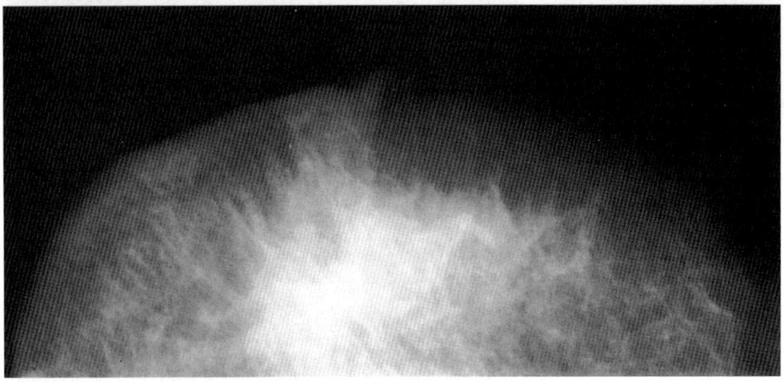

Fig. 16.**13 e** and **f** Two years after breast-conserving therapy, scar-induced cutaneous thickening in the medial half of the breast, ill-defined reticular markings. Because of edematous changes and dense parenchyma, it is difficult to assess. Eleven months later (**f**): clinically decreased size and increased consistency of the right breast. Corresponding increase in the mammographic density throughout the entire remaining parenchyma and progressing spiculation: diffusely growing recurrence

a

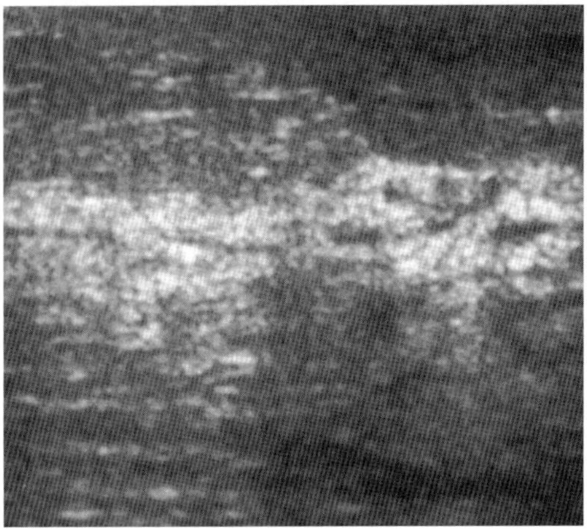

Fig. 16.**14 a–c** Sonographic presentation of the breast after tumorectomy (lumpectomy) and radiation
a Extensive lymphedema 3 months after completion of radiation therapy. Increased echogenicity is seen in the subcutaneous tissue as well as in the prepectoral fat, with loss of the demarcation between the subcutaneous soft tissue and thickened dermis as well as poor separation of parenchyma from fatty tissue

■ Focal Structural Changes

They can occur in context as

- Scar formation
- Fat necroses in the form of *oil cysts* or *lipophagic granuloma*

In its early stage, *the scar region*, similar to nonirradiated scars (see p. 287), often contains a seroma or hematoma; the resolution of either can be well-monitored sonographically. With increasing granulation tissue and fibrosis, small or large hypoechoic areas, and acoustic shadows—as also seen after surgery alone (see also Figs. 16.7 and 16.**15 c**)—can develop in the region of the scar and compromise the evaluation. Well-documented serial examinations may be helpful.

Oil cysts (compare p. 289) are in general correctly diagnosed only when the ultrasound is interpreted together with mammography.

A *lipophagic granuloma* is visualized as hypoechoic lesion with or without acoustic shadowing and cannot be sonographically distinguished from a primary or recurrent carcinoma.

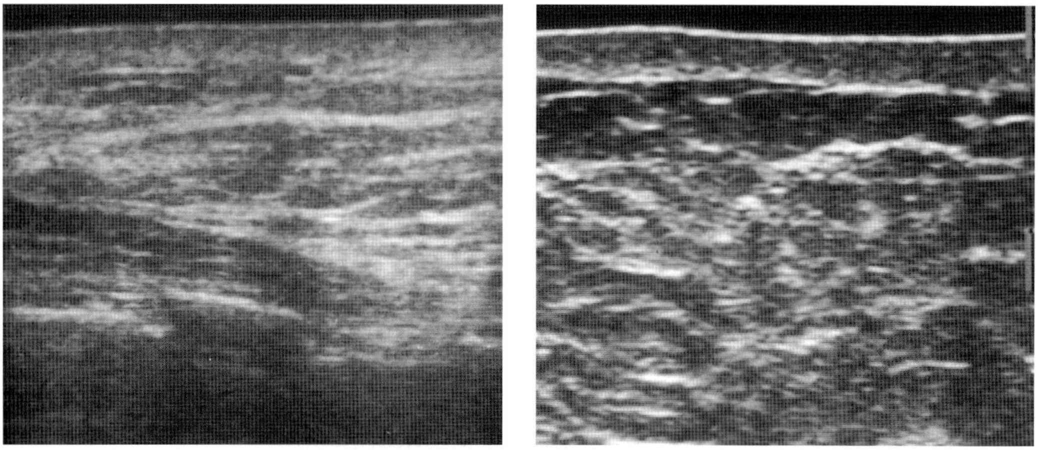

b c

Fig. 16.**14 b** and **c** Slow resolution of increased echogenicity of the fatty tissue with increasingly improved demarcation of the ligamentous structures 9 months (**b**) and 18 months (**c**) after therapy

■ Utility

In the follow-up of these patients, sonography

- Can be helpful to distinguish the mammographically visible or palpable hematoma from a mass, if doubts exist.
- Can be helpful to detect a recurrence (visible as persistent mass that does not resolve) if the breast tissue ist very dense. However, the policy regarding regular use of ultrasound in the follow-up of dense breasts after irradiation varies. Most consider it unnecessary.
- Is—as in other women—helpful in determining whether a new mass is due to a cyst.

More than 18 months after therapy, contrast-enhanced MRI is superior to sonography in the detection or exclusion of small recurrences and should be preferred if the mammographic evaluation is difficult.

Magnetic Resonance Imaging

■ Acute Stage

Immediately after radiation, as well as within the subsequent 12 months, the irradiated tissue and the scar generally show a moderate to markedly diffuse, but sometimes also patchy, enhancement. This enhancement usually decreases within the initial 12 months with considerable individual variation. About 12–18 months after radiotherapy, the irradiated tissue can still exhibit some diffuse, usually delayed enhancement.

Cutaneous thickening and enhancement usually regress more slowly than the parenchymal enhancement.

■ Late Stage

About 18 months after therapy, diffuse and delayed enhancement is only seen in individual cases. In the vast majority of cases only minimal (“absent”) enhancement exists. Residual skin thickening and focal, scar-related architectural distortion can be diagnosed as such by absent contrast enhancement and do not interfere with the evaluation by MRI (Figs. 16.**15 d** and **e**).

■ Utility

Within the first 12 months after radiotherapy, the information provided by MRI is considerably compromised by diffuse and often patchy enhancement. With increasing fibrosis, the enhancement markedly decreases. Beginning 12 months after radiotherapy, detection and exclusion of recurrent disease in irradiated tissue is considerably improved. Here, contrast-enhanced MRI can be employed in problem cases as a supplemental method.

Beginning 18 months after radiotherapy, the evaluation by MRI is generally excellent since the fibrosed parenchymal tissue enhances even less than normal mammary parenchyma. Supplemental MRI can detect very small recurrent

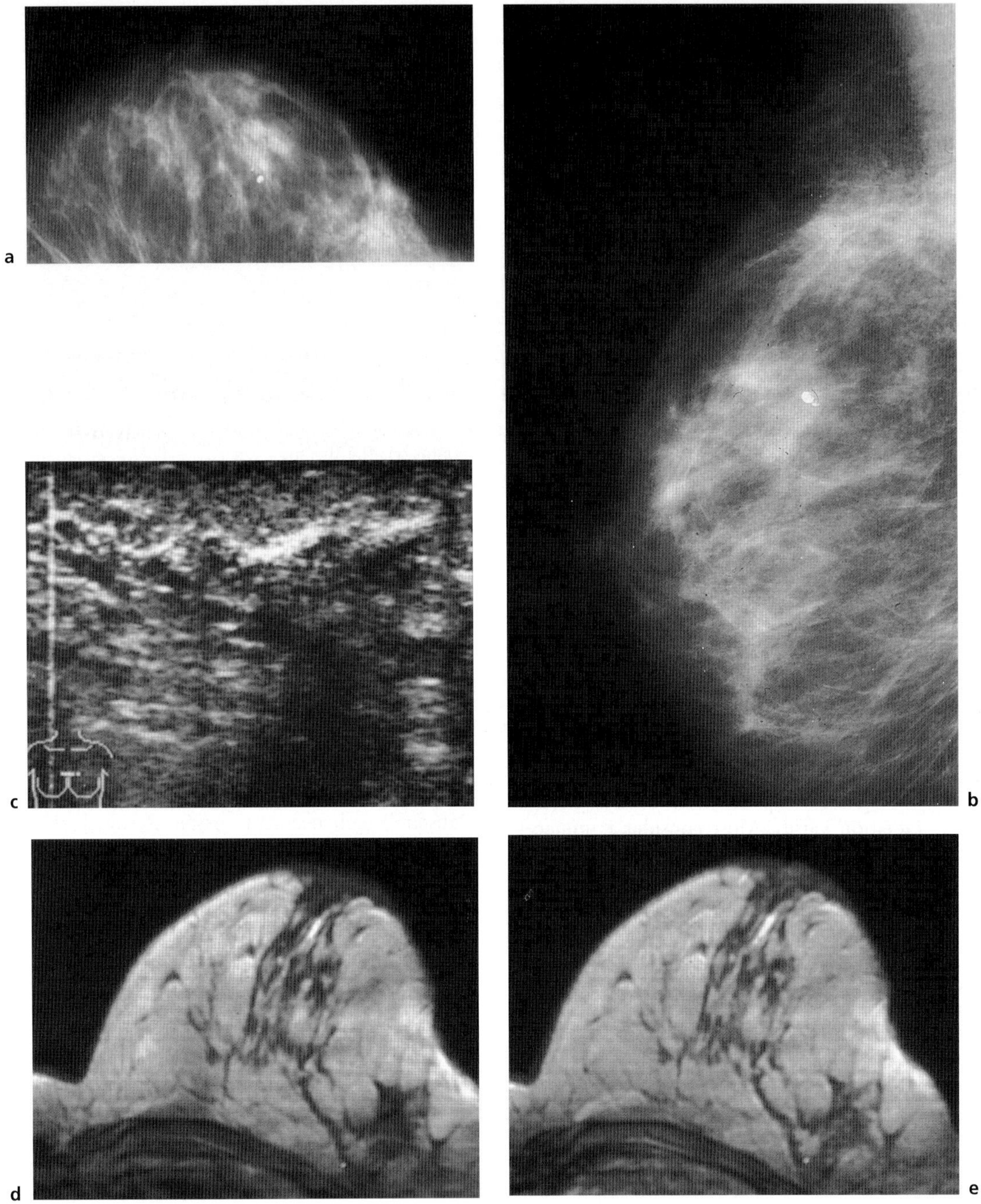

Fig. 16.**15 a–e** Indeterminate palpable finding in the region of the scar 14 months after breast-conserving therapy

a and **b** Craniocaudal and mediolateral views (suboptimal positoning due to extensive scar formation): the central radiolucency within the scar is consistent with a scar rather than a recurrent cancer

c Sonographically, the evaluation of the region of the scar is limited, showing acoustic shadowing

d Representative section through the scar region before administration of contrast medium

e The same section after i.v. administration of Gd-DTPA shows no appreciable enhancement: no evidence of a recurrence. Conclusion confirmed by clinical–mammographic follow-up for more than 3 years tumors in dense or even irregularly structured tissue with great sensitivity (Fig. 16.**16 a–d**) or excludes them with a high degree of certainty. Therefore, contrast MRI is the ideal method to complement mammography for otherwise difficult to evaluate tissue and for solving problems later than 12–18 months after breast-conserving therapy. However, mammography remains the modality of choice to detect suggestive microcalcifications, should they develop.

Percutaneous Biopsy

Percutaneous biopsy can be diagnostically helpful in the therapeutic decision, particularly since diagnostic excisional surgery on nonmalignant post-therapeutic changes should be avoided owing to the possibility of impaired healing.

Experience in this setting has been limited.

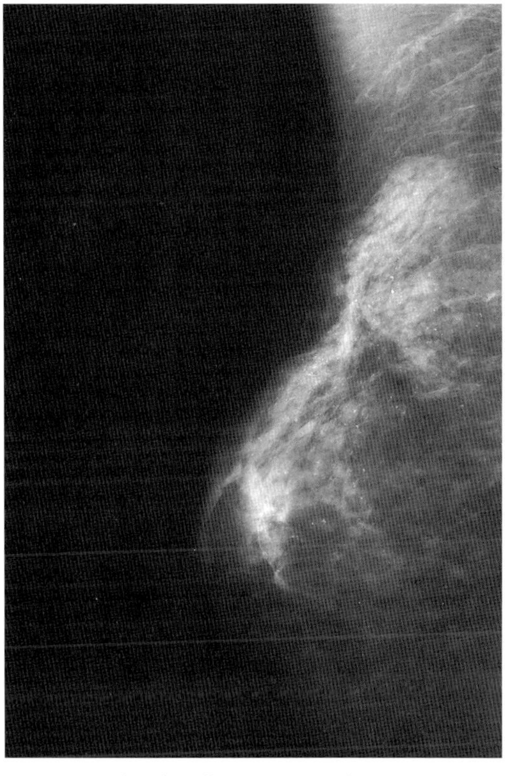
a

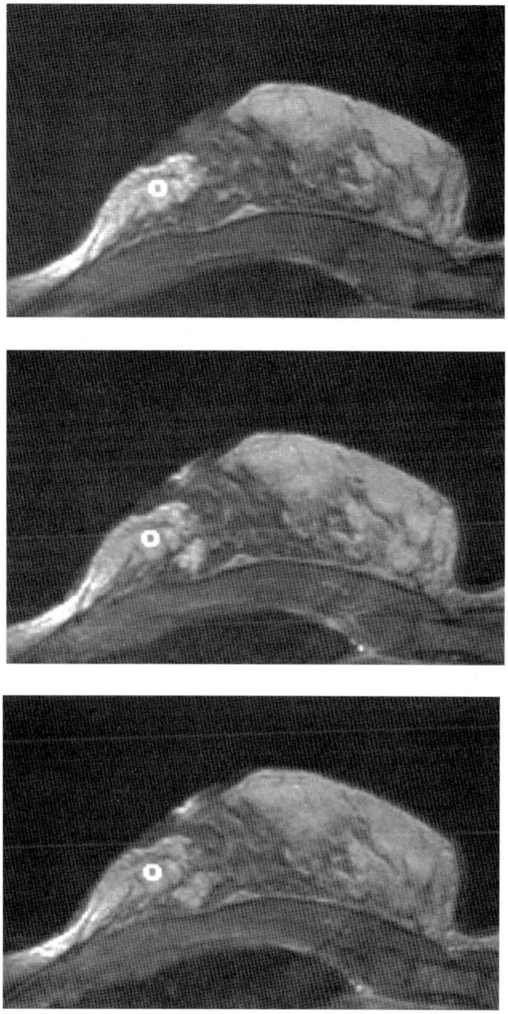
b
c
d

Fig. 16.**16 a–d** Clinically, status post breast-conserving therapy 5 years ago, unchanged palpable finding
a The mammogram shows spiculation in the upper half of breast at the lumpectomy site, unchanged since the previous examination. Diffuse microcalcifications known for years, unchanged (the primary tumor had no microcalcifications). Supplementary MRI was offered as part of a clinical trial
b–d MRI: representative section through the scar before (**b**) as well as immediately after (0–5 minutes) (**c**), and delayed (6–11 minutes) (**d**) after Gd-DTPA. Suggestive focal enhancement (arrow) is apparent in the scar region. It characteristically enhances early and shows so-called washout (**d**). The focus discovered by MRI was excised after MR-guided localization. *Histology:* recurrence of an invasive ductal carcinoma

Note:
- Accuracy can decrease in markedly fibrosed tissue due to needle deviation and due to insufficient or nonrepresentative tissue,
- Histologic accuracy may be reduced due to procuring smaller specimens in the presence of marked fibrosis or due to early post-therapeutic cellular changes (inflammation, necrosis)

Nonetheless, reported results in small numbers of patients have so far shown that needle biopsy is able to accurately differentiate recurrent cancer from fibrosis.

Summary

Depending on whether a hematoma, seroma, or fat necrosis is present, acute post-traumatic and postsurgical changes can have a variable mammographic presentation.
If a malignancy (residual tumor) has to be excluded in freshly traumatized or surgical tissue, mammography should always be used.
Scar-related changes in their late stage after trauma or surgery (more than 3 months) or after radiation (more than 12 months) can cause characteristic mammographic features (architectural distortion or spiculated areas mostly without central density, coarse, or ring-like dystrophic calcifications) or sonographic phenomena (acoustic shadowing or hypoechoic areas). Because of architectural distortion following surgery and increased density following radiation, the overall evaluation can be compromised, and the differential diagnosis can pose problems. For the scarred breast following (multiple) surgeries as well as for the breast with radiation changes, mammography remains the primary diagnostic method, together with clinical examination.
Next to the selected use of additional projections, coned-down compression, and magnification views, an important diagnostic role is given to serial mammograms, whereby the accuracy can be improved by keeping exposure conditions constant.
In the breast that is difficult to evaluate, the selected use of contrast-enhanced MRI is important. In particular, if the evaluation is impaired owing to increased density and scars, contrast-enhanced MRI permits a markedly improved and earlier detection of recurrence and a correct identification of scar-related fibrotic changes beginning 1 year after radiotherapy.
Percutaneous biopsy can be considered as an additional diagnostic step in problem cases.

Changes Following Reconstruction, Augmentation, and Reduction

Reconstruction

Definition

Reconstruction refers to the surgical reconstitution after mastectomy.

Surgical procedures

Breast reconstruction can be achieved by means of implants or myocutaneous flaps. The implant is placed underneath the pectoral muscle (subpectoral), generally preceded by implantation of an expander to create space for the prosthesis.

The submuscular implant is preferable to the subcutaneous implant because of its better cosmetic result and easier follow-up care. The silicone prostheses have frequently been used in this context. They come in different designs, the most important of which are (Fig. 16.**17**):

- *Single-lumen* entirely gel-filled *prosthesis*
- The usual *double-lumen-prosthesis*, with the *inner lumen filled with silicone gel* forming a silicone cushion, surrounded by the outer lumen filled with a saline solution
- The rarely used *double-lumen prosthesis*, with the *inner lumen filled with a saline solution* and the outer lumen filled with silicone gel

Familiarity with these types is pertinent because each type is visualized differently, affecting the evaluation of the surrounding tissue.

Reconstruction with autogenous tissue transfer is most frequently done with the help of pedunculated or free myocutaneous flaps. The flaps are most frequently taken from the latissimus dorsi and transverse rectus abdominis muscle (TRAM-flap).

■ Diagnostic Strategy

Imaging is used to

- characterize clinically suspicious findings that may be due to malignancy and
- detect a rupture of the prosthesis.

For asymptomatic patients, only the clinical examination is standard following mastectomy and reconstruction.

An abnormal palpatory finding can be further evaluated by mammography and sonography. MRI can be very helpful in patients with scarring around implants that is difficult to assess and in patients with increased risk (after previous recurrence, multifocal disease).

Mammography

■ Silicone Prosthesis

Because of the radiopacity of silicone gel, silicone prostheses obscure large portions of the surrounding subcutaneous tissue, muscles, and scars, and it is for this reason that these patients are usually followed clinically without imaging.

If breast tissue is around the implant, multiple views of the breast are necessary to image it. Imaging should include at least two orthogonal views including the chest wall and the displaced views, described by Eklund, to better image tissue anterior to the implant, if possible. Additional coned or tangential views, or both may be needed (see p. 55). Any palpable finding must be further evaluated by means of an oblique projection with appropriate tilting of the X-ray tube for tangential visualization of the tissue in question. Additional views should survey the remaining tissue surrounding the prosthesis to exclude, as far as possible, further areas of suspicion.

Normally, the prosthesis, which is surrounded by a thin rim of scar tissue, is covered by subcutaneous fat and skin. In submuscular implants, the muscle is visualized as a band-like density directly overlying the prosthesis. Only those tissues, which are imaged tangentially be-

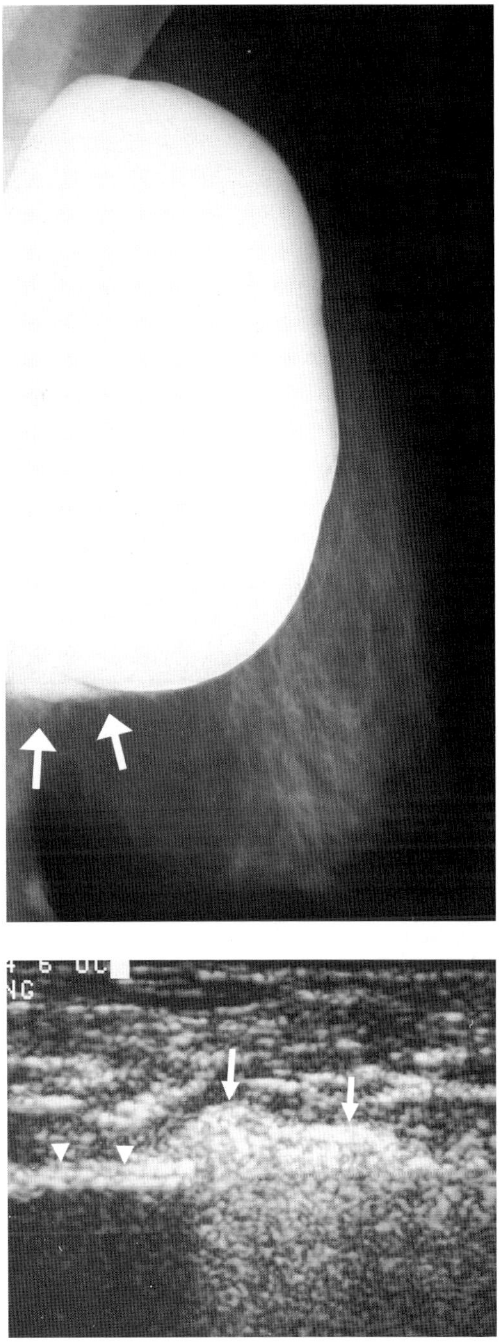

a

b

Fig. 16.**17 a–d** Presentation of implant rupture
a and **b** Extracapsular rupture
a Routine mammogram 17 years after augmentation shows an extracapsular rupture with silicone outside the implant (arrows)
b Sonographic image of this rupture shows echogenic silicone (arrows) beyond the homogeneous echo of the implant (arrowheads)

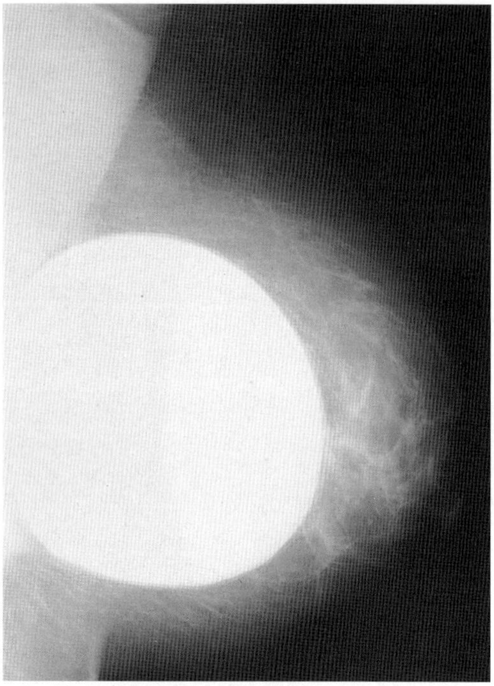
c

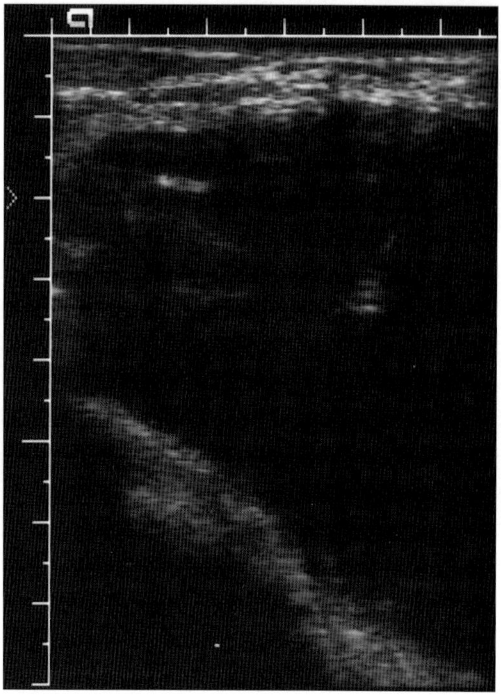
d

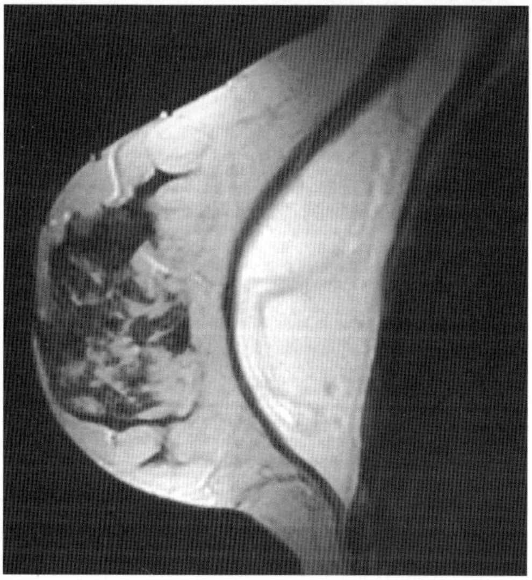
e

Abb. 16.**17 c–e** Intracapsular rupture
c, d Forty-nine-year-old woman 12 years after breast augmentation
c Mammographically, the silicone implant is intact
d Sonographically, multiple echoes, including several linear echoes, indicate an intracapsular rupture
e Intracapsular rupture on MRI (linguini sign). Low signal linear structures within the high signal silicone are due to the collapsed implant shell

side the implant, can be evaluated, while the rest is obscured by the radiopaque implant (Fig. 16.**18**).

Utility

Because of the partial mammographic visualization of the tissue surrounding the prosthesis, mammography plays a limited role in the evaluation of any scar formation or detection of recurrent disease.

The mammographic exclusion of malignancy, particularly if clinically suspected, is often impossible (exception: oil cysts). The role of mammography—in contrast to MRI—is mainly restricted to the detection of suspicious microcalcifications (Fig. 16.**19**).

■ Myocutaneous Flap

(Fig. 16.**20 a**)

In the United States, mammography is indicated for diagnostic evaluation of abnormalities. When performed after breast reconstruction with autogenous tissue transfer, it must be considered that the mammographic evaluation of areas with dense scars or muscle tissue is limited. Regressive dystrophic changes of the adipose

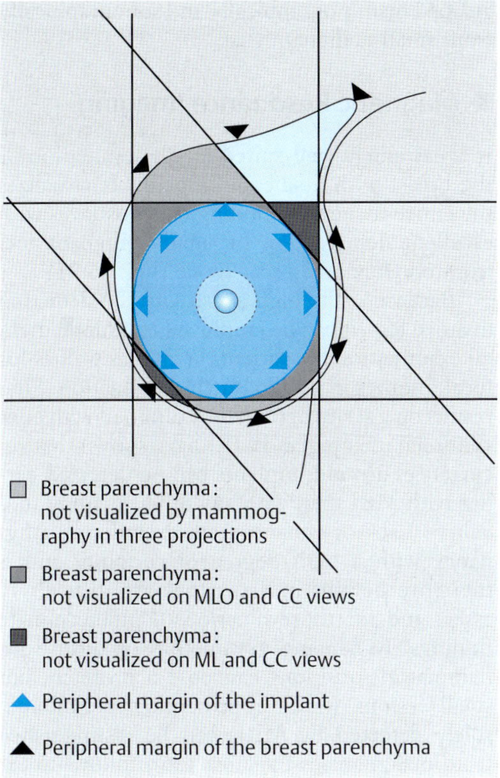

Fig. 16.**18** The different shading shows the parenchymal areas obscured by the implant on the standard projections (craniocaudad, mediolateral, and oblique views) (from Eklund and Cardenosa[3])

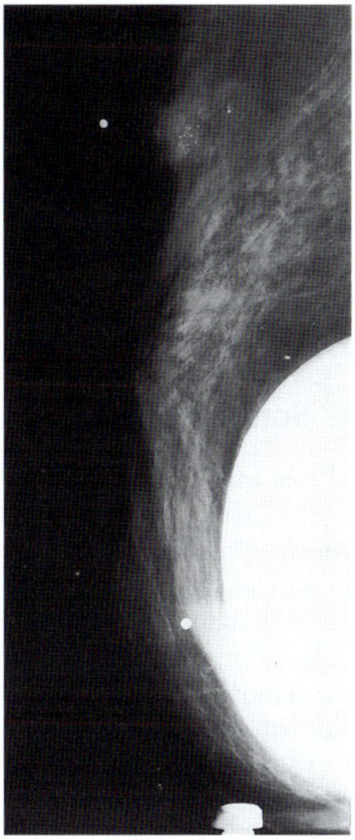

Fig. 16.**19** Recurrence in a patient with a submuscular prosthesis for breast reconstruction. Oblique mammography: an irregularly outlined focal density with suggestive calcifications is mammographically seen in the axillary parenchymal extension, corresponding to a palpable finding marked with a lead BB: recurrent intraductal and papillary endocystic carcinoma

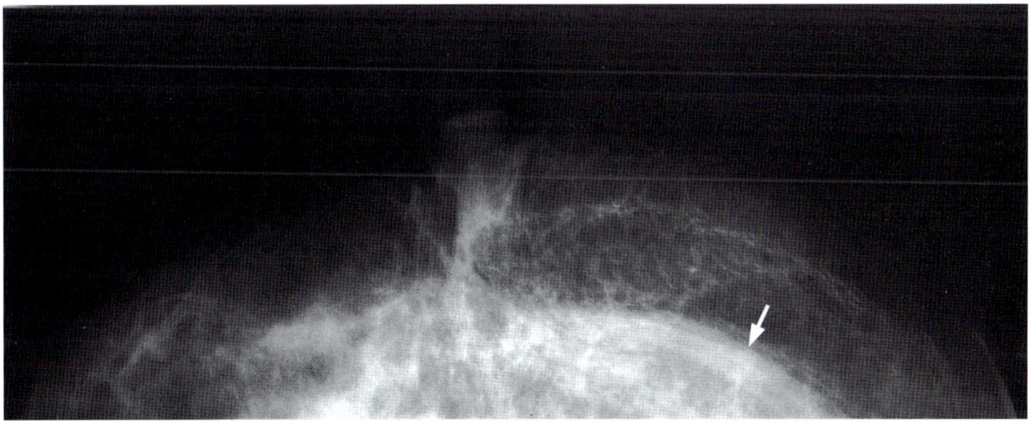

Fig. 16.**20** Myocutaneous flap.
The craniocaudad view delineates the coarse fascicular structure of the implanted myocutaneous flap in the upper outer quadrant as well as the coarse subcutaneous reticular connective tissue structure, in comparison with the other side

and connective tissue, such as oil cysts, are frequently found, producing clinically conspicuous palpatory findings. They can be positively diagnosed as benign by mammography. In general, the statement concerning postsurgical scars also applies to the evaluation of scars induced by reconstruction with autogenous tissue transfer.

Microcalcifications are reliably detected, as well as focal densities in fatty areas.

Sonography

While sonography is suitable for the evaluation of the tissue surrounding the prosthesis, it is not routinely used in asymptomatic patients with a prosthesis because of its limited accuracy concerning small nonpalpable findings and the difficult differentiation of changes caused by scar formation. Instead, it is used for further evaluation of palpatory findings. In selected cases, it can support the suspicion for a malignancy.

Even in the absence of mammographic and sonographic findings or in the presence of uncharacteristic findings, any clinical suspicion of malignancy cannot be dismissed. Aside from large silicone granulomas, which can produce a sonographically characteristic finding (see p. 206), small granulomas cannot be distinguished mammographically and sonographically from small malignant foci.

Magnetic Resonance Imaging

It is extremely well-suited for the evaluation of the breast with a silicone implant. It visualizes the entire tissue surrounding the prosthesis with excellent demarcation of small malignant foci from nonenhancing scar tissue (Fig. 16.**21**).

Because of its high sensitivity for detecting invasive foci, it can be employed as a supplemental examination for patients at risk, as well as for focal findings in need of further evaluation. First results on a series of patients examined with conventional imaging and MRI have shown that recurrences around implants can be detected earlier with MRI than with any other imaging modality.[5] Lack of enhancement excludes a malignancy with a high degree of certainty and is therefore helpful in areas that are difficult to assess and for the evaluation of indeterminate findings. Enhancing granulomas or diffuse inflammatory reactions can pose a problem, but small lesions (often representing granulomas solely detected by MRI) can be distinguished from malignancies by short-term follow-up examinations.

Percutaneous biopsy can only be used

a

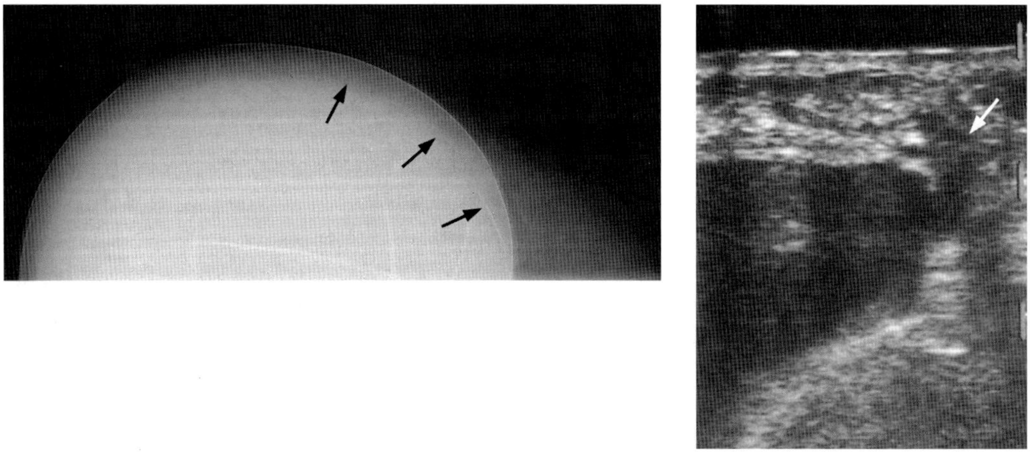

b

Fig. 16.**21 a–d** Detection of the carcinoma in the presence of a silicone prosthesis
a The mammographic evaluation is considerably compromised by the narrow mantle of tissue surrounding the prosthesis. The mobility is impaired because of scarring along the thoracic wall. No evidence of densities or calcifications suspicious for malignancy in several projections, with the craniocaudal view shown here (the arrows point at the outline of the inner compartment of the double-lumen prosthesis)
b Sonography: the small carcinomatous focus at the dorsolateral aspect of the outer margin of the prosthesis was not noted clinically or sonographically. It was apparently mistaken as part of the prosthesis itself. Only retrospectively could a corresponding area be identified (arrow)

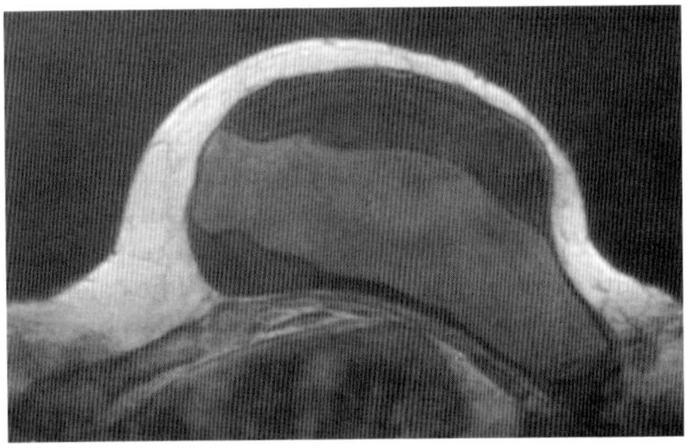

c

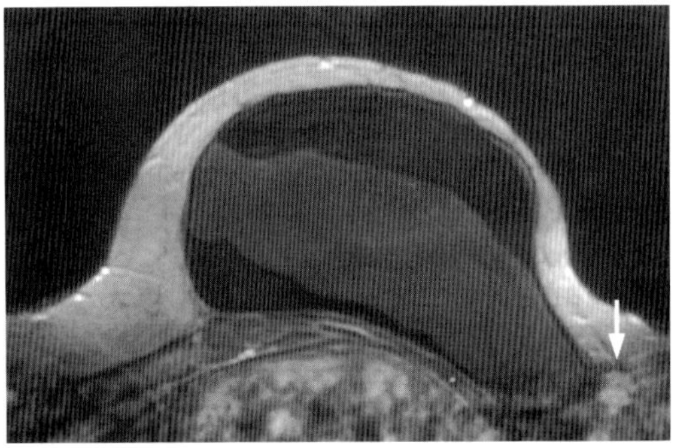

d

c Representative MRI section before administration of contrast medium at the level of subsequent suspicious enhancement (**d**)

d After application of contrast medium, highly suspicious enhancement adjacent to the prosthesis (arrow): *Histology:* recurrence of a ductal carcinoma (from Heywang-Köbrunner et al.[4])

selectively when the needle can be inserted parallel to the prosthesis without risk of damaging it.

Appendix: Evaluation of Defects of the Prosthesis

Leakage of silicone or tears in the breast prosthesis cannot be reliably recognized by mammography. Larger areas of silicone leakage that lead to the formation of silicone granulomas produce a rather typical sonographic finding (see p. 206). However, the sonographic evaluation of the integrity of the prosthesis and the sonographic differentiation between a tear with periprosthetic silicone deposition and folds of the prosthesis are difficult. For the detection of even small prosthetic defects, MRI (without contrast enhancement) has now become the method of choice. Using a combination of specific pulse sequences,[6,7,8,9,10] even small defects can be detected with high sensitivity (approximately 90%) and specificity (approximately 90%).

Augmentation

Definition

Augmentation refers to enlargement of the breast for the correction of congenital or acquired anisomastia or micromastia, or for cosmetic reasons.

Surgical Procedures

Prostheses containing silicone gel or saline or both are used to enlarge the breast. Because of the risk of the development of fibrotic changes or contractures, submuscular prostheses are preferred to retroglandular prostheses. The prosthesis is implanted using a laterocaudal (along the inferior mammary fold) or perimamillary approach. Direct silicone injections are prohibited, as are injections of wax and autogenous adipose tissue.

Diagnostic Strategy

In the presence of submuscular prosthesis, the visualization of most of the parenchymal tissue can sometimes be achieved by two views using the technique described by Eklund. If this is not feasible, more views in additional projections are necessary. Retroglandular prostheses usually require a combined mammographic technique (Eklund views and supplemental views).

If the parenchymal tissue can be visualized free of any superimposition of the implant, the diagnostic approach for detecting or excluding malignancies is identical to that used for the nonaugmented breast.

Portions of the parenchyma that cannot be evaluated despite combined mammographic techniques can be further evaluated by supplemental sonography or contrast-enhanced MRI. Large defects of the prosthesis are rarely mammographically visible but are generally seen

19. Screening

■ **Definition**

Screening refers to examinations performed regularly on an asymptomatic population group with the goal to detect clinically occult breast cancer at an early stage. Its task is searching, not diagnosing.

Results of International Studies

■ Randomized Studies

The HIP (Health Insurance Plan of Greater New York) study is the oldest randomized study. Between 1963 and 1970, 31 000 women between the ages of 40 and 64 years were allocated to have a two-view mammogram together with a clinical examination, followed by three annual follow-up mammograms. This screening was not offered to the control group of 31 000 women. Five years after commencement of the study, a 50% reduction in mortality was found in the screened women aged 50 to 64 years. Reduced mortality was still found after 18 years but declined to 23% since women could only participate for 4 years. For women ages 40 to 49 years, a mortality reduction was only evident after a longer follow-up; it now is at 24.6%.

Three randomized trials were conducted in Sweden. The first (two county study) trial was undertaken in the counties of Kopparberg and Östergotland. About 77 000 women were in the screening group and 56 000 women in the control study, i.e., passive study group. Single-view mammography without clinical examination was performed on women aged 40 to 49 years at 2-year intervals, for the older women at intervals of 33 months. The mortality reduction was 40% in women ages 50 to 74 years. Up to 12 years after the initiation of the study, no statistically significant reduction in mortality was observed in women aged 40 to 49 years.

The 2nd Swedish trial in Malmö included 21 000 women older than 45 years who had a two-view mammogram for the first two screening examinations, followed by three single-view mammographic screenings, without clinical examination. The intervals were 18 to 24 months. In comparison with the control group, a reduction in breast cancer mortality of 19% could be achieved over a period of 12 years. For the correct interpretation of the rather disappointing data, it should be mentioned that 24% of the women in the control group had at least one mammogram, and this was obtained in 13% of the women aged 65 to 69 years and 34% of the women aged 45 to 49 years, and that 20% of the breast carcinomas were also mammographically diagnosed in the control group. Considering that 26% to 30% of the women in the study group had no mammography, the lack of any detectable benefit for the women aged 45 to 49 years should not be surprising.

The 3rd Swedish randomized study in Stockholm began in 1981. Single-view mammography without clinical examination was performed on 40 000 women aged 40 to 64 years at 2½-year intervals. The reduction in mortality rate 7 years after initiation of the trial was 30% for all patients and 43% for patients older than 50 years.

Additional randomized studies were carried out in Scotland (Edinburgh) and Canada (Table **19.1**).

The Edinburgh study included 23 000

Table 19.**3** Results of the BCDDP multicenter study conducted: cancers of 280000 women, tabulated according to patient age and tumor stage

Histology	Breast Cancer Detection Demonstration Project (BCDDP), Number of Cancers (%) 40–49 years	50–59 years	60–69 years	Total
In situ	166 (15)	232 (15)	130 (13)	528 (15)
Invasive	742 (75)	1180 (76)	761 (76)	2683 (75)
N–	544 (54)	866 (56)	599 (60)	2009 (56)
N+	198 (20)	314 (20)	162 (16)	674 (19)
Unknown	96 (10)	148 (9)	110 (11)	354 (10)
Total	1004 (100)	1560 (100)	1001 (100)	3565 (100)
Tumor size				
< 10 mm	78 (12)	117 (11)	106 (16)	301 (13)
10–19 mm	211 (32)	362 (35)	269 (40)	842 (35)
20–49 mm	181 (27)	286 (27)	144 (21)	611 (26)
> 50 mm	27 (4)	49 (5)	25 (4)	101 (4)
Total	663 (100)	1046 (100)	674 (100)	2382 (100)

some believe that statistical confirmation is still lacking. The often considerable differences of the results of the individual studies can be attributed to differences in trial design (mammography alone vs. mammographic–clinical screening, single-view vs. two-view mammography, intervals of 1 to 3 years, randomization vs. case control study, etc.).
All things considered, these studies document excellent effectiveness. No other diagnostic or therapeutic measure so far can show a comparably high reduction in the mortality rates. By further optimizing the image quality and physician training, by employing regular two-view mammography, combined with physical examination whenever possible, and by selecting shorter examination intervals, further improvements can be expected.

Benefit–Risk/Benefit–Costs

■ Benefit–Risk

Our knowledge of the carcinogenic effect of radiation on the breast is based on populations that have been subjected to considerably higher dose levels (1–20 Gy) in comparison to the current mean absorbed parenchymal dose levels of about 2.5 mGy delivered by mammography in two projections. These populations include survivors of the atomic bomb explosions of Hiroshima and Nagasaki, women who had fluoroscopic exposure to one hemithorax exceeding that of the contralateral hemithorax to monitor the therapy of their tuberculosis (Massachusetts, Canada), and women who underwent anti-inflammatory radiation for therapy of mastitis (New York, Sweden).

Any mention of the radiation risk of mammography refers to the *estimated hypothetical and theoretical risk*. These estimates depend on the dose, fractionation, and age at the time of the exposure, as well as on the dose–effect model and latent period, i.e., it is a complex interaction of factors. The most recent report from the National Research Council Committee on the Biological Effects of Ionizing Radiation (BEIR) in 1990 is based on the results of atomic-bomb survivors, fluoroscopic studies performed in

Canada and Massachusetts, and mastitis studies conducted in New York. The latent period is stated as 10 years after the exposure, and the assumption is based on age dependence and a linear dose effect relationship because this model encompasses the higher theoretical risk. This implies that repair mechanisms characteristically operative with solar and cosmic radiation remain excluded. Thus, the resultant estimates represent a worst-case scenario.

The estimates are as follows: If 100 000 women had a mammogram (2.5 mGy) at the age of 45 years, at the most one breast carcinoma (that is fatal in about 50%) could be induced throughout the entire life span of these women. This lifelong fatal risk corresponds to the risk of dying from smoking three cigarettes.

This has to be balanced against the fact that 1500 of each 1 million women ages 45 years will develop a breast carcinoma per year owing to the natural incidence of breast carcinomas and that 50% of them will succumb to it. In other words, 750 breast cancer deaths can be expected annually in 1 million women. If these women were subjected to a single screening examination and if a 20%, 40%, and 60% mortality reduction, respectively, is assumed, 150, 300, and 450 breast cancer deaths could be avoided with two-view mammography. A baseline mammogram at the age of 35 years and an annual screening mammogram beginning at the age of 40 years would increase the theoretical risk of a women developing a breast carcinoma in her lifetime from 9.3% (natural incidence) to at most 9.32 to 9.4%.

Therefore, the *theoretical radiation risk* as a disadvantage of regular screening mammography can be *ignored* by the individual woman if she considers the tremendous advantage of early detection, which, in addition to reducing her mortality, can offer her the possibility of breast-preserving therapy as well as possible avoidance of adjuvant therapy. As long as there is neither a primary prevention of breast cancer nor a 100% cure, screening for breast cancer by means of mammography and physical examination is the only and best method to exert a beneficial influence on the biologic course of this disease.

Benefit–Costs

Mammographic screening has made it possible to save lives. Even though the value of a woman's life saved from breast cancer cannot be expressed as a benefit–cost estimate, it is necessary to make benefit–cost calculations to obtain the financial support from society necessary to implement screening programs.

A realistic estimate of the costs expressing the benefit in relation to the calculated numbers of years saved is extremely difficult since many of the determining factors are quite variable and are different to asses.

The following factors are included in the calculation:

- The actual costs of the mammographic screening (costs for the material of single-view and two- view mammography, costs for equipment depreciation, wages for technologists and fees for physicians, frequency of screening examinations, e.g., annually, biannually, triennially).
- The costs of additional examinations (imaging, needle aspiration, surgical excision) performed because of suggestive or unclear findings on the screening examination. In all screening programs, the number of findings requiring further evaluation is considerably higher than that of the ultimately confirmed carcinomas. Thus the costs of workup strongly depend on the false positive rate of the initial screening.
- The effectiveness of the achievable early detection (number of carcinomas actually detected by screening, compiled from the distribution of the stages of the carcinomas and from the stage-dependent survival rates).
- Natural prevalence and mortality of breast carcinoma in the examined population.
- Compliance rate: Since most costs are caused by the examination itself as well as by the ensuing costs of workup mentioned above, the compliance rate has only limited influence on calculating the cost-effectiveness.
- Costs of primary therapy of the carcinoma (percentage of the performed breast-conserving therapies). Unfortunately, breast-conserving therapies, which have increased due to improved early detection, are more expensive than mastectomy and consequently are a cost-raising factor.
- The costs saved by reducing the number of cost-intensive therapies needed for advanced stages of the disease.
- Effect of years gained on the gross national product, on income, and on taxes (cost savings only for years gained before reaching retirement age).

Depending on the healthcare system, these factors vary from country to country.[1] From the above considerations, it is also apparent that the most cost-effective screening program unfortunately will not be the one with the highest detection rate of breast carcinoma. (For instance, more and earlier carcinomas are detected by annual screening in comparison to biannual screening. The number of detected carcinomas, however, increases less than the cost increments due to the additional screening examinations). The technical quality as well as the interpretive quality are of great importance. Both determine not only the number of prognostically favorable carcinomas detected at an early stage but also the false positive rate with its resultant cost-intensive additional examinations performed for confirmation. There are studies that show high fluctuations of the false positive rate from country to country as well as markedly reduced false positive rates for centralized screening.[2, 3]

Currently, the most cost-effective screening programs appear to be in the Netherlands and Great Britain.[4, 5] But even there, the costs (the screening itself, the ensuing examinations, and the expensive breast-preserving therapies) by far exceed the cost-savings (reduced expenses due to fewer palliative therapies). This means that approximately $3000 to $5000 is spent for each year of patient-life gained. Though these costs are considerable, they can compete with other health-related costs in our society, considering that screening for cervix carcinoma in the same countries is about three times as expensive.[6]

As already mentioned, these results of the Netherlands and Great Britain are not directly applicable to other countries with different populations and, above all, differently structured healthcare systems.

All things considered, the costs of screening and early diagnosis cannot be compensated by cost-savings in palliative therapy. This means that the screening programs, depending on their effectiveness, may induce costs for each year of a woman's life gained. However, in comparison to other healthcare costs, these costs are within an acceptable range. It can therefore be hoped that more countries implement lifesaving screening programs.

Recommendations on the Basis of the Trials

A consortium of American medical organizations including the American Cancer Society has issued the following recommendation: Between the ages of 40 and 49 years, women should undergo a physical examination and mammography every year or two. Women older than 50 years should have an annual physical examination as well as a mammogram.

In Europe, the recommendations for the respective national screening programs differ from country to country. In England, women between the ages of 50 and 64 years are examined by single-view mammography every 3rd year. In the Netherlands, women between the ages of 50 and 70 years are examined every other year, with two-view mammography initially and single-view mammography thereafter. In Sweden, the screening interval is a year and a half for women ages 40 to 54 years and 2 years for women ages 55 to 74 years. The initial screening examination consists of two-view mammography, followed by single-view mammography. In Finland, women ages 50 to 62 years undergo a two-view mammography at 2-year intervals. In Iceland, the same scheme is used for women ages 40 to 69 years.

In general, screening should only be performed with the highest standard of quality. The intervals should be adapted to the individual risk, the expected tumor doubling time and the incidence. Since breast carcinomas with high growth potential can develop between the ages of *40 and 49 years*, women in this age group should have an annual physical examination and mammography for optimal early detection. *Beginning at the age of 50 years*, the incidence of breast carcinoma increases linearly. This is the reason for annual mammography and physical examination in these age groups. For older women (65 or older) as well as for women with partial or complete parenchymal involution, some have suggested that the intervals be increased to 2 years. For diagnostic reasons (markedly improved accuaracy, fewer patient recalls because of diagnostic uncertainties), mammography should be performed in two views and combined with a physical examination. This can be concluded from the interval cancer rates reported by centers with single-view mammography.

Scientific studies have not established the upper age limit for screening.

References

1. v. Ineveld BM, v. Oortmarssen GJ, de Koning HJ et al. How cost-effective is breast cancer screening in different EC countries? Eur J Cancer. 1993;29(a/12):1663
2. United Kingdom Trial of Early Detection of Breast Cancer Group. Specificity of screening in United Kingdom trial of early detection of breast cancer. Br Med J. 1992;304:346
3. Kopans DB, Swann CA. Observation on mammographic screening and false positive mammograms. AJR. 1988;150:785
4. Forrest P. Breast cancer screening. Report to the Health Ministers of England, Wales, Scotland and Northern Ireland. London; 1986
5. de Koning HJ, v. Ineveld BM, v. Oortmarssen GJ et al. Breast cancer screening and cost-effectiveness; policy alternatives, quality of life considerations and the possible impact of uncertain factors. Int J Cancer. 1991;49:531
6. v. Ballegooijen M, v. Habbema JDF, v. Oortmarssen GJ et al. Preventive papsmears: striking the balance between costs, risks and benefits. Br J Cancer. 1992;65:930

Suggested Reading

Andersson L, Aspegren K, Janzon L et al. Effect of mammographic screening in breast cancer mortality in an urban population in Sweden. Results from the Malmö mammographic screening trial (MMST). Boston Med J. 1988;297:943

Chu KC, Smart CR, Tarone RE. Analysis of breast cancer mortality and stage distribution by age for the Health Insurance Plan clinical trial. J Natl Cancer Inst. 1988;80:1125

v. Fournier DV, Anton HW, Junkermann H et al. Brustkrebsscreening. Wissenstand und Einführung als Vorsorgeleistung. Radiologe. 1993;33:227–35

Frischbier HJ. Beitrag zur kontroversen Einschätzung des Mammographie-Screenings bei asymptomatischen Frauen zwischen dem 40. und 50. Lebensjahr. Geburtshilfe Frauenheilkd. 1994;54:1–11

Frisell J, Eklund G, Hellstrom L et al. Randomized study of mammography screening—preliminary report on mortality in the Stockholm trial. Breast Cancer Res Treat. 1991;18:49

Nyström L, Rutqvist LE, Wall S et al. Breast cancer screening with mammography: an overview of the Swedish randomized trials. Lancet. 1993;341:974

Roberts MM, Alexander FE, Anderson TJ et al. Edinburgh trial of screening for breast cancer: mortality at seven years. Lancet. 1990;335:241

Sickles EA, Kopans DB. Deficiencies in the analysis of breast cancer data. J Natl Cancer Inst. 1993;85:1621–4

Schreer I, Heywang-Köbrunner SH. Brustkrebsfrüherkennung. Gynäkologe. 1994;27:12

Smart CR, Hartmann WH, Beahrs OH, Garfinkel L. Insights into breast cancer screening of younger women: evidence from the 14-year-follow-up of the Breast Cancer Detection Demonstration Project. Cancer. 1993;72:1449

Tabar L, Fagerberg G, Suffy SW et al. Update of the Swedish two-county program of mammographic screening for breast cancer. Radiol Clin North Am. 1992;30:187

Tabar L, Duffy SW, Warren-Burhenne L. New Swedish breast cancer detection results for women aged 40–49. Cancer. 1993;72:1437

20. Additional Diagnostic Evaluation of Screening Findings and Solving of Problems in Symptomatic Patients

Pathognomonic Findings

(Table 20.**1**)

■ Definition

The term pathognomonic refers to findings that, without further tests, are diagnostic of a certain histology and consequently do not require surgical confirmation.

■ Incidence

Pathognomonic findings are rare. Most fibroadenomas, for instance, fail to show the mammographically typical calcifications.

■ Typical Findings and Diagnostic Strategy

Pathognomonic findings have to be distinguished from typical findings, which are strongly suggestive of the underlying histology but cannot unequivocally prove it. For probably benign findings, comparison with previous examinations or follow-up mammography at half-year intervals is generally adequate. Malignant findings should be confirmed histologically by surgical or percutaneous biopsy before any therapy is initiated.

Table 20.**1** Pathognomonic images

Histologic diagnosis	Characteristic mammographic findings
Lipoma	Focal, round, or oval lesion of fat density with delicate rim (capsule
Hamartoma	Focal, smoothly outlined lesion containing areas of lipomatous and water density
Oil cyst	Focal radiolucency with surrounding rim (capsule) without/with eggshell-like calcifications
Lymph node	Focal, oval, smoothly outlined density, with — depending on the projection — central or marginal, round radiolucency
Galactocele	Focal, smoothly outlined lesion, composed of fatty components and water-equivalent structures (layering possible), history of pregnancy or lactation
Calcified fibroadenoma	Smoothly outlined, focal density with/without halo, oval, or polylobulated, if containing characteristic calcifications
Cyst containing milk of calcium	Smoothly outlined, focal, rund density with calcifications that project centrally in the craniocaudad view and layer inferiorly on the mediolateral view
Verruca	Smoothly outlined mass exhibiting a cauliflower-like structure (multilobulated) and frequently very sharp borders (soft-tissue–air)
	Characteristic sonographic findings
Cyst	Anechoic, smoothly outlined thin-walled lesion with good distal acoustic enhancement and good compressibility

Differential Diagnosis and Diagnostic Work-up

Smoothly Outlined Density

(Fig. 20.**1**)

■ Diagnostic Question

A smooth outline of a density generally speaks for a benign lesion.

Smoothly outlined localized findings seen on screening mammography most frequently represent cysts or fibroadenomas, but 2–7% of all breast carcinomas can be expected to present as a nodule with a partially well-circumscribed margin and 2% with a well-defined outline.

Owing to displacement of surrounding fat by their growth, medullary, papillary, or mucinous carcinomas can give the impression of a capsule and even might have a halo sign (see Fig. 14.**2e**). In some medullary carcinomas (Type I), the same phenomenon can result in a demarcating capsule-like zone of connective tissue. Furthermore, intracystic carcinomas, metastases, involved lymph nodes, lymphomas, or sarcomas can present as smoothly outlined focal lesions.

■ Diagnostic Strategy

1. The first step of the evaluation addresses the question: Is the lesion within or outside the parenchyma?
   - This can sometimes be answered by inspection, palpation, or routine imaging.
   - If this cannot be unequivocally answered, the tangential coned-down view should be obtained after marking the skin (Fig. 20.**2**).
     Concerning skin changes, see Chapter 17.
   - Overlying structures such as the incidentally visualized contralateral nipple (Fig. 20.**3**) or even the tip of the nose (Fig. 17.**1f**) are typical artifacts seen as semicircular density in one view only.
2. The smoothly outlined intraparenchymal lesion is further evaluated as to radiodensity.
   - Fat-containing lesions are pathognomonic (lipoma, oil cyst, hamartoma, galactocele, lymph node) and do not require any further diagnostic evaluation.
   - Solitary, smoothly outlined lesions are pathognomonic as long as they exhibit calcifications characteristic of fibroadenomas. But this is only applicable to a small number of patients. They are observed by follow-up mammography with the intervals determined by the overall observation period available. If no previous films exist, follow-up is usually recommended after 6, 12, 24, and 36 months.
3. The well-circumscribed or fairly well-circumscribed lesion of soft-tissue density needs further evaluation.
   - The simplest approach is the comparison with previous mammograms.
   - If a lesion is stable for more than 3 years, no special diagnostic evaluation is necessary. For lesions with shorter observation periods, further follow-up is indicated. Since some smoothly outlined malignancies can grow slowly, it is advisable to check a newly discovered lesion at 6, 12, 24, and 36 months to establish stability for a period of 3 years. During this follow-up, it is advisable to always compare with the initial films as well, and not only with the most recent films.
   - A growing lesion or a new well-circumscribed lesion should be evaluated by sonography to determine if it is a simple cyst.
   - If sonography proves a cyst, no further evaluation is needed.
   - If the cystic nature is equivocal, aspiration is indicated.
   - If a sonographically solid lesion is well-circumscribed on mammography and more than 75% of its contour clearly visible without superimposition, short-interval follow-up mammograms are adequate.
   - For the other smoothly outlined solitary lesions found to be solid, further evaluation is needed. Most masses, especially those larger than 5 mm in diameter, should be subjected to percutaneous biopsy for histologic evaluation. If the histology is compatible with a benign entity, further mammographic observation or routine following is adequate.
   - Multiple somoothly outlined lesions

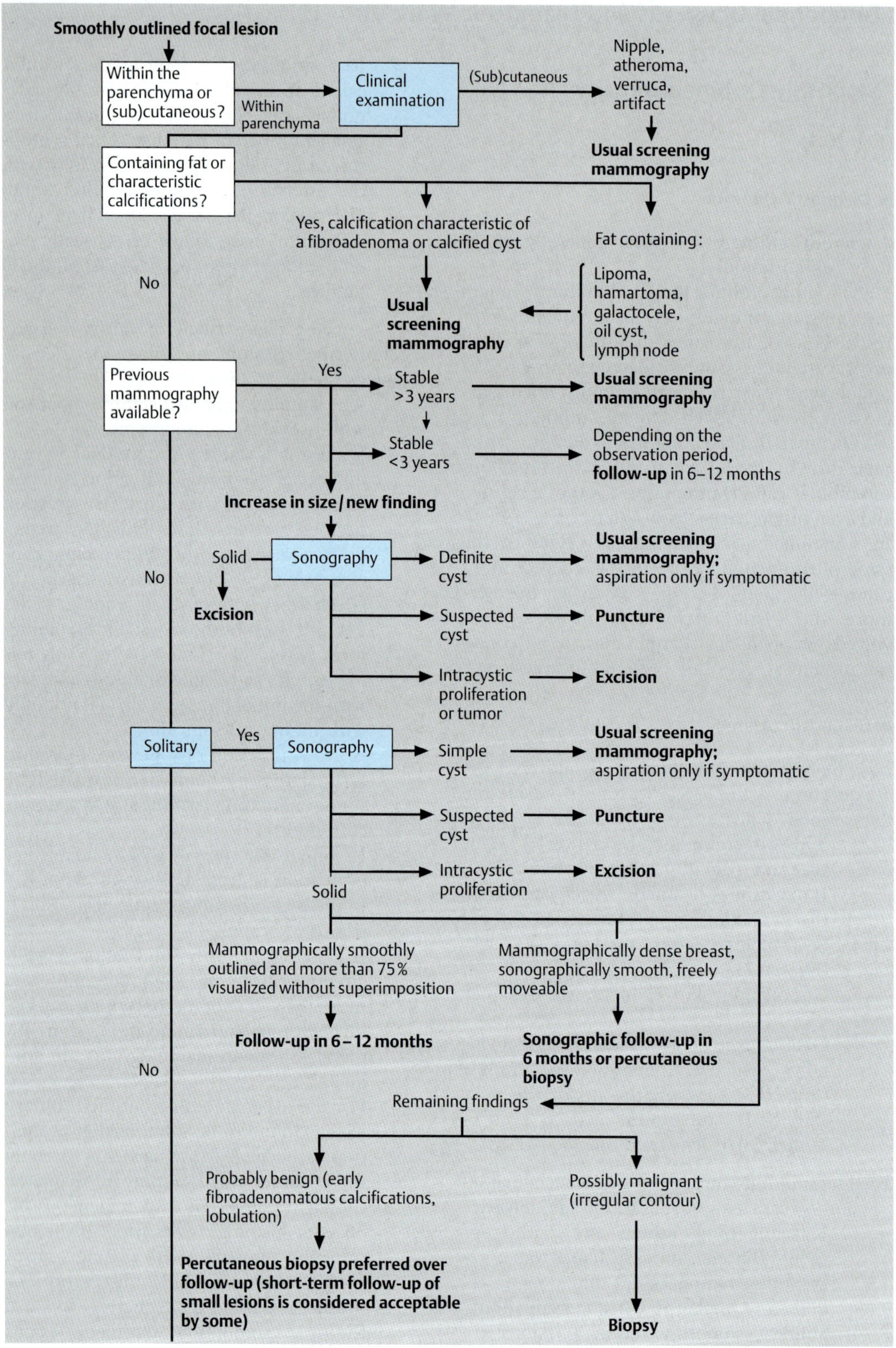

Fig. 20.**1** The smoothly outlined focal finding (continued on p. 341)

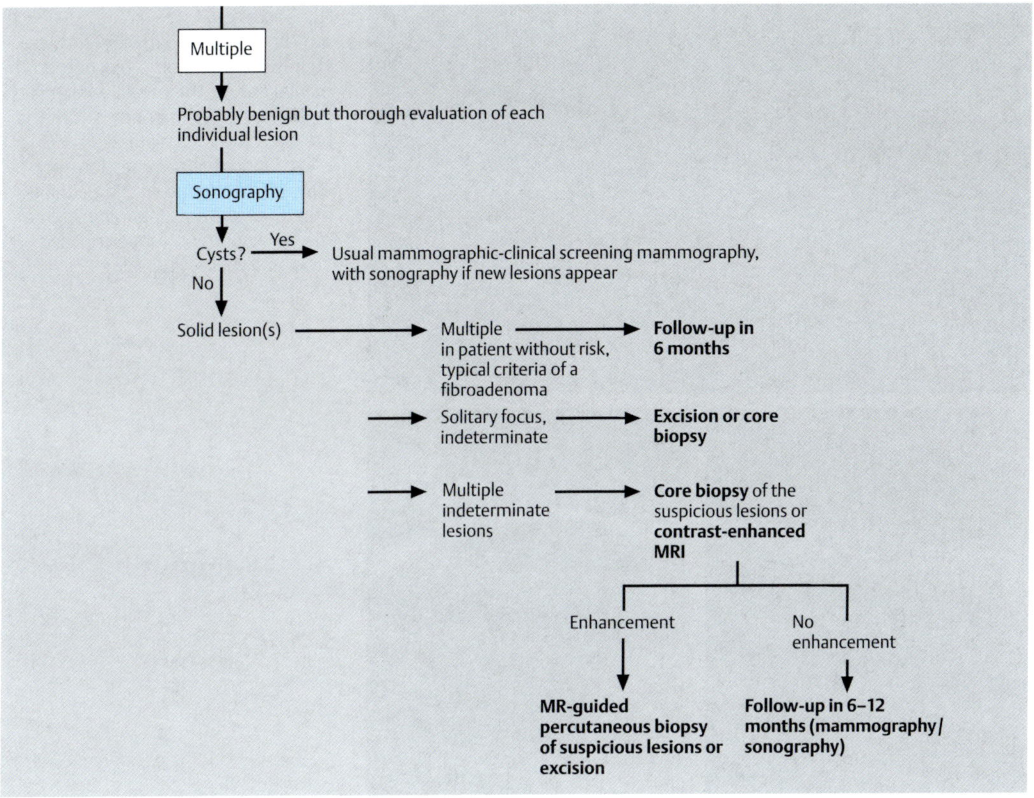

Fig. 20.**1** (Cont.)

speak for benignity, but this is not definitive since nodular lesions can, albeit rarely, be the manifestation of multicentric or metastatic disease. Moreover, thorough mammographic–sonographic analysis should be conducted so that a carcinoma is not overlooked amidst multiple benign lesions (Fig. 20.**4**). In individual cases with multiple lesions of concern, MRI may be helpful in demonstrating absence of enhancement (in fibrous fibroadenomas) or in guiding biopsy to the most suspicious lesion (Fig. 20.**5a–d**).

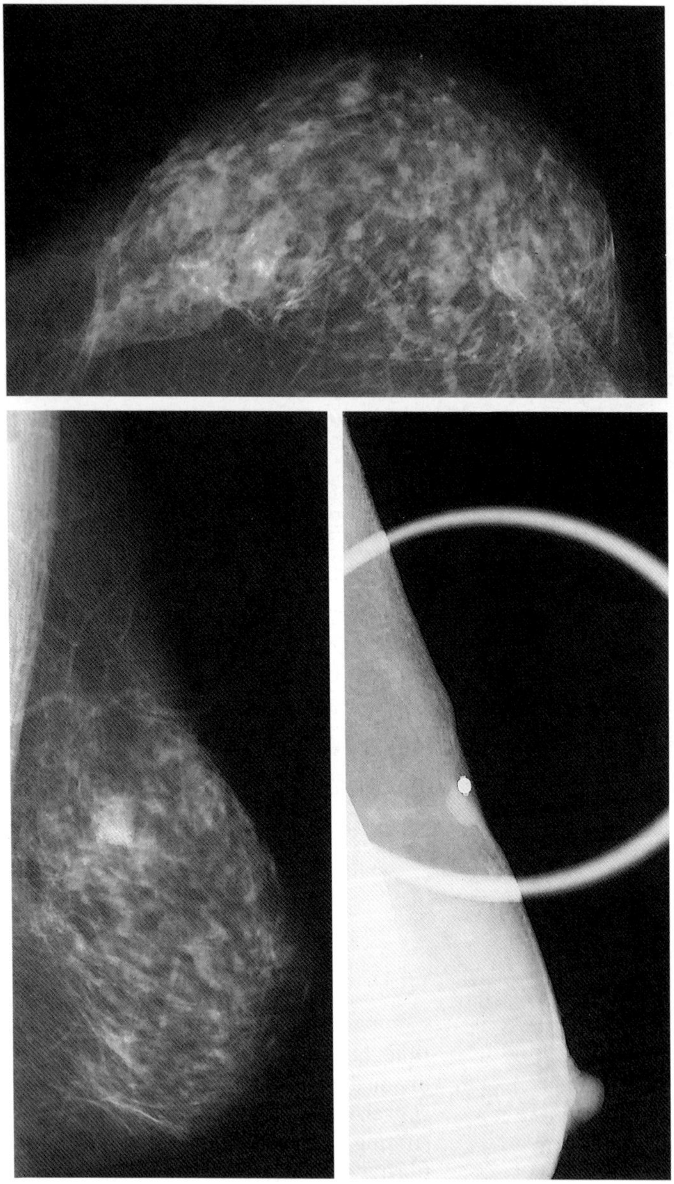

a b c

Fig. 20.**2a–c**
a The craniocaudad view shows a 10 mm round lesion projecting on the medial half of the breast, which can be localized in the upper half of the breast in the mediolateral view (**b**)
c A tangential compression spot view after marking of the palpable atheroma shows superimposition of marker and lesion (underexposed view to visualize the skin)

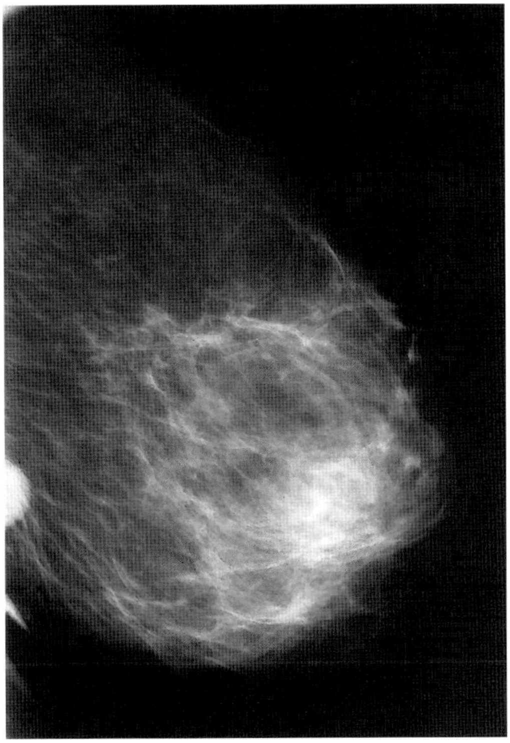

Fig. 20.3 Incidental visualization of the contralateral nipple, seen as convex density close to the chest wall (mediolateral view)

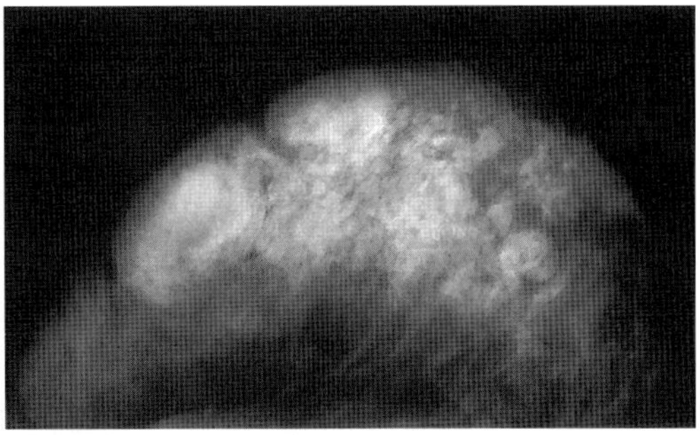

a

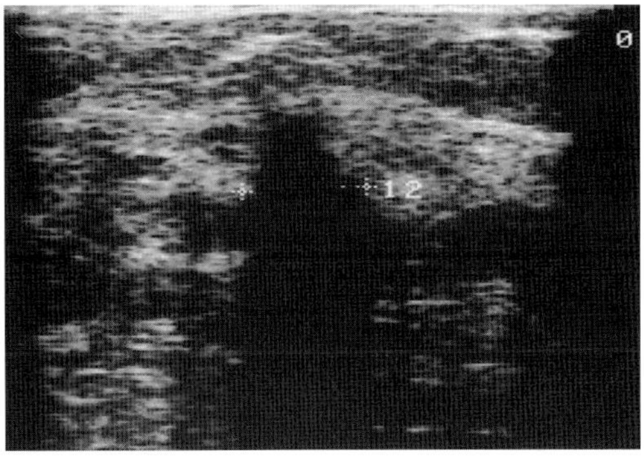

b

Fig. 20.4a and b
a Patient with known fibrocystic changes. Mammography shows lumpy, dense breast tissue unchanged since films. The lumps could be confirmed as representing simple cysts by sonography
b In addition, an irregularly outlined hypoechoic lesion with distal shadowing, measuring 9 mm in diameter, is visualized sonographically within dense surrounding tissue. *Histology:* infiltrating lobular carcinoma

Fig. 20.5a–d Multiple round lesions. This patient had supraclavicular nodal metastases and came for primary tumor search
a and **b** Mammographically (craniocaudal view), several indeterminate masses are seen in the outer quadrants

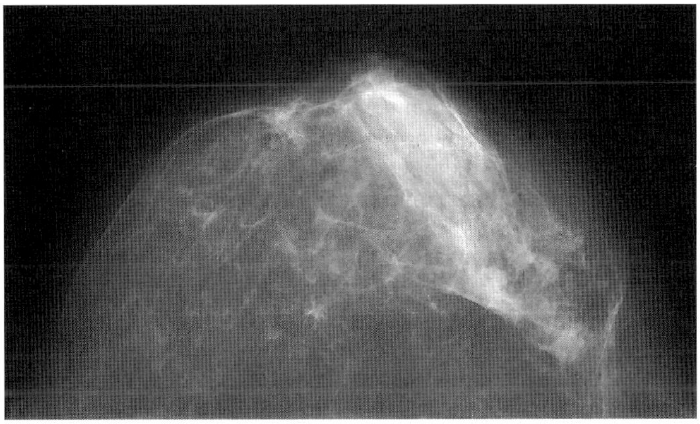

a

- Any increase in size mandates further evaluation.

3. Before unnecessary surgery is recommended, it should be determined if a lesion could be hormone–induced.
   - In postmenopausal patients, hormone replacement therapy can induce the growth of cysts or fibroadenomas otherwise not observed in this age group. After hormone therapy has been discontinued, the hormone-stimulated parenchyma very rapidly undergoes involution, usually accompanied by a mammographically visible decrease in size and density of the hormonally induced focal finding.
   - If the focal finding persists after discontinuation of the hormone therapy, biopsy is indicated to establish the diagnosis.
4. Clinical history and physical examination determine whether the findings are post-traumatic or post-therapeutic. In the presence of scarring, the following approach is recommended:
   - As long as clinical and mammographic findings concur, follow-up examinations are adequate.
   - If serial examinations reveal an increase in size, progressing radial configuration, or suspicious microcalcifications, biopsy is indicated.
   - In case of questionable findings or impaired mammographic evaluation or both, MRI can be very helpful since it is able to detect tumor, even within severe scarring, and since it can readily differentiate between tumor and fibrosis.

Architectural Distortion

(Fig. 20.**7**)

■ Diagnostic Questions

Architectural distortion may be the only sign or an early sign of a carcinoma. Tubular carcinomas characteristically present as a spiculated mass. Absence of a central density is not a reliable sign of benignity. Neoplastic changes must be distinguished from summation effects caused by crossing Cooper's ligaments and from radial structures secondary to post-traumatic/post-therapeutic scarring. Differentiation from radial scars (synonym: infiltrating epitheliosis), which represent a special manifestation of fibrocystic and proliferative changes, requires excisional biopsy since these can coexist with DCIS, tubular carcinoma, or invasive carcinoma.

■ Diagnostic Strategy

(Fig. 20.**8** and 20.**9**)

1. First, a scar should be excluded by clinical history and physical examination. Even small incisions for abscess drainage can induce intraparenchymal scars.
   - If clinical and mammographic findings do not completely agree with this diagnosis, previous examinations, including preoperative mammograms, should, if possible, be obtained for comparison. Knowing the original location of an excised finding is helpful. Periareolar scars are usually not helpful in localizing the site of prior breast surgery.
   - If previous mammograms are not available, if the region of interest is not included, or if the radial structure does not unequivocally coincide with the scar, contrast-enhanced MRI may be helpful (Fig. 20.**9**).
   - An evolving or progressing spiculation is an indication for biopsy. In addition to a carcinoma, post-traumatic fat necrosis must be considered, which can also be manifested as an ill-defined mass or as architectural distortion with or without central density.
2. Architectural distortions that cannot be explained by scarring should be biopsied, even if previous mammograms reveal stability. The reason is that several malignancies, especially tubular carcinoma and carcinoma in situ, present as architectural distortion that can be stable for a long time or can grow very slowly.
3. If architectural distortion is seen in one projection only, superimposition of structures must be excluded by spot compression views or by rolled views. If it is reproducible and remains undetectable in a second or third projectional plane, it must be searched for by spot compression or magnification views in additional projections.

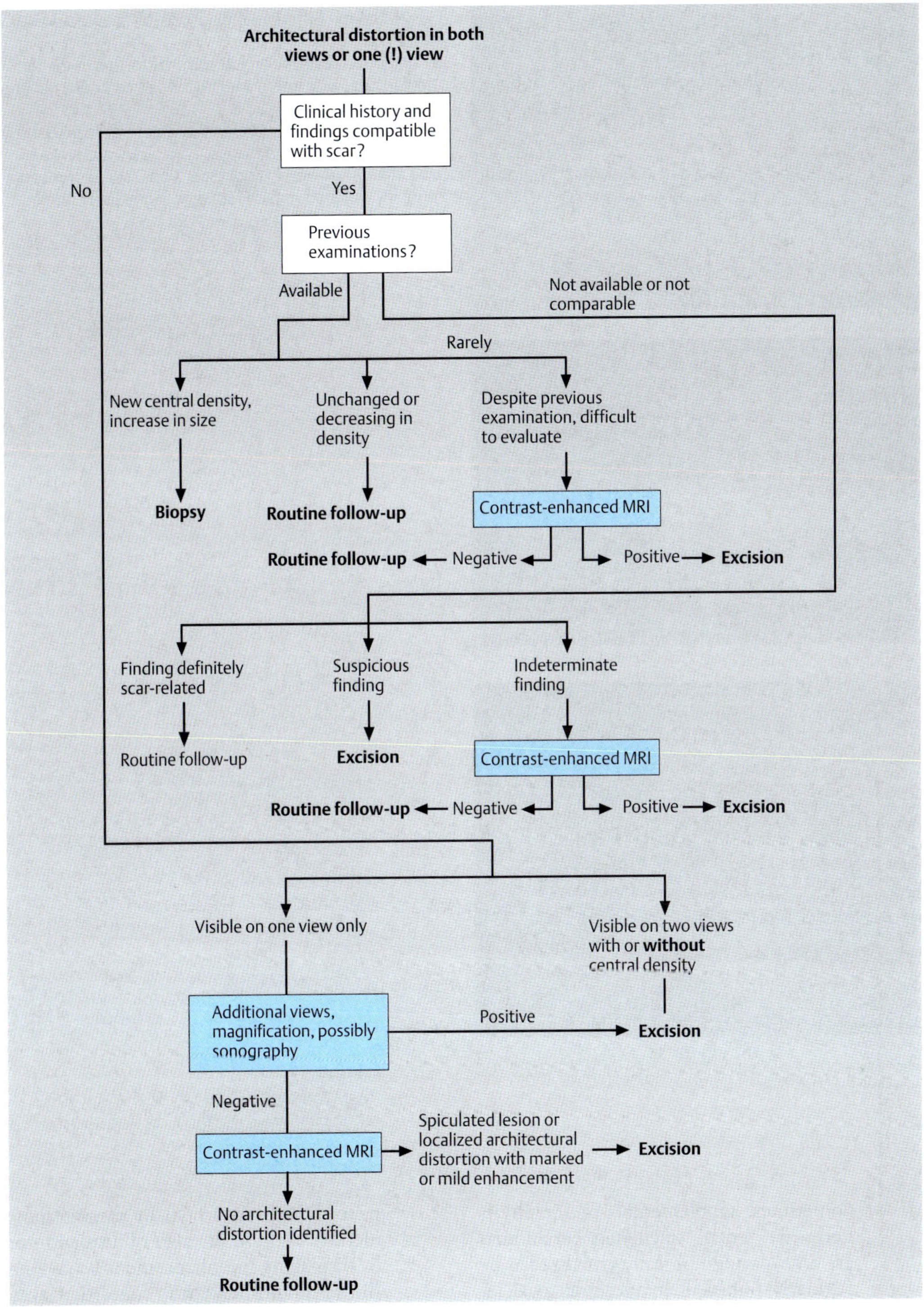

Fig. 20.**7** Architectural distortion

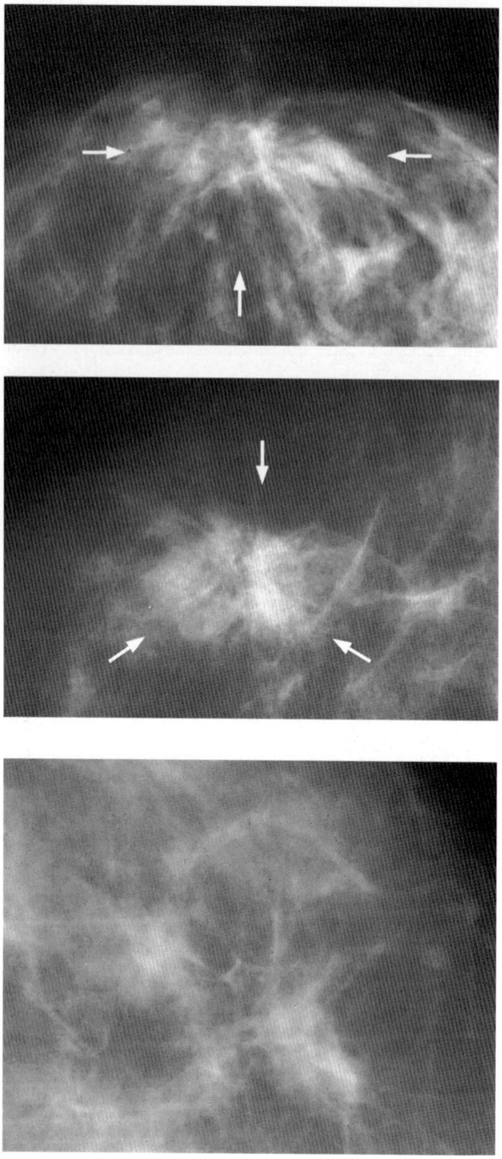

a b c

Fig. 20.**8a–n** Differential diagnosis of architectural distortion

a Patient A: delicate architectural distortion in the retroareolar area, with interposed fat lobules centrally: periareolar scarring.

b Patient B: architectural without central focal density. *Histology:* sclerosing adenosis

c Patient C: relatively thick extensions radiate from an irregularly outlined mass. *Histology:* regressively altered fibroadenoma

▷

- Sometimes, supplemental sonography is necessary. Small spiculated carcinomas are often sonographically visualized as irregularly outlined, hypoechoic focal lesions with or without distal acoustic shadowing.
- If the exact location of an architectural distortion remains unclear, contrast-enhanced MRI may help by tomographic identification of the area of distortion or by displaying its enhancement behaviour. But it should be kept in mind that even faintly enhancing spiculated structures should be excised since radial scars can harbor carcinomas in situ that might not show strong enhancement.[1]

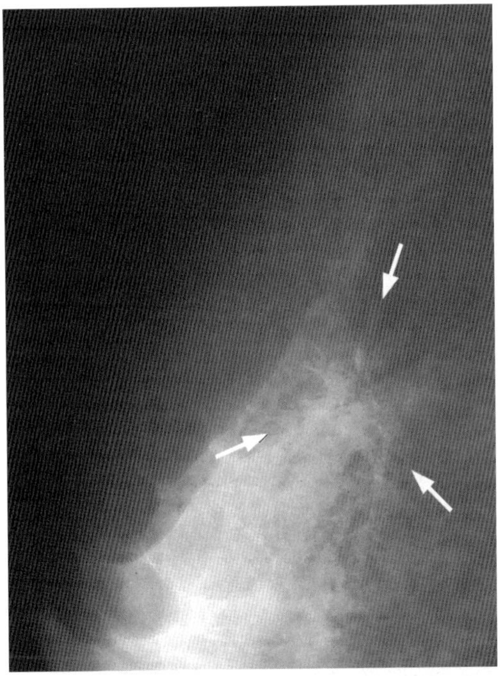

d

Fig. 20.**8d** Patient D: delicate radial structural transformation without central focal density. *Histology:* tubuloalveolar variant of an infiltrating carcinoma, measuring 8 mm in diameter.
e and **f** Patient E

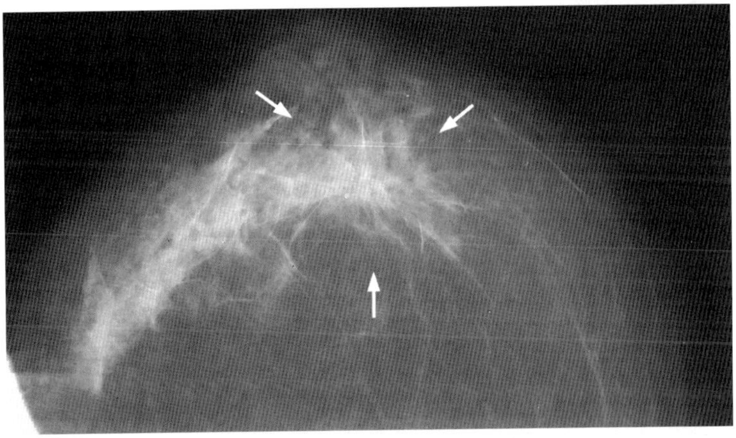

e

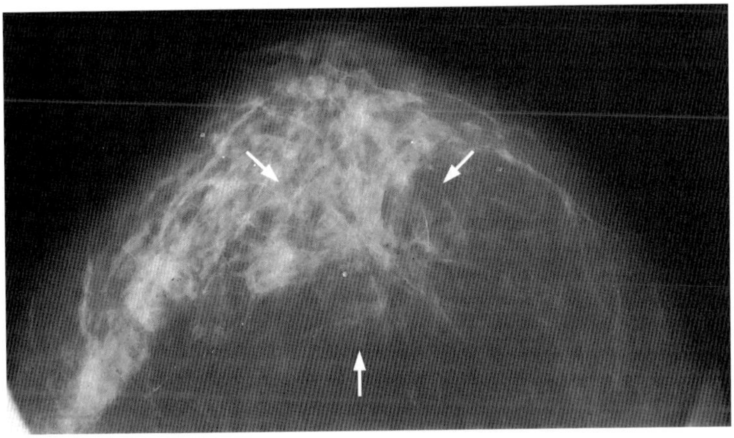

Fig. 20.**8e** Clinically, no palpable abnormality. Mammographically, marked architectural distortion
f The same patient, mammography 6 years later. The radial extensions are longer. *Histology:* radial scar

▷

Fig. 20.**15d** ML view, left breast. Outside mammography, which was obtained without clinical suspicion, reveals no evidence of malignancy and would not have prompted any further investigation. Retrospectively reviewed, sonography reveals no focal finding. *Histology:* ductal carcinoma

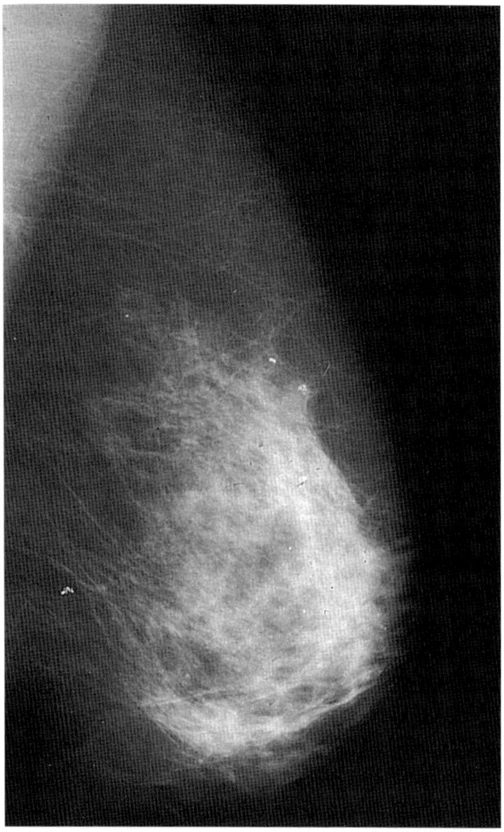

d

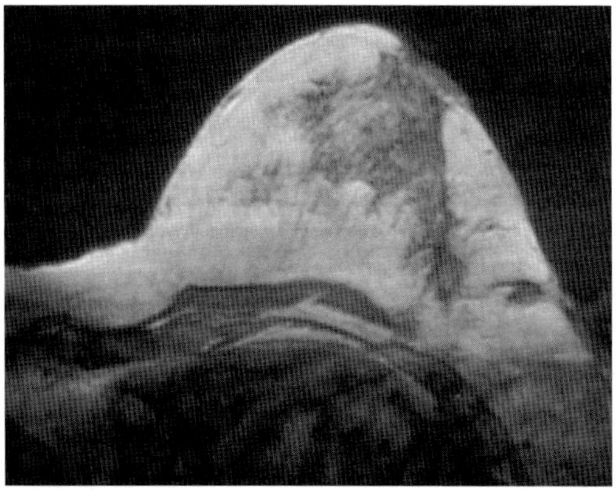

a

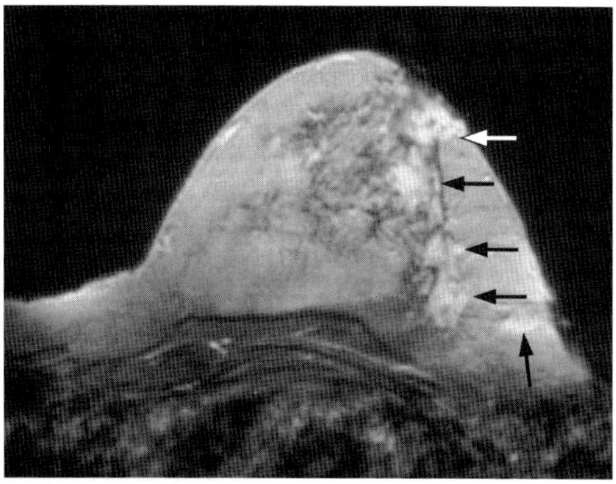

b

Fig. 20.**16a–f** Assessing extent of and detecting additional foci in the mammographically dense breast. *Histology:* multifocal papillary carcinoma

a and **b** In this patient with two small mammographically suspicious foci in the region of a palpable finding in the upper outer quadrant (Fig. 14.**2i** and **k**), only the contrast-enhanced MRI discloses the true extent of involvement

a Representative transverse slice through the level of the mammographically suspicious lesions before administration of contrast medium

b After administration of Gd-DTPA, multiple additional lesions (arrows) are disclosed in the retroareolar area as well as in further quadrants (not shown here), indicating more widespread disease than initially suspected

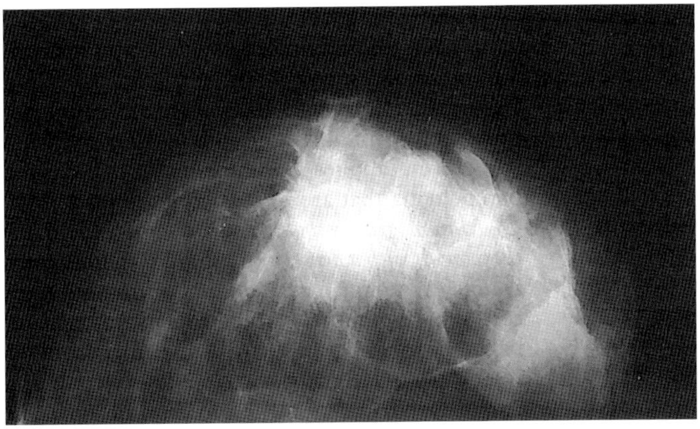

c

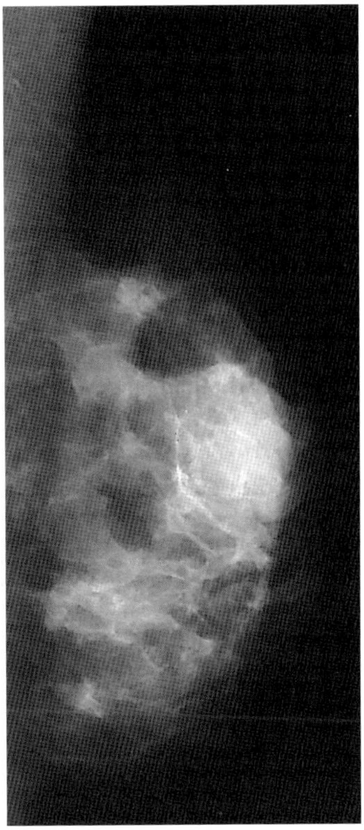

d

Fig. 20.**16c–f** Patient with a suspicious palpable finding behind and medial to the nipple following excisional biopsy of a benign lesion 3 years ago. Though the area is sonographically hypoechoic and thus considered suspect, supplemental MRI was ordered because of impaired evaluation of the surgically altered retroareolar region
c and **d** Mammography, CC, and oblique views show very dense tissue with cicatricial retraction

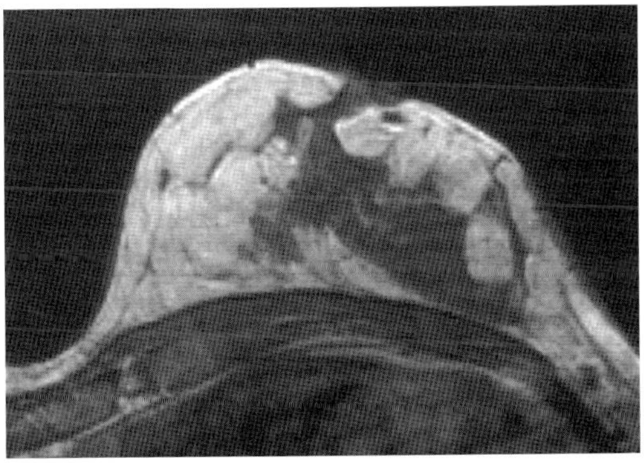

e

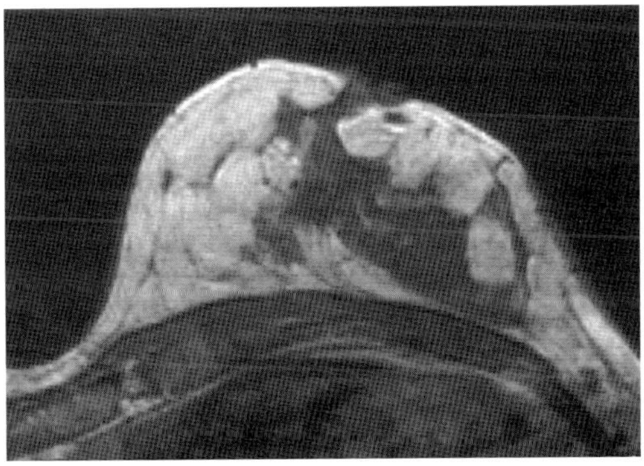

f

Fig. 20.**16e** MRI section at the level of the palpable finding in the region of the scar before administration of Gd-DTPA
f The same level after Gd-DTPA shows highly suspicious enhancement in the palpable finding (arrow). Also visualized are several additional foci of suspicious enhancement, neither suspected clinically nor by any other method

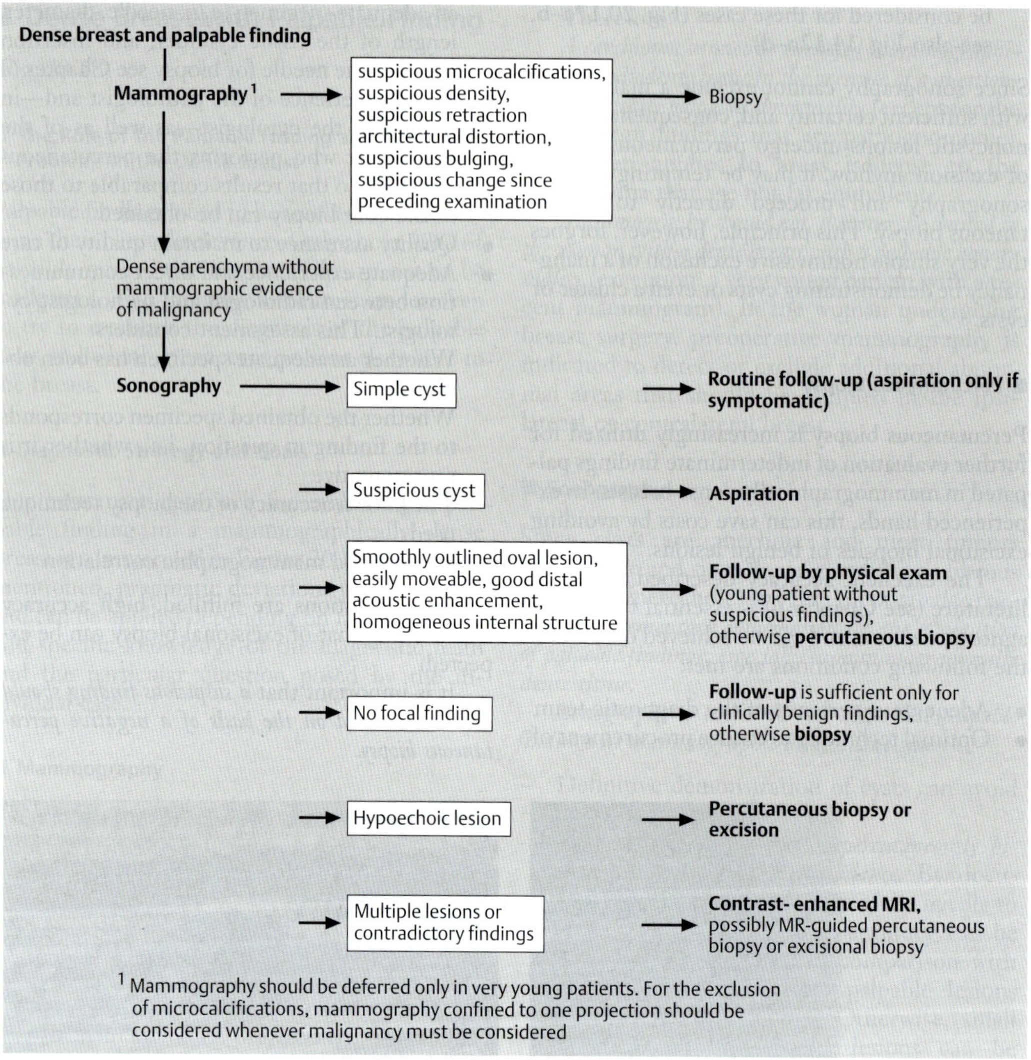

Fig. 20.**18** Approach to the dense breast with palpable finding

Contrast-enhanced MRI

Though the combination of mammography and contrast-enhanced MRI is highly sensitive and detects even small carcinomas, contrast-enhanced MRI should not be considered the primary method to supplement mammography in the evaluation of a palpable finding in the dense breast. The reasons are the considerably higher false positive rate of contrast-enhanced MRI in comparison with percutaneous biopsy and the relatively high proportion of patients (about 25%) with diffuse enhancement that precludes a definitive diagnosis, as well as the high cost of the examination.

The use of contrast-enhanced MRI is appropriate in patients with:

- Extensive scars and unclear palpable findings (status post surgery, implants, or radiation). A false positive diagnosis of cancer when the lesion represents old scar tissue (except for cases with fat necrosis) is rare with MRI. Small recurrences can be detected early.
- Multiple questionable findings, in particular when the results of other modalities are con-

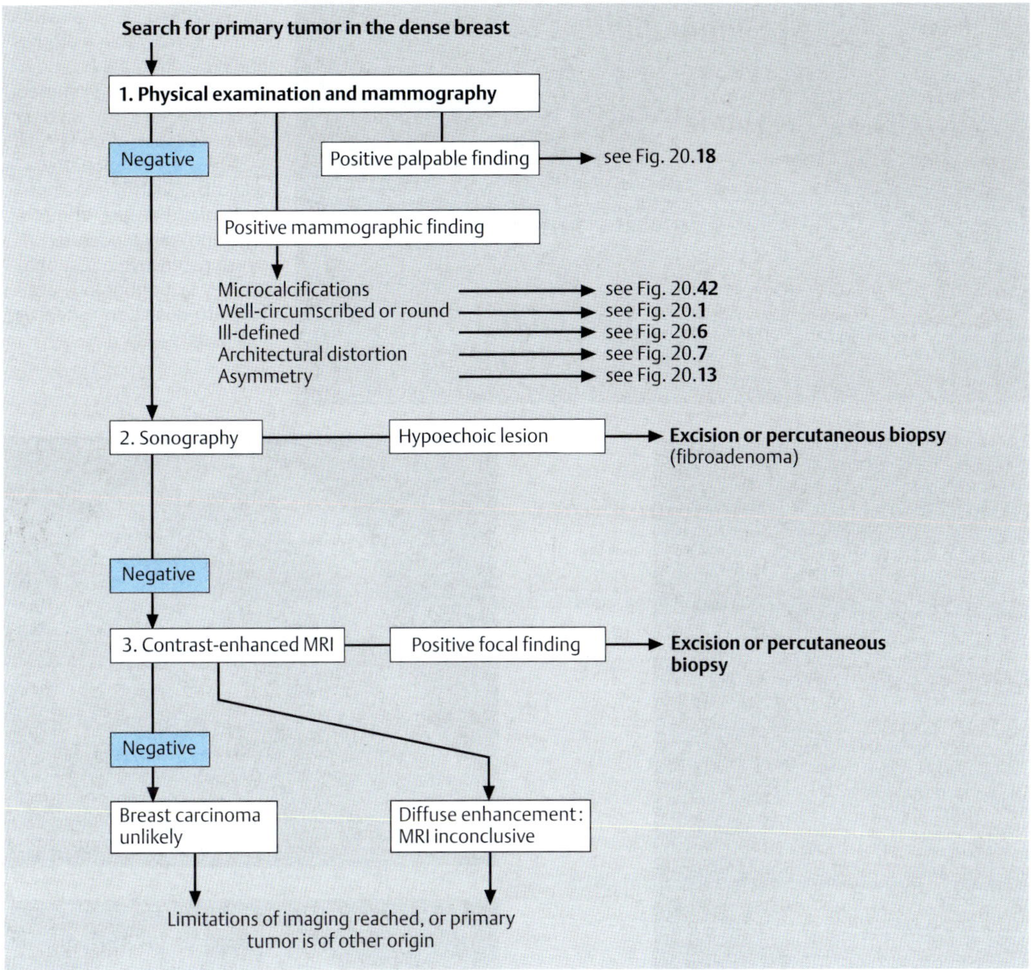

Fig. 20.**19** Search for the primary tumor in the mammographically dense breast

tradictory. The pattern of enhancement can serve to find or select suscipious areas for a targeted percutaneous biopsy.

Dense Breast and Special Considerations

Pain

Pain, especially when it varies with the menstrual cycle, is a frequent manifestation of fibrocystic alteration. It usually is bilateral and more severe in the upper outer quadrants. If a thorough mammographic and clinical evaluation is negative, the patient should be informed of the probable hormonal cause and be reassured. In general, this pain is not a manifestation of a malignancy.

If the patient complains of localized pain, experienced as “crawling ants” or a “creeping sensation” and it appears essentially unrelated to the menstrual cycle, it should be taken seriously and deserves further evaluation just like a palpable abnormality.

Search for Primary Tumor

In the woman with an axillary nodal metastasis and no palpable lesion in the breast to suggest a primary mammary carcinoma, clinical imaging in the usual order is indicated.

If mammography fails to identify the primary lesion in the breast, supplemental methods, such as sonography and particularly contrast-enhanced MRI, can be helpful (Figs. 20.**19** and 20.**20a–d**).

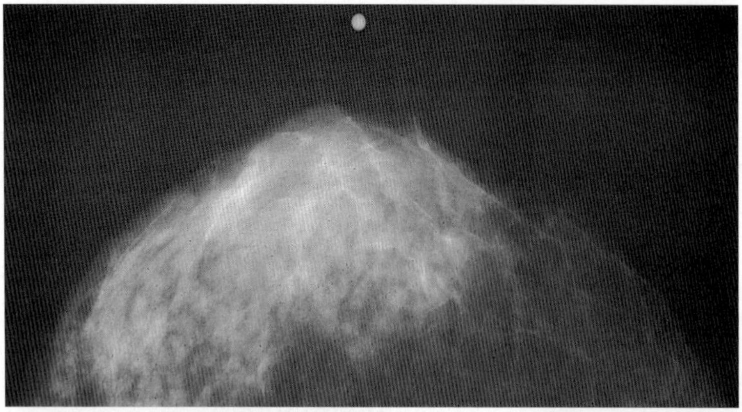

a

Fig. 20.**20a–d** This patient with unremarkable mammographic, sonographic, and clinical findings was referred to MRI for search of a primary tumor because of metastatic axillary lymphadenopathy
a and **b** Slightly impaired evaluation because of mammographically moderately dense parenchyma (CC and ML views). Sonography also failed to detect any underlying malignancy

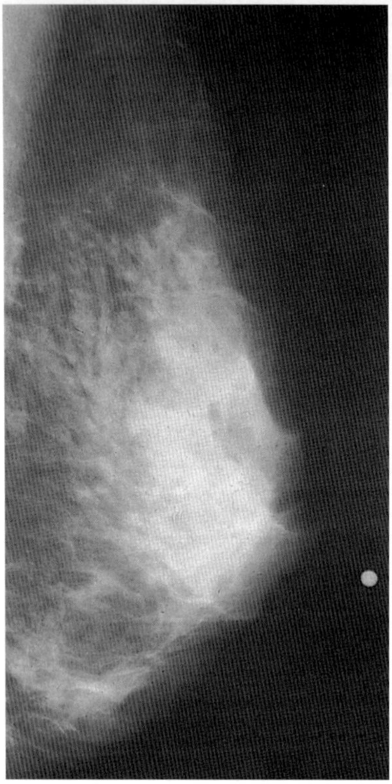

b

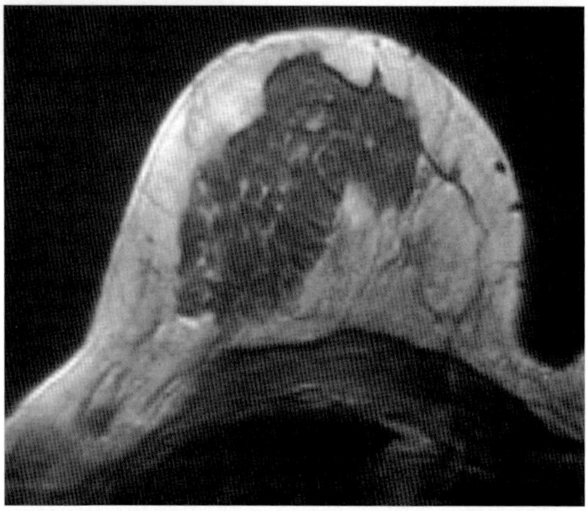

c

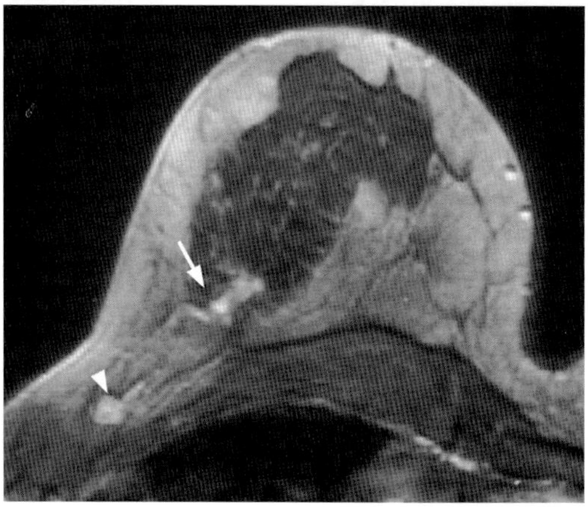

d

Fig. 20.**20c** Representative section before administration of Gd-DTPA
d The same section as shown in (**c**) after administration of Gd-DTPA discloses within the nonenhancing parenchyma a highly suspicious, strongly enhancing lesion (arrow). An additional second strongly enhancing lesion with small extensions is noted in the prepectoral region. Both MRI-suspicious lesions were localized for the surgeon under MR-guidance. Histologically, a small ductal carcinoma (arrow) could be confirmed as well as an involved intramammary lymph node (arrow head) (from Heywang-Köbrunner et al.[13])

Fig. 20.**21a–d** This 61-year-old patient came for screening mammography. The patient had noticed the unilateral nipple retraction "for a long time." No evidence of a palpable finding or discharge
a Oblique view
b Craniocaudal view
A discrete architectural distortion was suspected in the retroareolar region on the cc-view only. Because of this finding and the unilaterality of the nipple retraction, magnification views in two planes were performed

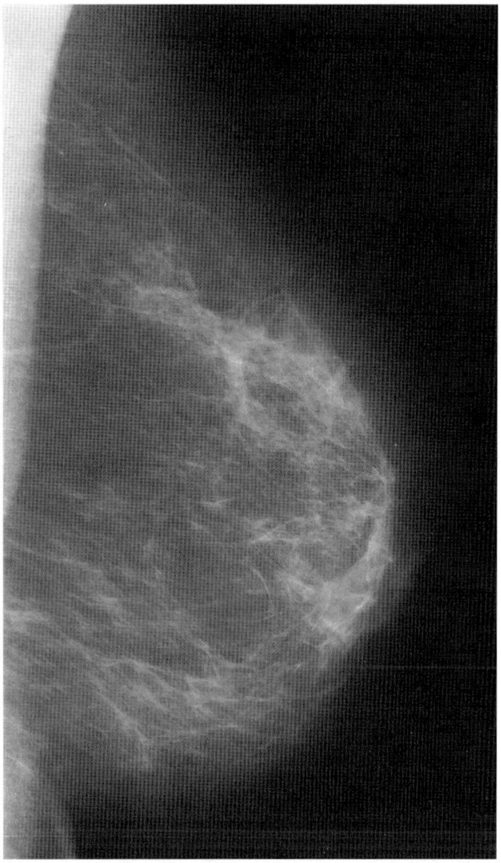
a

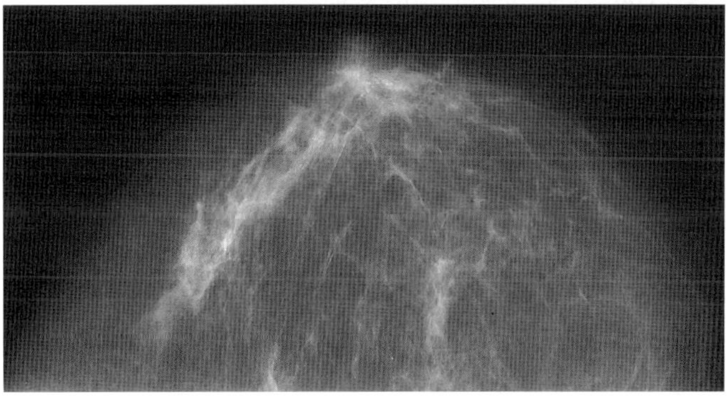
b

Fig. 20.**21c** u.**d** ▷

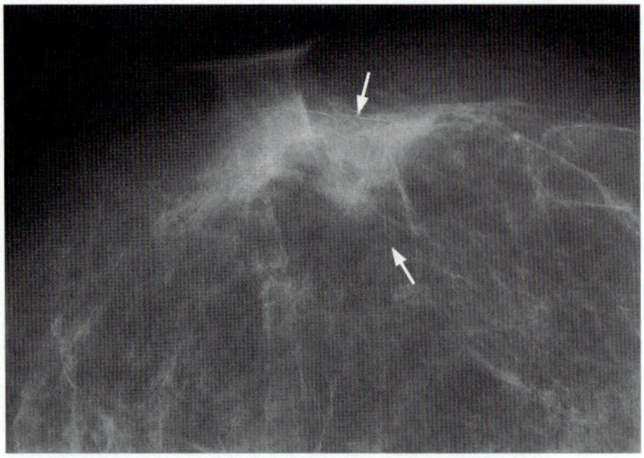

c

Fig. 20.**21 c** The spot compression clearly discloses the carcinoma as typical spiculated lesion

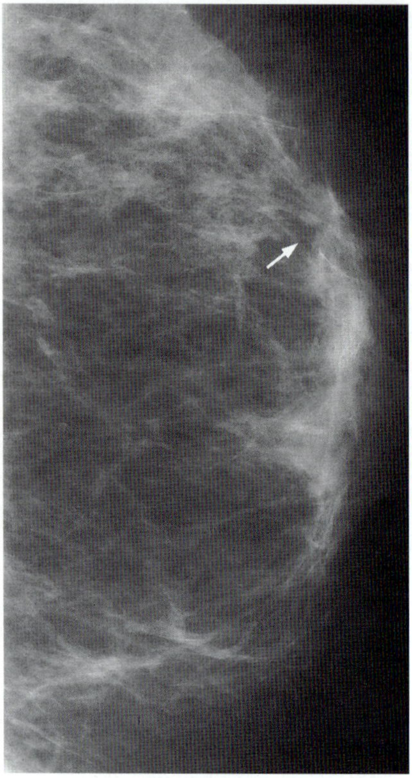

d

Fig. 20.**21 d** Only the magnification view in the oblique projection can positively localize the carcinoma (cranial) in the second plane. *Histology:* ductal carcinoma (mammography by Dr. D. Breuer, Halle, Germany)

If contrast-enhanced MRI is negative or inconclusive because of diffuse enhancement, breast imaging has reached its limitation, or the primary tumor is not in the breast. In the majority of these rare cases, the primary tumor is indeed found in other organs and, consequently, searching for a primary tumor in other organs is appropriate in the presence of an axillary nodal metastasis. This also applies to adenocarcinomatous or even hormone-receptor positive metastases. (Depending on the method used for hormone-receptor analysis, carcinomas of other origin, rarely even lymphomas, can be hormone-receptor positive).

Nipple Retraction

Nipple retraction has to be evaluated carefully. Since a high percentage of new, unilateral nipple retraction is induced by an underlying carcinoma, supplemental methods, above all contrast-enhanced MRI, should be employed generously. (Figs. 20.**21** and 20.**22**, see also Fig. 14.**4b–e**).

Discharge

Discharge of the dense breast is guided by the same differential diagnostic considerations as discharge found in the breast of normal parenchymal density (see p. 389).

Microcalcifications

(Fig. 20.**42**)

Possibilities and limitations of diagnostic methods

Mammography

Mammography is the only diagnostic method that can reliably detect calcifications suggestive for malignancy. Detecting calcifications is of great importance because about 30–40% of carcinomas harbor microcalcifications and since these carcinomas, because of the microcalcifications, are often discovered in a very early stage,

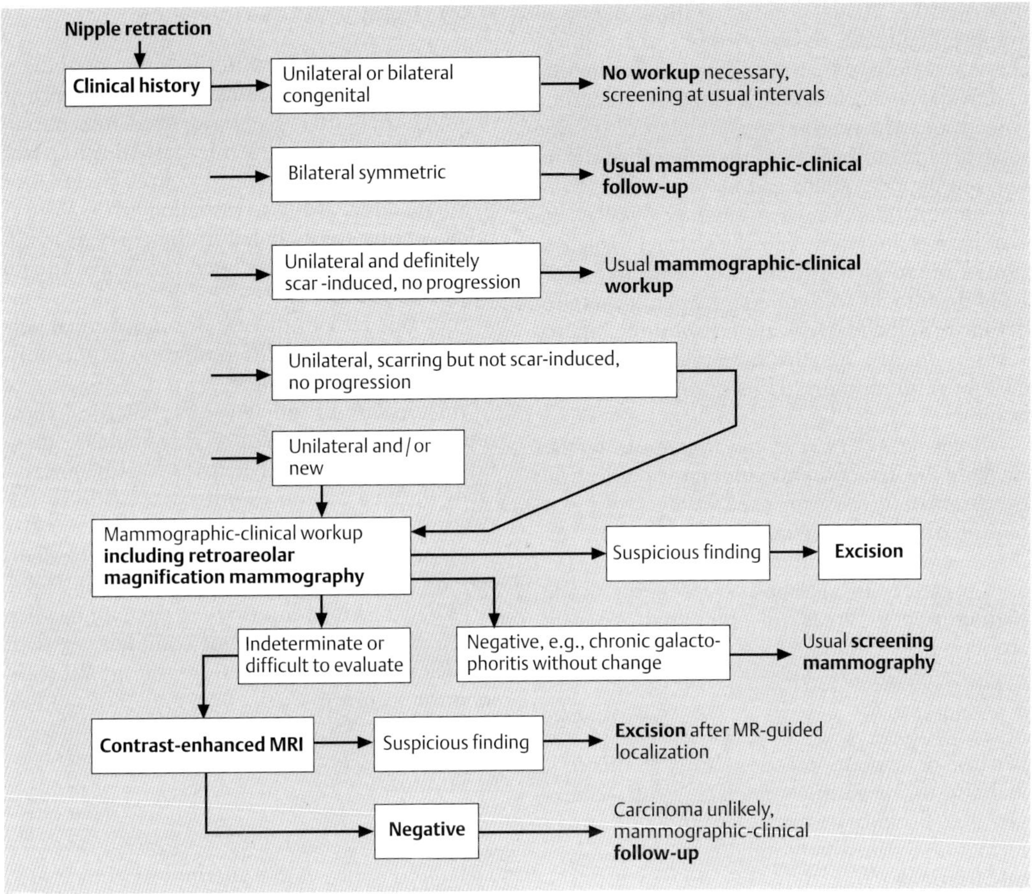

Fig. 20.**22** Nipple retraction of the mammographically dense breast

frequently in a preinvasive stage (DCIS). The problem, however, is that a *considerable number of benign changes also contain microcalcifications.* The indiscriminate excision of all microcalcifications would yield a carcinoma in only every 10th to 20th specimen. Such a high number of diagnostic biopsies can be justified neither medically nor economically. Therefore, the presence of microcalcifications should not invariably lead to a recommendation to biopsy.

Technical Requirements for Mammographic Detection and Differential Diagnosis of Microcalcifications

Correct exposure is particularly important since underexposure can render microcalcifications undetectable within dense tissue (see p. 22).

Adequate compression is equally important since it improves sharpness and contrast (see p. 18).

Magnification mammography. Its use yields a better morphologic evaluation and often the detection of additional fine calcifications. Thus, it improves the differentiation between calcifications judged to be benign or suscipious for malignancy, increases the identification of carcinomas, and helps to reduce the number of unnecessary biopsies. Moreover, *determining the exact extent* of the carcinoma may be decisively improved by magnification mammography.

Future Technical Improvements

The continued development of *digital imaging* may result in better visualization of microcalcifications in the future. Digital imaging plates can improve the image contrast within mammographically dense tissue through their linear characteristic curve and by largely eliminating underexposures. New image detectors hopefully will advance the presently insufficient resolution to an acceptable degree, so that the other advantages of digital systems can be implemented.

The introduction of *X-ray tubes with microfocus* has resulted in noticeably sharper visualization of microcalcifications, even if located away from the film, by minimizing the penumbra. Together with the magnification technique, microfocus technique has the potential to solve the current resolution problems of digital mammography.

Computer-aided image analysis should further increase the detection rate of microcalcifications by eliminating misses caused by decreasing attention of the radiologist. For this purpose, very sensitive computerized detection would be used for prescreening. Such a program could highlight any areas of potential concern, attracting the radiologist's attention.

Sonography

Because of its poor detection of DCIS due to its inability to image microcalcifications, sonography does not provide any relevant diagnostic information to the differential diagnosis of microcalcifications.

Individual cases of microcalcifications with sonographic visualization of thickened ducts or of the larger microcalcifications have been reported in the literature, but this does not justify the conclusion that sonography can diagnose microinvasive or carcinomas in situ.

Magnetic Resonance Imaging

MRI does *not* appear to be suitable for the differential diagnosis of microcalcifications.

The reason is that most proliferative changes associated with microcalcifications enhance with a pattern similar to that of carcinomas in situ with microcalcification and are therefore indistinguishable. Furthermore, it can be assumed that only 80% to 85% of carcinomas in situ show enhancement (which can be uncharacteristic, i.e., delayed or diffuse).

Core Biopsy

The role of core biopsy in the differential diagnosis of microcalcifications is still the subject of ongoing trials. It is to be expected that not all carcinomas in situ with microcalcifications are included in the specimens procured by FNA or by single cores owing to sampling error. Even if calcifications are included in the cores, it is not guaranteed that an associated carcinoma in situ will be included.[14]

For this reason, the use of conventional percutaneous biopsy for differentiation of microcalcifications may be limited.

In the case of indeterminate microcalcifications, percutaneous biopsy may increase diagnostic confidence and help to avoid unnecessarily delayed diagnoses otherwise made by follow-up examinations only.

A negative core biopsy of suscipious calcifications, however, cannot replace surgical biopsy.

The latest techniques using vacuum needles, which allow the removal of complete areas of suspicion, promise a further significant improvement of accuracy.

Summary

Mammography is the method of choice for the detection and differential diagnosis of microcalcifications.
Meticulous analysis of mammographically visualized microcalcifications is the prerequisite for

- Accurate detection of carcinomas
- Best possible assessment of the extent of carcinomas
- Avoiding high numbers of unnecessary biopsies of benign changes with microcalcifications

Analysis of Microcalcifications

The goal of analyzing calcifications is the categorization of calcifications as:

- Highly suspicious for malignancy
- Definitely benign
- Indeterminate

■ Microcalcifications Suggestive of Malignancy

■ Principal Classification

The systematic investigations of Lanyi and other authors[15–18] have shown that typically malignant microcalcifications arise almost exclusively in *invasive and noninvasive ductal carcinomas*, while lobular carcinomas calcify only very rarely and fail to develop a mammographically typical calcification pattern. These observations form the basis for considering calcifications that are ductal in distribution and configuration and are suggestive of malignancy.

Calcifications are analyzed as to

- Their location (malignant calcifications are implicitly intramammary)
- Their individual shapes
- Their distribution pattern

■ Typical Morphologies of Calcifications Suggestive of Malignancy

The following individual shapes are typical of carcinomas:

Linear and Branching Calcifications (Casting)

(Fig. 20.**23a–c**)

These calcifications, which can branch and assume *V-shapes or Y-shapes*, correspond to calcified casts of the small lactiferous ducts and are frequently a manifestation of a *comedo-type DCIS* or an *invasive ductal carcinoma* (see also p. 195). Their margins are irregular.

These calcifications are to be differentiated from the needle-like or branching calcifications of the so-called plasma cell mastitis (Figs. 20.**24b** and 20.**25**) that are generally larger and may have smooth parallel walls. Because the branching and casting microcalcifications are a frequent sign of carcinoma, the suspicion of malignancy should be raised whenever such calcifications are observed *within* a cluster of microcalcifications.

Pleomorphic and Larger Granular Calcifications

These microcalcifications are very variable in size, shape, and density and have been described as resembling crushed stone. The individual calcification within a group can be extremely *irregular*, sometimes even bizarre in shape (Figs. 20.**26a** and **b**) and ranges from fine to 2 mm in size. Usually each calcification is different from the others.

These calcifications have to be differentiated from the bizarre calcifications in fibroadenomas, which usually (but not always) are larger and coarser, frequently exhibit a different distribution pattern, and often are associated with a large, coarse dystrophic calcification. If such calcifications are contained in a completely well-circumscribed soft-tissue mass, this can be diagnostically helpful by indicating a fibroadenoma. However, any less characteristic soft-tissue density around microcalcifications is generally not helpful (see p. 375). In addition to fibroadenomas, the larger granular calcifications can be observed in certain proliferative fibrocystic

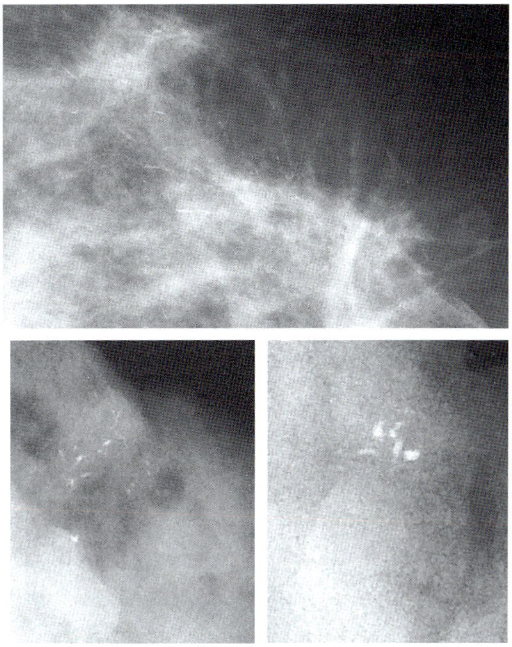

a b c

Fig. 20.**23a–c**
a Multiple needle-like and fine microcalcifications in a ductal distribution (magnification view). *Histology:* DCIS, comedo-type
b Group of microcalcifications including several elongated or v-shaped calcifications: highly suspicious. *Histology:* DCIS, comedo type with microinvasion
c Group of elongated and very polymorphic, suspicious microcalcifications. *Histology:* DCIS, comedo-type

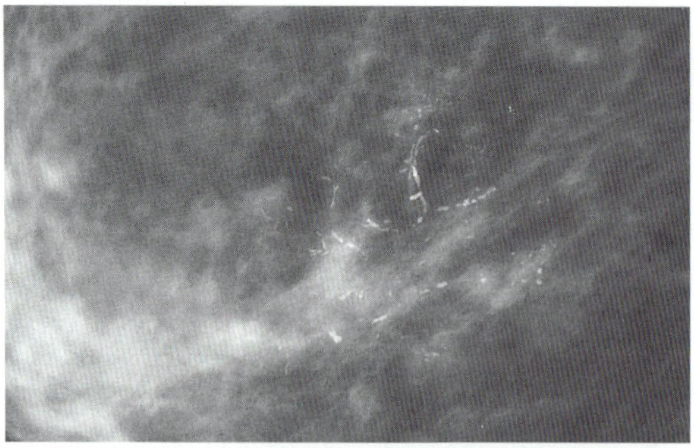
a

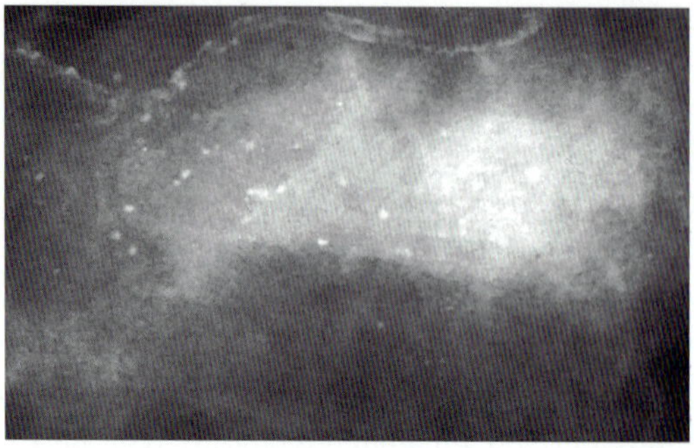
c

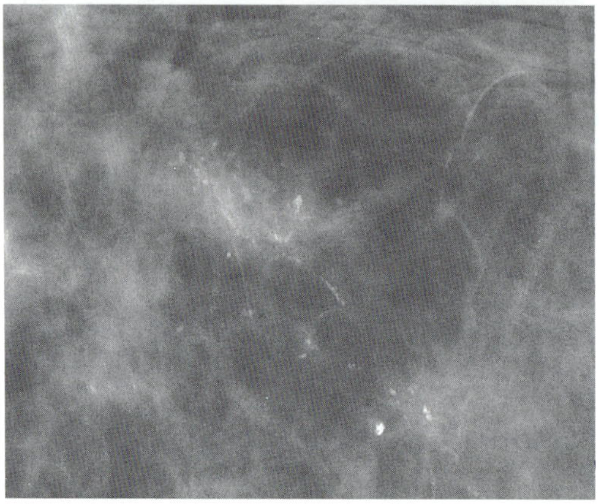
b

Fig. 20.**24a–c** Though pleomorphic, linear calcifications must be considered strongly suggestive of malignancy, smooth, linear calcifications can be a manifestation of a benign condition

a Relatively coarse, elongated, partially v-shaped or y-shaped casting calcifications that grow along the ducts. In addition to these coarse calcifications, fine and tiny microcalcifications suggest the correct diagnosis: DCIS

b Calcifications with similar morphology and distribution as in (**a**). *Histology:* so-called plasma cell mastitis, no malignancy

c Diffusely distributed microcalcifications with slight polymorphism including individual elongated forms. *Histology:* fibrocystic disease including secretory type calcifications

changes (Fig. 20.**27**) and analyzing the distribution pattern may contribute to the differential diagnosis (see below).

Fine-granular Calcifications

Fine-granular calcifications can occasionally be a manifestation of a carcinoma if they are extremely delicate and typically clustered in *small groups* or *segmentally distributed* (see below) (Fig. 20.**28a** and **b**). These distribution patterns suggest fine-granular calcifications in noncomedo DCIS. In the micropapillary and cribriform subtypes of the noncomedo DCIS and in the corresponding invasive carcinomas, these very fine-granular calcifications precipitate in the secretion-filled interspaces between the papillary or cribriform cellular proliferations.

Since fine-granular calcifications are frequently associated with benign changes, these calcifications have to be considered uncharacteristic of carcinoma. They should only raise a

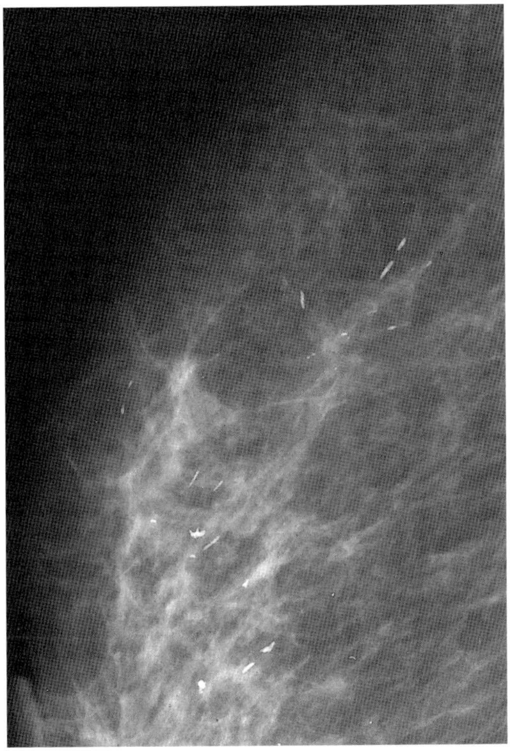

Fig. 20.**25** Coarse needle-shaped calcifications, following the ducts and oriented toward the nipple: "Plasma cell mastitis"

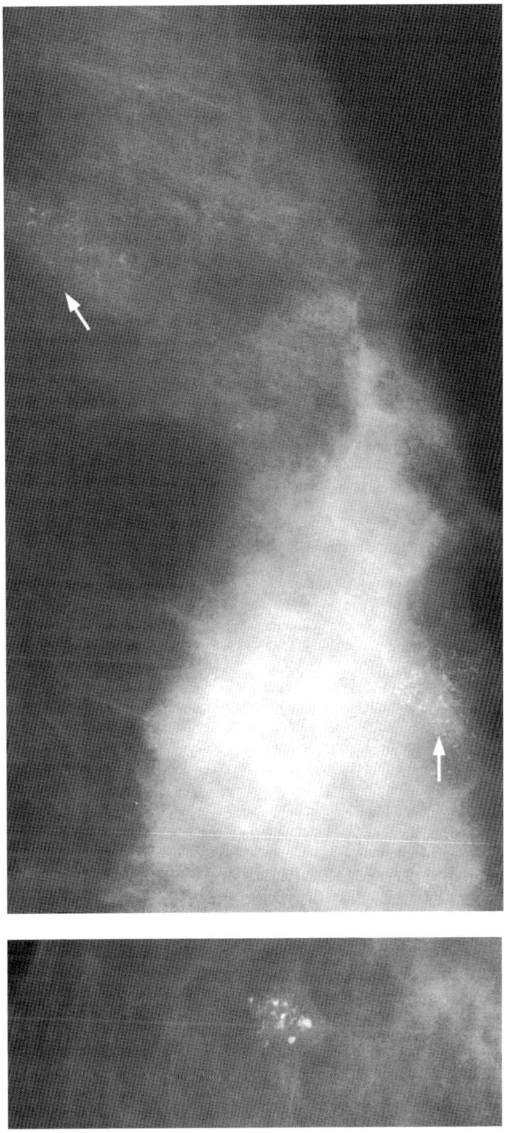

a

b

Fig. 20.**26a** and **b** Pleomorphic microcalcifications suggestive of malignancy can be both very fine and very coarse (> 1 mm)

a The mediolateral view shows two groups of very fine pleomorphic microcalcifications, 4 cm apart, in the lateral aspect of the breast: multicentric DCIS

b Delineation of a small group of considerably coarser pleomorphic calcifications, so-called granular mircrocalcifications. Despite the accompanying soft-tissue density, these calcifications should not be mistaken for bizarre calcifications of a fibroadenoma. Furthermore, the somewhat irregular contour of the accompanying soft-tissue density should be noted. *Histology:* DCIS

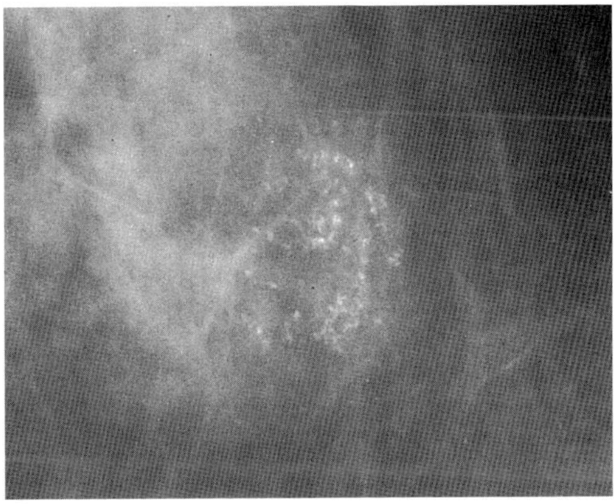

Fig. 20.**27** Large group of polymorphic and casting microcalcifications highly suspicious. *Histology:* DCIS ▷

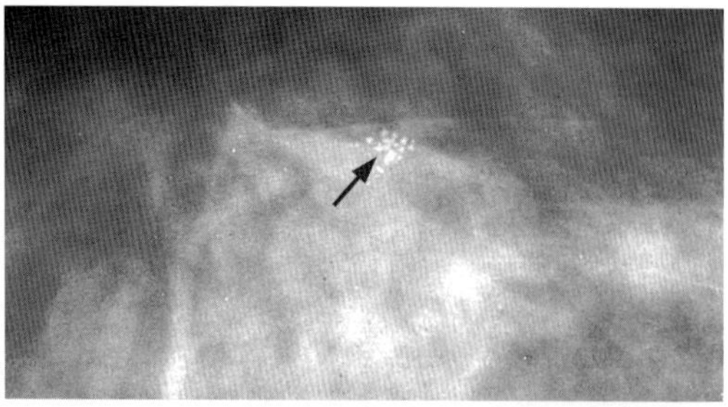
a

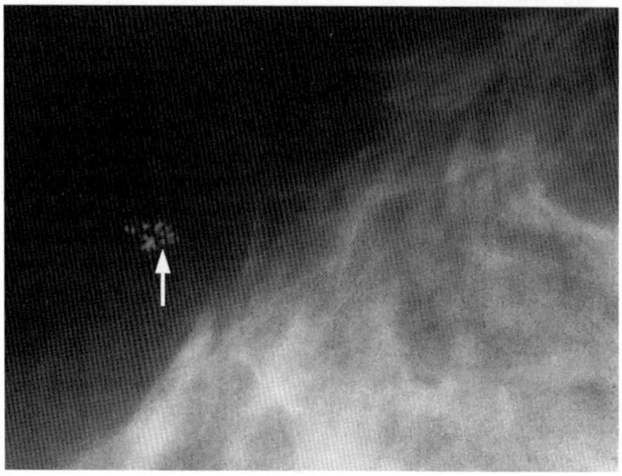
b

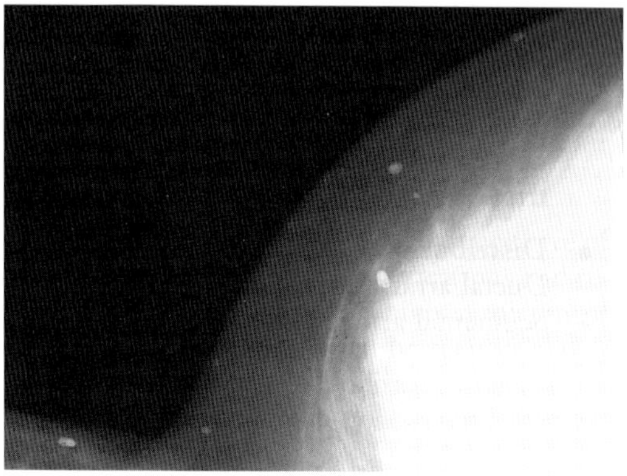
c

Fig. 20.**31a–c**
a The craniocaudal view shows several round calcifications close together in the retroareolar region (arrows)
b These calcifications are projected over the subcutaneous region (arrow) in the tangential view
c Underexposed film copy of the tangential view with cutaneous calcifications of another patient. The relative underexposure (**b, c**) is necessary to illustrate the cutaneous location of the calcifications

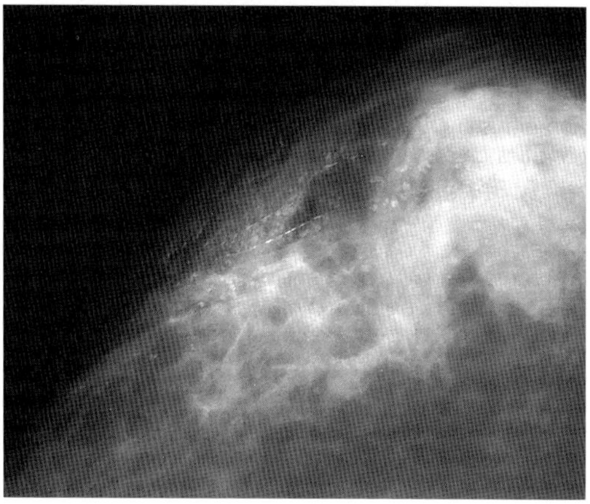

Fig. 20.**32** Artifacts caused by ointment applied to the skin

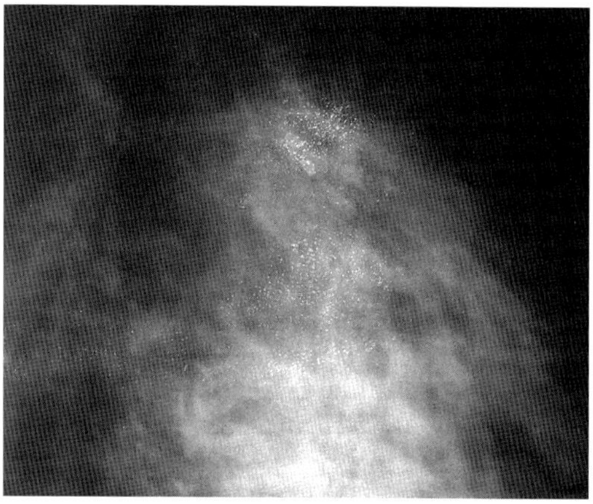

Fig. 20.**33** Artifact of the intensifying screen: fingerprint.

on the intensifying screen caused by fingerprints, dust, and defects of the screen. Furthermore, dot-like or linear artifacts can be imprinted on the film by the rolls in the automatic processor.

■ Benign Intramammary Calcifications

The analysis of the shape and distribution determines the correct diagnosis of benign intramammary calcifications.

Typical Morphology of Benign Calcifications

(Figs. 20.**34**–20.**40a–c**)

Large (> 1 mm), rounded calcifications with or without central radiolucency can develop in scars or fat necroses (subcutaneous without trauma, usually bilateral with calcifying liponecrosis), "plasma cell mastitis," and calcified fibroadenomas or papillomas (whereby the soft tissue density may or may not be visible). *They are invariably benign.*

Semicircular or shell-like calcifications around radiolucent lesions can develop in oil cysts, scars, and fat necrosis, as part of a foreign-body reaction around droplets of silicone or wax injected for augmentation, in calcifying liponecrosis, and in "plasma cell mastitis."

They also are *always benign.*

These calcifications have to be distinguished from *shell-like calcifications along the periphery of lesions of soft-tissue density.*

They occur:

- *In fibroadenomas or papillomas.* Together with other evolving calcifications confined to an oval or round area or within a smoothly outlined soft-tissue density, the evolving peripheral calcification is relatively characteristic of fibroadenomas or papillomas. Since small peripheral calcifications are not absolute proof, follow-up examinations at 6-, 12-, 24-, and 36-month intervals should be obtained for confirmation, showing progression to typical coarse calcifications.
  In the case of additional suspicious findings (e.g., indistinctly outlined surrounding density), further evaluation of individual cases is indicated.
- *In cysts.* Calcifications in the wall can develop in oil cysts or milk of calcium cysts but can also indicate a complex cyst. If an oil cyst (radiographically visualized central radiolucency) or a simple milk of calcium cyst ("teacups" on ML mammogram or, in the case of large cysts, sonographically moveable sedimentations) has been documented, further diagnostic steps are unnecessary. Otherwise, further workup (aspiration or biopsy) is needed. The reason is that particularly hemorrhagic cysts, which can be a manifestation of a papilloma or carcinoma, have the tendency to form mural calcifications.
- *As a foreign-body reaction around deposits of silicone or wax* that have been injected for augmentation. These shell-like calcifications are *definitely benign.* The usually increased density due to fibrosis, silicone, and calcifications, however, compromises the overall evaluation of the breast tissue (Fig. 20.**37b**).

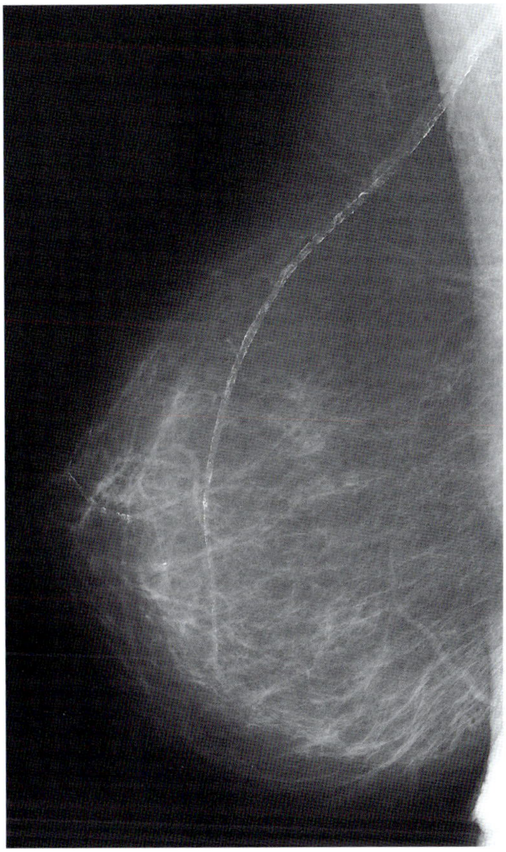

Fig. 20.**34** Linear and round calcifications directly following a narrow, vascular structure: arteriosclerosis

Coarse, popcorn-like, or bizarre calcifications larger than 2 mm can be found in fibroadenomas and papillomas. The larger these calcifications are, the more characteristic they are. Such *characteristic popcorn-like or bizarre calcifications support the diagnosis of a fibroadenoma or papilloma with a high degree of certainty.*

Only *if (very rare!) calcifications suggestive of malignancy are found next to these calcifications* or if coarse calcifications are surrounded *by an irregularly outlined density* must the differential diagno-

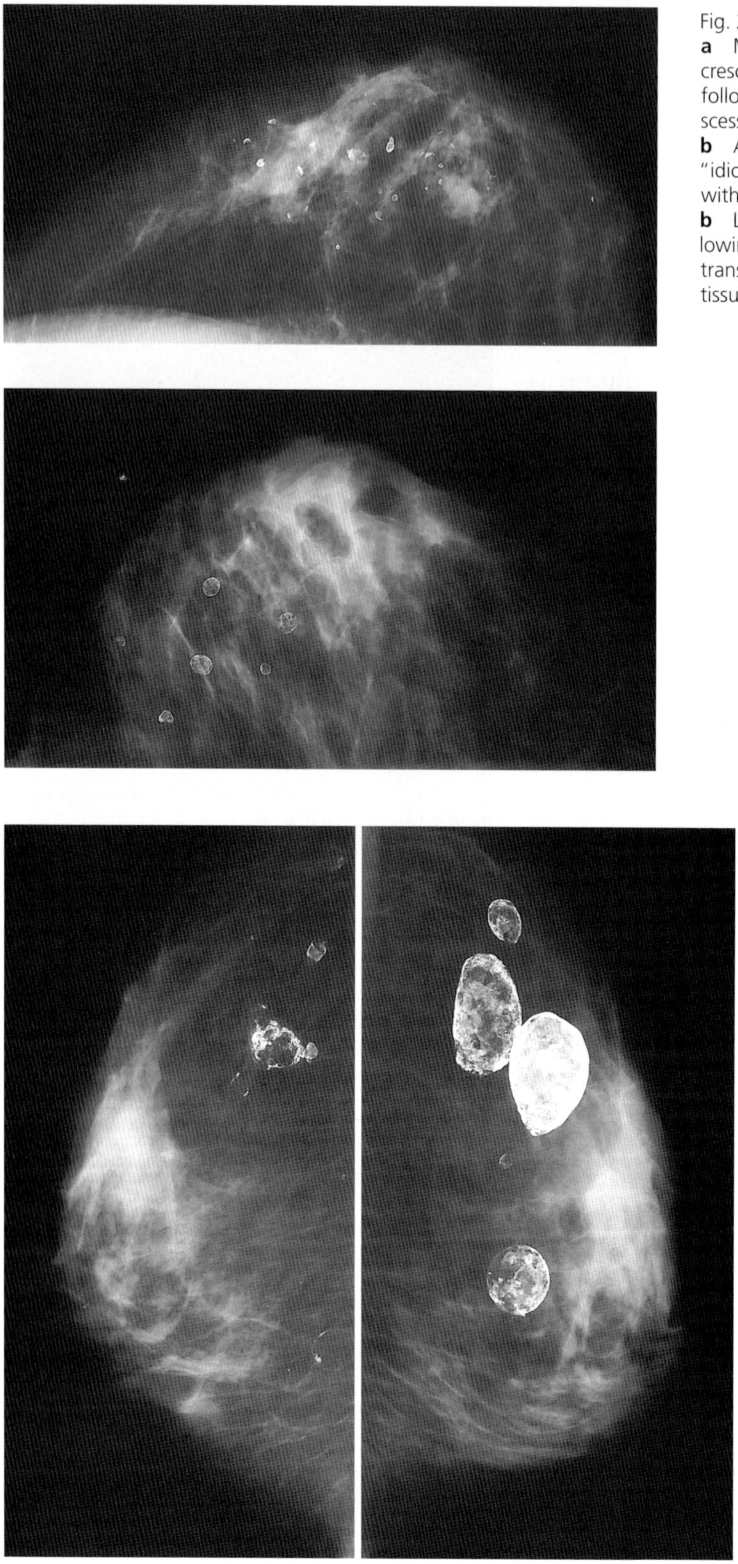

a

b

c

Fig. 20.**35a–c**
a Multiple elongated, curved, crescentic, and ring-like calcifications following recurrent mastitis with abscess incision and drainage
b Almost symmetrically arranged "idiopathic" calcifying liponecrosis without known preceding trauma
b Large calcified fat necrosis following breast augmentation with transplanted autogenous adipose tissue (ML view)

sis consider *necrotic calcifications in a carcinoma* or *a calcified fibroadenoma* surrounded by a carcinoma.

It is also important to keep in mind that *bizarre fibroadenomatous calcifications smaller than 2 mm can resemble pleomorphic granular calcifications found in carcinomas.*

Consequently, bizarre calcifications can only establish the diagnosis of a fibroadenoma if they are large enough and show an arrangement uncharacteristic of malignancy.

Coarse, needle-like calcifications can occur:

- *In so-called plasma cell mastitis.* Like ductal calcifications, they follow the ductal system. Histologically, they are intraductal and periductal. *Despite a ductal or segmental, V-shaped and Y-shaped arrangement, they can be clearly identified as benign as long as they are large, coarse, and smooth.* A central radiolucency within the needles or a combination with round, coarse calcifications with or without radiolucency is considered definitive proof. Caution is advised when evaluating *needle-like, fine* calcifications since the differentiation between a primary ductal carcinoma and "plasma cell mastitis" can be difficult (Fig. 20.**24a**).
- *In scars.* Mainly, *coarse needles* and *bizarre linear calcifications* are characteristically seen along the scars. Again, caution should be taken when evaluating *delicate* calcifications and possible ductal distribution since a new or residual carcinoma within or adjacent to the scar has to be excluded.

Parallel microcalcifications are characteristic of vascular calcifications. They do not follow (in two projections) the course of ductal structure. Even if these calcifications appear amorphous or fragmented, the correct diagnosis can usually be established as long as the outer border of the calcifications form two *parallel* lines that resemble railroad tracks. The outer contour of the lines is smooth, but the lines need not be completely calcified. The vascular nature is further supported when the vessels are delineated as tubular soft-tissue densities within the surrounding adipose tissue.

Small calcifications *that are round, punctate, or stippled and have a uniform shape* are *characteristically* associated with various forms of fibrocystic changes. Most calcifications are diffusely distributed or are in a rosette-like arrangement (see below). Only with additional suspicion (existence of adjacent suspicious microcalcifications or masses) must malignancy coexisting with fibrocystic changes be excluded.

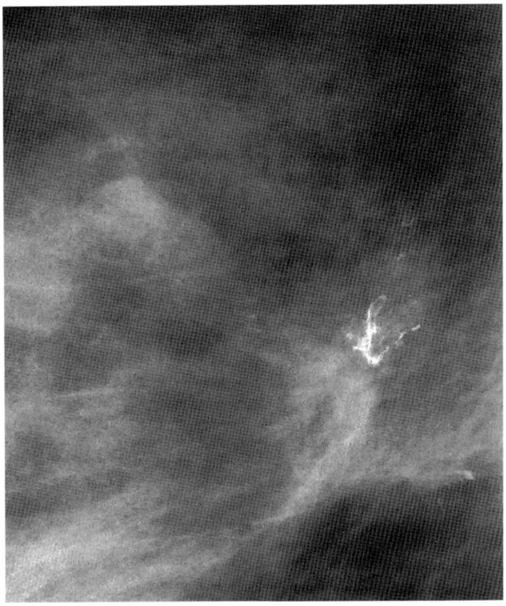

Fig. 20.**36** Elongated, in part linear, dystrophic calcifications within scar-induced architectural distortion

Calcifications that show a *teacup phenomenon* are characteristic of fibrocystic changes (Fig. 20.**39**).

The teacup phenomenon is caused by sedimentation in microcysts (cysts containing milk of calcium) (see also p. 147). Since the teacup phenomenon may be detectable only on the 90° lateral view, *obtaining a 90° lateral view—if possible, with magnification—is mandatory for the assessment of indeterminate microcalcifications.*

In the craniocaudal view, these calcifications frequently appear amorphous, and accurate diagnosis cannot be made on this view. The teacup phenomenon is usually seen in some of the microcalcifications only. The diagnosis of a benign process can be made with a high degree of certainty if *neither calcifications suggestive of malignancy nor suspicious masses* (as evidence of a carcinoma that *coexists* with the described benign changes) are observed amidst these calcifications (Fig. 20.**41**).

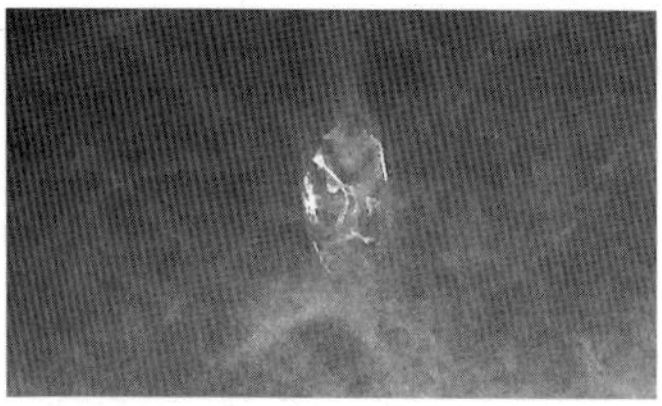

a

Fig. 20.**37a** and **b**
a Fine eggshell-like calcifications projected over an oval radiolucency: calcifying oil cyst
b Subtle shell-like (in part, punctate) calcifications around drop-like deposits of wax, injected for augmentation

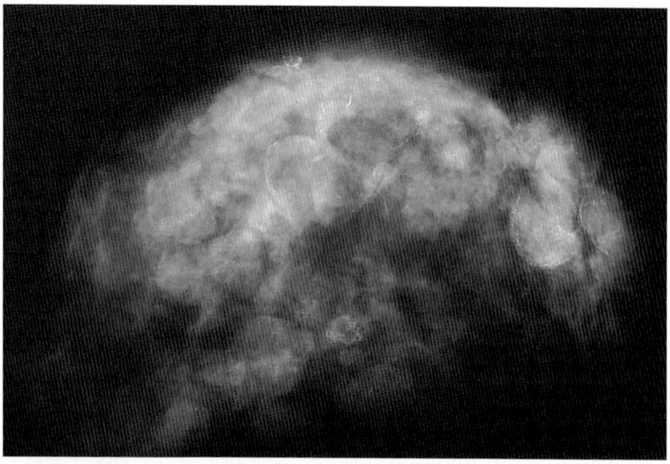

b

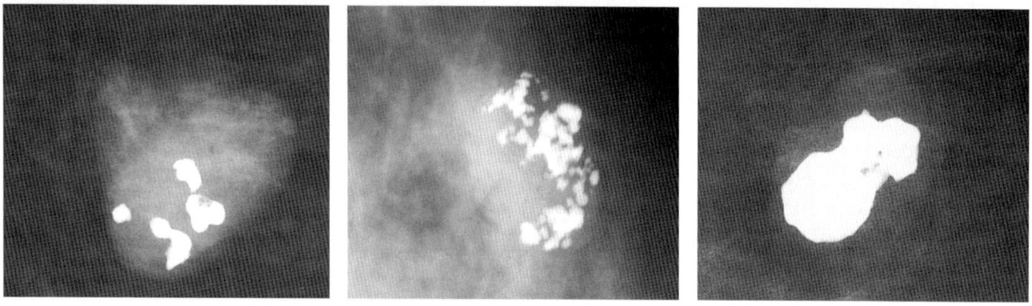

a b c

Fig. 20.**38a–c**
a Several coarse, irregularly outlined calcifications within a lobulated lesion: typical fibroadenoma
b Barely discernible oval density with typical coarse bizarre fibroadenomatous calcifications
c Macrocalcifications of an almost completely calcified fibroadenoma

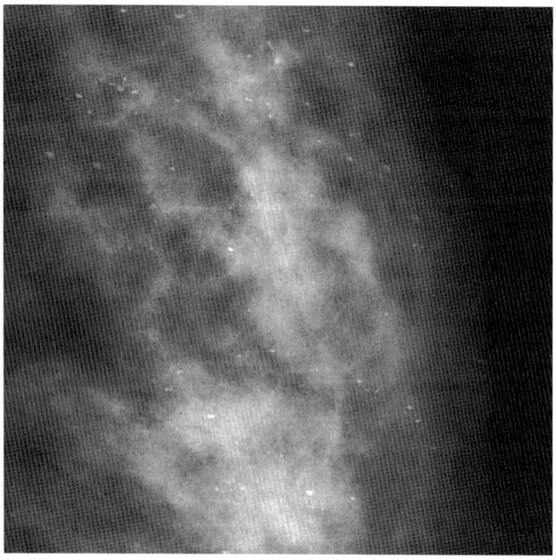

Fig. 20.**39** In part round, in part linear and multiple crescentic, teacup calcifications due to sedimentation of calcific particles within milk of calcium cysts, only seen in the mediolateral view

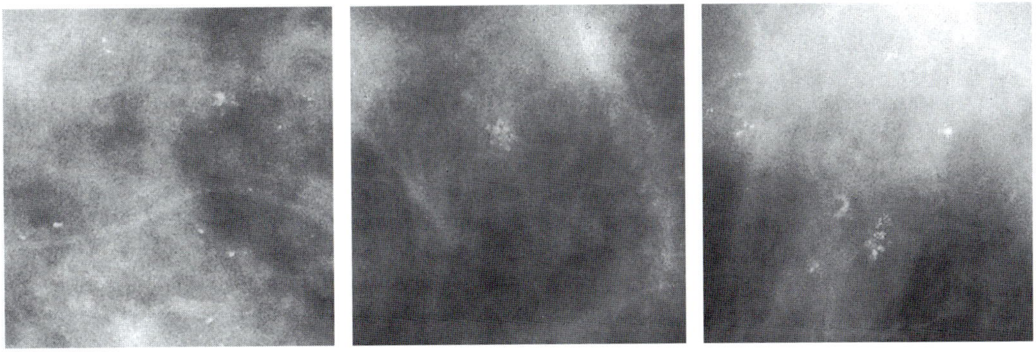

a b c

Fig. 20.**40a–c**
a Punctate scattered calcifications in blunt duct adenosis
b Several punctate, clustered calcifications in a round group (morula-like): small cystic adenosis
c Typical image of multiple, morula-like calcifications with intralobular distribution in sclerosing adenosis

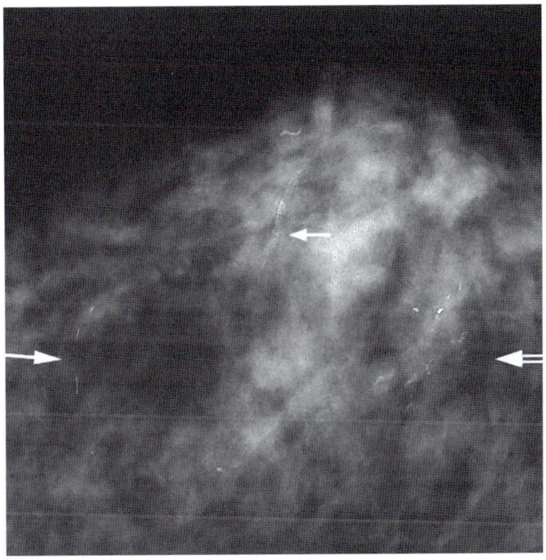

Fig. 20.**41** Long arrow: calcifications as part of a plasma cell mastitis
Short arrow: vascular calcification
Open arrow: segmentally arranged, pleomorphic calcifications of DCIS

Typical Distribution of Benign Calcifications

Solitary calcifications are characteristically benign. Several solitary calcifications can be observed in one or both breasts.

Diffuse (evenly distributed throughout the parenchyma, see also Fig. 20.**40**) **and symmetric distribution** favors benignity. Diffusely distributed, mostly symmetric calcifications are typically associated with certain types of fibrocystic changes, mainly sclerosing adenosis. As proven by Lanyi, the symmetric appearance of malignant microcalcifications is extremely rare.

The calcifications in benign changes are frequently punctate, stippled, or round.

If amorphous calcifications show a symmetric distribution, a predominantly monomorphic appearance and, in particular, the teacup phenomenon, the diagnosis of fibrocystic changes is supported.

It is important that *no branching or pleomorphic calcifications* are seen among *these calcifications* and that *segmental distribution* cannot be identified. Otherwise, a malignancy coexistent with benign changes must be considered.

Clustered calcifications should be carefully evaluated.

To determine whether microcalcifications are clustered, the cluster must be visualized *in two pro-*

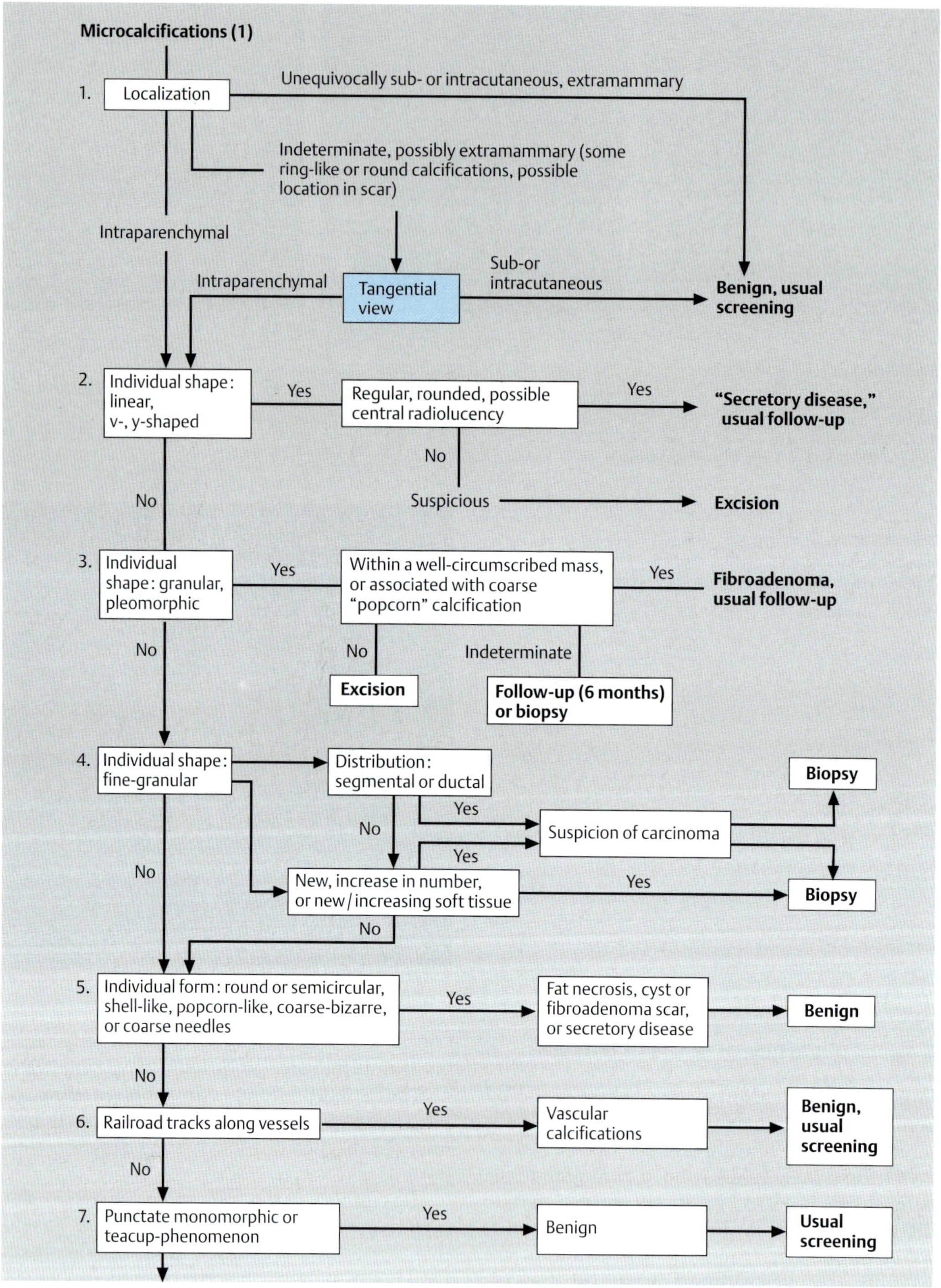

Fig. 20.**42** Microcalcifications

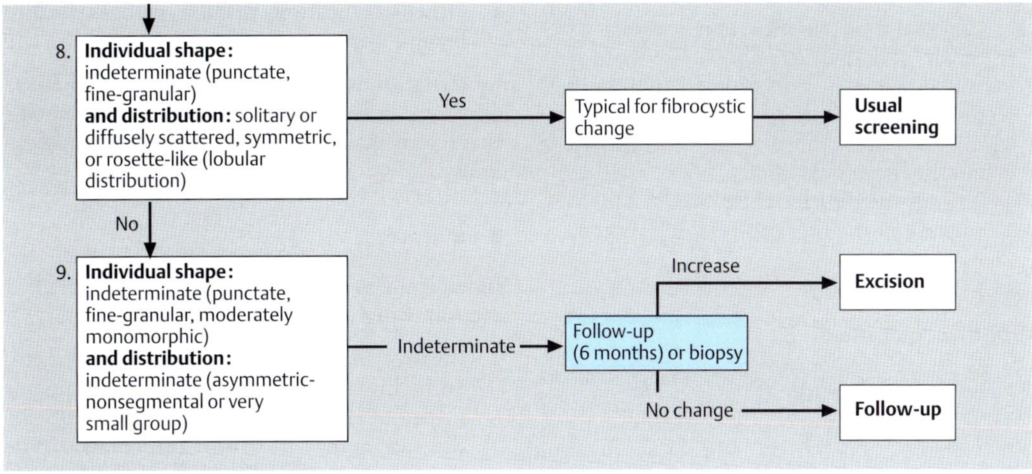

Fig. 20.**42** (Cont.)

jections. Only an evaluation in two projections can separate a true cluster from a coincidental superimposition of calcifications that are at different locations but seen next to each other in one view. Such *"pseudogroups"* are *not indicative of malignancy*.

Typical benign groups can be observed:

- In *calcifying liponecrosis* and subcutaneous calcifications. Benignity can be proved by documenting the subcutaneous location (tangential view) or by identifying a central radiolucency or round configuration.
- In a confined small area corresponding to a *fibroadenoma or papilloma* and exhibiting a typical morphology of the calcifications (see above) or, if the calcifications are within a smoothly outlined (see definition p. 169) soft-tissue density.
- *Along scars* as typical individual forms (coarse needles, ring-like, round calcifications) and lacking any malignant forms and distribution pattern.
- *In microcystic adenosis* (Figs. 20.**40b** and **c**). These calcifications characteristically are close to each other in a round, *rosette-like or morula-like* arrangement. They are in the lobule and, *because of their lobular location, are not indicative of malignancy*.
  The diagnosis of benignity is further supported by the *multiplicity and symmetry* of such small groups and by relatively uniform morphology. Additional casting or pleomorphic calcifications in a ductal or segmental distribution have to be excluded. Otherwise, a carcinoma must be considered.

Track-like calcifications along vessels are definitely benign (see above).

Summary

(Fig. 20.**42**)

Extramammary calcifications, with their location proven by tangential views, are benign. Artifacts mimicking microcalcifications have to be excluded.
Intramammary calcifications are benign if they exhibit the following calcification pattern:

Morphology

- Coarse, with or without central radiolucency.
- Semicircular or shell-like calcifications around lesions with a central area of radiolucency. Examples: oil cysts, fat necrosis, calcifying liponecrosis.
- Relatively typical also are peripheral calcifications of fibroadenomas and papillomas.
- Coarse, popcorn-like, and large bizarre calcifications (in general >2 mm). Examples: fibroadenomas, papillomas, "plasma cell mastitis," scars.

- Railroad track vascular calcifications.
- Small and tiny calcifications that are round, punctate, or stippled monomorphic. Distribution: symmetric, diffuse, or in individual morula-like groups. Example: fibrocystic changes.
- Teacup calcifications. Examples: milk of calcium in microcystic benign changes.

Distribution Pattern

- Solitary calcifications.
- Diffuse and symmetrical distribution.
- Groups can be observed in the following conditions:
  - Calcifying liponecrosis (typical subcutaneous in location and ring-like or round in morphology).
  - In fibroadenomas and papillomas with typical shapes or with a typical surrounding well-circumscribed soft-tissue density.
  - In scars.
  - In blunt duct adenosis with typical lobular configuration: rosette-like and closely packed.
- Along the course of vessels.

Indeterminate Microcalcifications

Definition

Indeterminate microcalcifications are calcifications that are classified as not unequivocally benign or as suspicious because of

- Their location
- Their morphology
- Their distribution

These mainly include:

- Fine-granular and amorphous calcifications that do not follow a typical distribution pattern
- Calcifications with mild to moderate pleomorphism (Fig. 20.**43**)
- Calcifications that do not show a typical segmental or lobular arrangement, appear asymmetric to the contralateral side, are found in one location only (Fig. 20.**44**) or appear to form groups
- Other calcifications that are neither typically benign nor typically malignant

In terms of numbers, indeterminate calcifications are unfortunately at least as frequent as characteristically benign or suspect calcifications.

Incidence

Indeterminate calcifications can be expected in the following conditions:

- Invasive *carcinoma* and *carcinoma* in situ: Some invasive carcinomas, most carcinomas in situ of the noncomedo type, and 20% of the carcinomas in situ of the comedo type show no characteristic microcalcifications or no microcalcifications at all.
- Since benign fibrocystic changes frequently represent an amalgamation of different proliferative changes of *ductal as well as lobular origin* and since the lobules themselves can be involved in sclerosing processes, the described typical benign forms and arrangements of microcalcifications are only found in a certain percentage. This means that pleomorphic or elongated shapes as well as worrisome distributions can be encountered in benign changes. Since these calcifications cannot be differentiated from malignant calcifications with sufficient certainty, a gray zone exists in which an unequivocal classification of the analyzed calcification cannot be achieved.
- With beginning *calcification of fibroadenomas*, small bizarre, linear, or punctate calcifications can appear. They cannot always reliably be differentiated from suspicious microcalcifications.
  Location of uncharacteristic calcifications *within a smoothly outlined soft-tissue mass* can be helpful in the differential diagnosis.
- Rare differential diagnostic problems arise when the calcifications in plasma cell mastitis are relatively delicate.
- Furthermore, calcifications in *fat necroses and scars* can occasionally be pleomorphic, containing elongated and more characteristically curved shapes. If the microcalcifications are still small or appear in groups, they cannot invariably be differentiated from suspicious ductal calcifications.

General Aspects of the Differential Diagnosis of Indeterminate Microcalcifications

In principle, it is not possible to detect *all* invasive carcinomas or carcinomas in situ, because only some of the invasive and even fewer of the carcinomas in situ contain microcalcifications. Some carcinomas only display indeterminate calcifications. Furthermore, typically benign calcifications can occasionally be associated with carcinomas when the carcinoma arises in an area of benign disease. Such individual cases should not lead to the uncritical removal of all microcalcifications.

It is inappropriate to resect all uncharacteristic calcifications because only a small portion of the biopsies will be positive for malignancy. Diagnostic biopsies of benign calcifications will not only raise the costs to unacceptably high levels but also will compromise the outcome of future evaluations because of scarring secondary to multiple surgeries. Furthermore, too many diagnostic excisions of benign lesions will lead to a loss of confidence in diagnostic imaging and a loss of compliance.

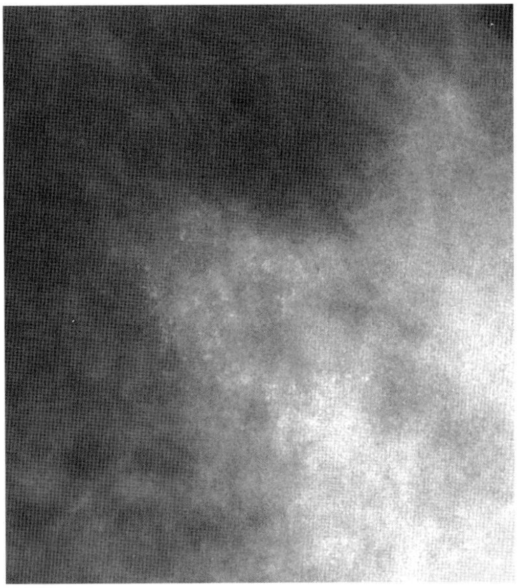

Fig. 20.**43** Punctate, linear, and pleomorphic microcalcifications in the upper outer quadrant (magnification mammography). *Histology:* Parenchyma containing matrix microcalcifications

Considerations as to the Differential Diagnosis of Indeterminate Calcifications in the Individual Case

The diagnostic decision, which should include a recommendation of how to continue with the workup, must *always* be *individualized.*

When deciding between *biopsy* and *follow-up examination*, it must be considered that calcifications in a carcinoma in situ can remain *stable* over several years. If situated within dense tissue, an associated mass might not be recognized. In general, follow-up examinations obtained at *6-month* intervals are considered totally adequate.

The decision process must incorporate:

- An assessment based on a meticulous analysis of the microcalcifications (location, individual form, distribution pattern)
- Supplemental information as to the surrounding soft tissue structures (asymmetries, retraction, prior surgeries, scars, etc.)
- Clinical history (family history, patient history as to previous breast cancer and other risk factors, prior surgery, scars, etc.)
- Clinical findings, e.g., discharge, retraction, scars, as well as palpable abnormalities, review of the mammographic findings
- Serial changes if previous mammograms are available

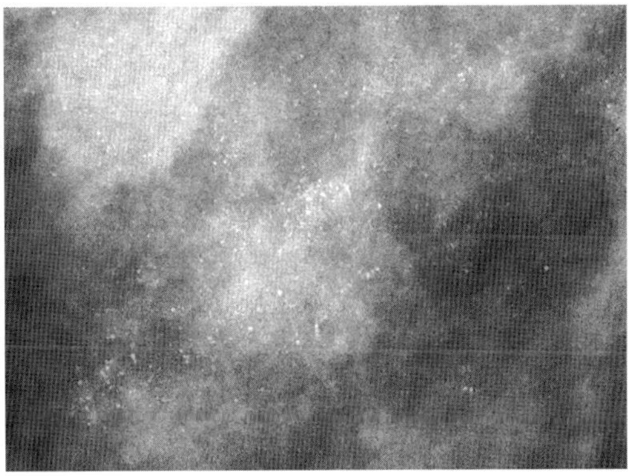

Fig. 20.**44** Unilateral, relatively monomorphic, fine microcalcifications without typical distribution. *Histology:* simple fibrocystic changes without proliferations containing psammomatous calcifications

The radiologist should recognize that:

- New or increasing microcalcifications and a new or increasing contiguous soft-tissue density are an indication for biopsy
- Failure to observe any appreciable changes for less than 1–2 years raises the likelihood of a benign diagnosis only slightly

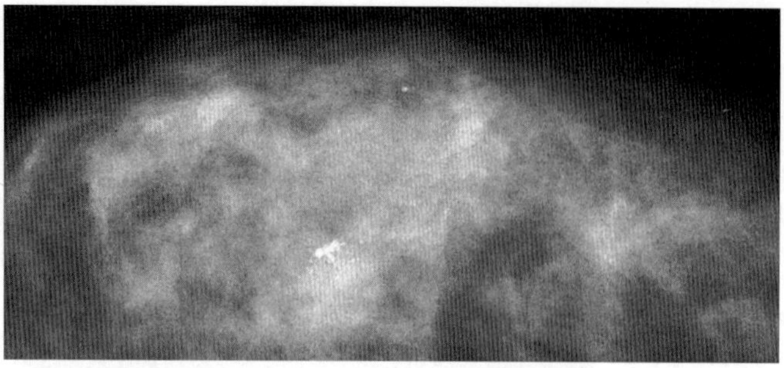
a

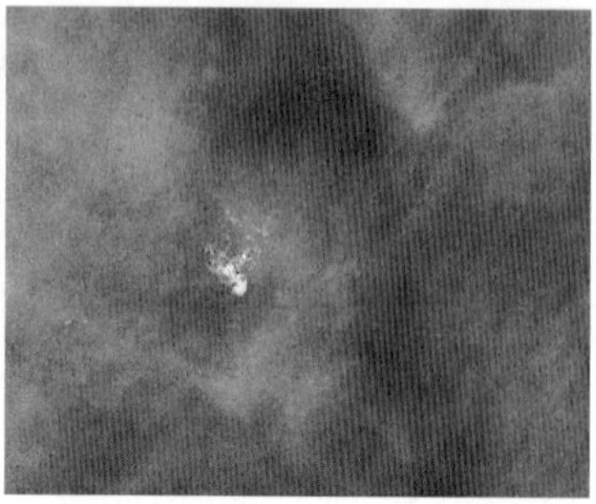
b

Fig. 20.**45a** and **b**
a Very fine calcifications as well as a coarse calcification with a bizarre outline are seen within a barely discernible round density measuring 7 mm located within dense parenchyma
b Magnification mammography. Diagnosis: fibroadenoma, confirmed by increasing coarseness of the calcifications on follow-up

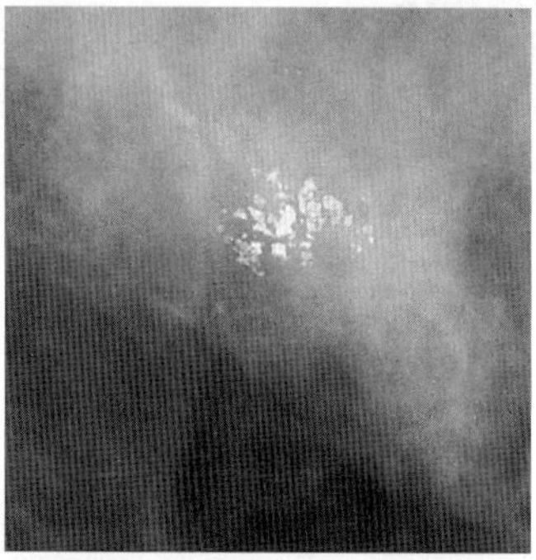
a

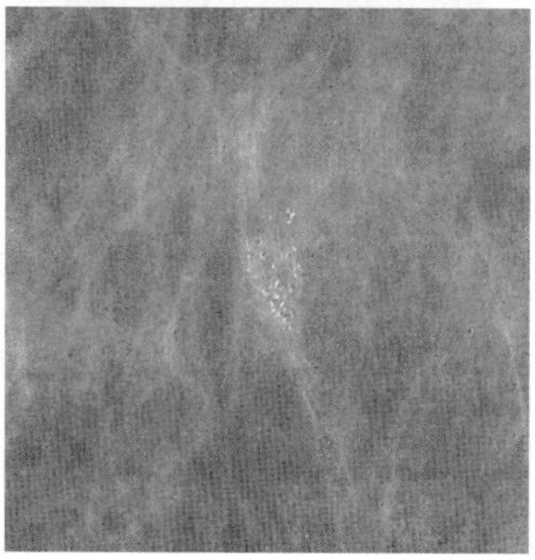
b

Fig. 20.**46a** and **b**
a Pleomorphic bizarre calcifications in a subtle oval area. *Histology:* fibroadenoma
b Granular and irregular linear calcifications forming an oval group with a pointed extension. Note the calcifications outside the soft-tissue density. *Histology:* DCIS

The decision to proceed with follow-up examinations, core biopsy, or excisional biopsy has to incorporate all available data.

Considerations include:

- Follow-up examinations are advisable only when the compilation of all findings suggest a benign lesion with a high degree of certainty
- That the accuracy of percutaneous biopsies for the evaluation of microcalcifications depends on the ability to sample calcifications at the time of biopsy

The presence of microcalcifications in cores should be documented with specimen radiography. Adequate material has to be obtained (> 5 core specimens, 14 gauge needle, length of the specimen core > 1.5 cm). The core biopsy can confirm a presumed benign or malignant finding. A negative core biopsy should not be used to dismiss a suspicion raised by clinical imaging. The excisional biopsy is considered the most reliable method to evaluate continued suggestive or possibly malignant findings.

The newly developed percutaneous vacuum needle biopsy promises to provide even higher accuracy, considering that surgical biopsies do not include the lesion in a small percentage, while removal of the area under suspicion can be monitored mammographically during vacuum needle biopsy.

■ Appendix: Differential Diagnostic Significance of a Soft Density Surrounding Microcalcifications

(Figs. 20.**45**–20.**49**)

A surrounding or accompanying soft-tissue density is often not helpful. Presence or absence of a soft-tissue density can by no means substitute a meticulous analysis of the mircocalcifications.

A surrounding soft-tissue density is **contributory** if:

- It is identifiable as a vessel (best if seen in two projections) with beginning mural calcifications
- It is round and entirely smooth in outline:

this can also be considered as quite reliable evidence of a fibroadenoma

- It is ill-defined or spiculated and consequently unequivocally suspect
- It is of fat density and consequently has a pattern diagnostic of a benign entity, e.g., oil cyst

Less contributory is:

- Finding uncharacteristic densities around microcalcifications, since they may be caused by infiltration, reactive changes, uncharacteristic benign changes, or superimposition.
- Finding nodular densities around microcalcifications. They can—unless unequivocally smooth in outline—suggest an early calcifying fibroadenoma or papilloma. But this is not conclusive because invasive carcinomas or carcinomas in situ can be nodular and calcify.
- Finally, presence or absence of a soft-tissue density around microcalcifications permits no reliable differentiation between invasive carcinoma and carcinoma in situ. On one hand, a soft-tissue density accompanying an invasive carcinoma can be overlooked amidst surrounding dense parenchyma. On the other hand, a reactive fibrosis can produce a soft-tissue density around a pure carcinoma in situ.

Nipple Discharge

(Fig. 20.**50**)

■ Definition

A pathologic discharge refers to a spontaneous, usually unilateral, nonmilky secretion from one or a few lactiferous ducts.

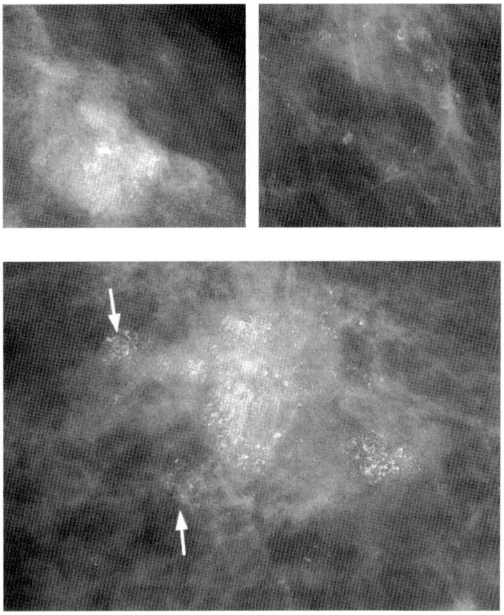

a b c

Fig. 20.**47a–c**
a Specimen radiography. Round lesion measuring 8 mm, with multiple, somewhat pleomorphic calcifications that are closely aggregated: papilloma
b Specimen radiography. Multiple tiny round groups, almost forming a circle, of punctate calcifications: papillomatosis
c Specimen radiography. Multiple groups of microcalcifications are delineated within an indistinctly outlined soft-tissue density, with two groups unmistakably punctate. In addition, there are many granular, pleomorphic calcifications: papillary carcinoma

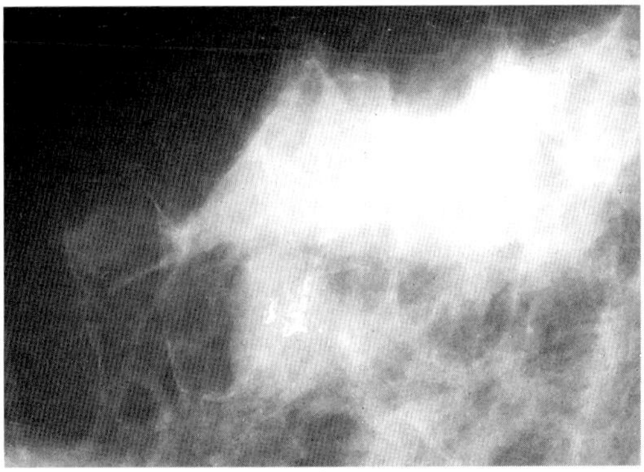

Fig. 20.**48** Oval, partially sharply outlined lesion measuring 11 mm, with relatively large, pleomorphic, bizarre calcifications centrally. Despite the relatively coarse structure, not a fibroadenoma but an intraductal carcinoma

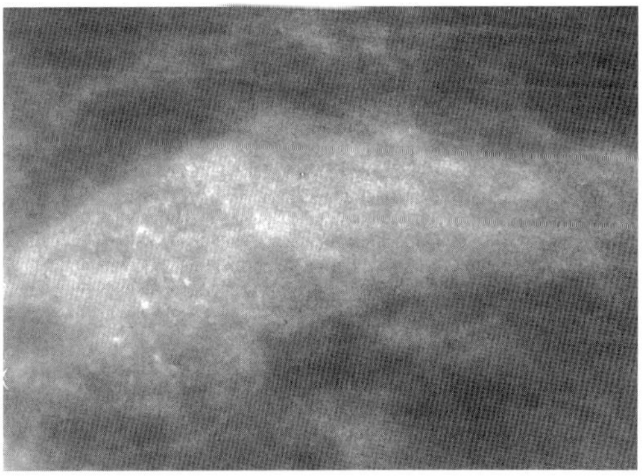

Fig. 20.**49** Multiple fine-granular microcalcifications. Biopsy recommended because of suggested segmental distribution (magnification × 3): DCIS

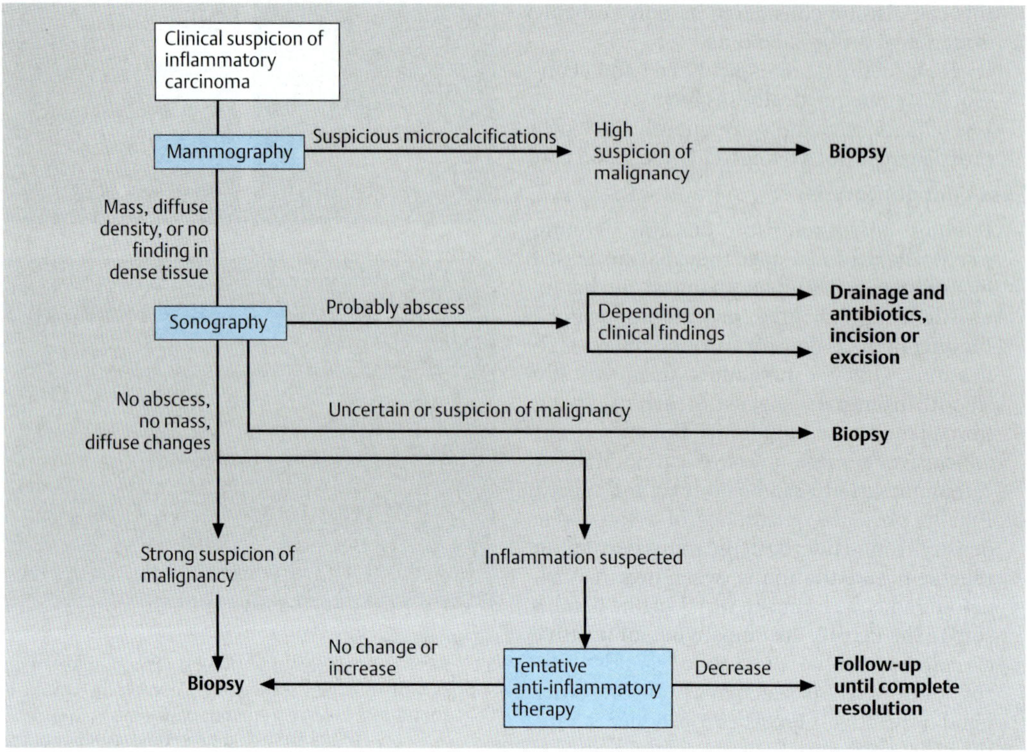

Fig. 20.**50** Inflammatory changes

■ Diagnostic Problems

An intraductal lesion presenting with nipple discharge can be localized and its extent determined by galactography. Neither galactography nor other imaging methods can ascertain the histopathology of the process. Therefore, any galactographically detected intraductal lesion must be surgically explored.

■ Diagnostic Strategy

1. Bilateral nonmilky discharge is generally a manifestation of a hormonal dysfunction and consequently not an indication for galactography. Only the case of a bilateral hemorrhagic or cytologically suggestive secretion warrants further evaluation. As a rule, any discharge calls for a cytologic smear. Only a positive cytologic smear is diagnostically useful. A negative cytologic smear can never exclude malignancy.
2. Unilateral discharge must be further evaluated whenever one or several lactiferous ducts secrete, whenever the color of the discharge may indicate malignancy (see below), or the cytologic smear is positive:
   - A serous discharge from several ducts usually has a hormonal cause, and checking the status of the endocrine system is recommended. If the cytology of the discharge is questionable or suggestive, one duct after the other has to be canalized for galactography.
   - If the discharge is brownish, greenish, or hemorrhagic, galactography is indicated.
   - Any unilateral discharge from one duct should be galactographically evaluated.
   - Any cytologically suggestive discharge is an indication for galactography.
3. Any filling defect with or without irregularities of the ductal wall or any truncated duct is a manifestation of an intraductal process that must be excised after prior localization. For galactographically documented ductectasia or a normal ductal system, follow-up mammography at the age-specific intervals is adequate.

Inflammatory Changes

■ Definition

If localized erythema or diffuse changes with erythema or hyperthermia, or both are noticed clinically, the differential diagnosis must center around the differentiation between malignancy (carcinoma with inflammatory component, inflammatory carcinoma, and, rarely, hematologic malignancy or metastases) and inflammation (mastitis, abscess).

■ Diagnostic Problems

Above all, the differentiation between subacute or chronic inflammatory processes can be difficult.

■ Diagnostic Strategy

The diagnostic approach is summarized in Figure 20.**50**. The possibilities and limitations of the individual methods can be briefly outlined as follows.

The *clinical history* speaks for an inflammatory origin in context with a pregnancy, with lactation, or with prior or recurrent inflammations. In the presence of nipple discharge, the microbiologic and cytologic examination of the discharge can be helpful.

Mammography is of special importance here. It is true that malignancy and inflammation generally cannot be distinguished in a focal mass or diffuse density without microcalcifications, but if suspicious *microcalcifications* can be indentified, a malignancy is very probable.

Sonographically demonstrated hypoechoic or anechoic spaces with fluctuation would speak for an inflammatory process. An abscess, which is characterized by a relatively smooth inner wall, has to be distinguished from a carcinoma with central necrosis, which usually exhibits nodular thickening and an irregular inner surface.

Without conclusive evidence provided by mammography or sonography, *anti-inflammatory therapy* can be tried if an inflammation is suspected clinically. The resolution of the finding has to be monitored until it becomes undetectable. The necessary short-term follow-up can be performed sonographically/clinically.

Finally, it should be mentioned that some inflammatory processes fail to elicit any clinical inflammatory signs, as found in so-called cold abscesses (TB, fungus) and in some granulomatous conditions, as well as in chronic inflammations that may occur in association with fibrocystic changes. Their diagnosis is generally only established histologically after biopsy of a lesion that was discovered as a palpable finding or mammographic density.

The Young Patient

■ Special Considerations and Problems

Diagnosis of breast cancer can be more difficult in young patients (below 35–40 years) than in those who are older

There are several reasons for this:

- Very low incidence of breast cancer in this age group
- High incidence of benign breast disease (lumpiness, fibroadenomas)
- Decreased sensitivity of mammography in some of these patients due to dense tissue
- Minimal but increased radiation risk at a young age[19]

These factors have lead to an increased rate of delayed diagnoses of carcinoma among young patients compared to older patients. Furthermore, the positive biopsy rates (the number of carcinomas per recommended biopsies) are much lower in younger patients.[20–23]

Few women in this age group undergo mammographic screening. This is usually limited to women with first-degree relatives with premenopausal breast cancer, a history of treatment for Hodgkin disease, a prior breast biopsy revealing a high-risk lesion, or a previous history of breast cancer. In younger women, most cancers present as clinically evident masses, which need to be distinguished from the numerous benign masses and lumps detected in the young patient. These should be viewed with suspicion and the workup of these lesions individually tailored to each patient. The screening for the detection of lesions in these women is approached as in older women. A sensitivity to the real or perceived risk of radiation-induced cancer should be part of the treatment of these younger women. Even in pregnant women, however, suspicious lesions should be appropriately worked up.

Breast Changes in the Young Patient and Their Histology

The appearance of the normal breast starting from childhood to adult age has been reviewed in Chapter 8. Based on age-related physiologic changes, the breast of the young patient on palpation is denser and lumpier than that of older patients (> 50 years). This higher consistency or lumpiness in itself does not imply disease. It does, however, impair clinical and—if performed—mammographic evaluation. Large individual variations exist; sometimes the breast of even very young patients (in their twenties) can contain ample amounts of fat.

The following benign entities are typically found in young patients.

Fibrocystic changes, hyperplastic and proliferative changes can occur. When proliferative changes with atypia are detected, this entity is associated with an increased risk of malignancy (see Chapter 9), as it is in older women.

Fibroadenomas. Even though fibroadenomas have a wide age distribution, the greatest incidence is in women between the ages of 25 and 35, and the fibroadenoma is the most frequent breast mass in children. Both pericanalicular and intracanalicular types are seen. In young patients, they largely consist of ample myxoid stroma with a high water content and are vascular. Some are cellular and adenomatous. Fibrosed fibroadenomas usually do not occur in young women. Multiple fibroadenomas are frequently encountered.

The juvenile fibroadenoma or *giant fibroadenoma* is a special type of fibroadenoma that occurs almost exclusively in young patients (maximum incidence around menarche). It is a well-circumscribed tumor, typically with rapid growth. Histologically, it consists of proliferating stroma and often epithelial hyperplasia. It is completely benign and not associated with an increased risk of malignancy.

The *phyllodes tumor* (see Chapter 15) is much rarer in the young patient than the juvenile fibroadenoma. It can, however, be encountered, albeit rarely, in the young patient as well as a rapidly growing, well-circumscribed mass.

Papillomas can occur in young patients.

Juvenile papillomatosis is an infrequent finding, which is typically diagnosed in adolescents and young women. Histologically, the lesion, which generally becomes apparent as a palpable mass or nipple discharge, is characterized by ductal papillomatosis, papillary apocrine hyperplasia, multiple (micro)cysts, often cellular atypia, and sometimes even necrosis. About 30–40% of the cases are associated with a family history of breast carcinoma. Local recurrence and bilaterality have been reported. Whether the individual risk of breast carcinoma is increased is debated. An association of juvenile papillomatosis and juvenile secretory carcinoma has been reported.[24–27]

Overall *malignancy* is less frequent in young patients than in the patient above 40 years of age. Various types of malignancy, including breast carcinomas, hematologic malignancy, and sarcomas, have been encountered.

During pregnancy the following benign and malignant entities can also be encountered: *Benign.* The fibroadenoma is the most frequent benign mass occurring during pregnancy. It is followed by papillomas, fibrocystic disease, galactocele, abscess, puerperal mastitis, and (see Chapters 10 and 12, respectively), rarely, breast infarct or phyllodes tumor.

Many fibroadenomas increase in size during pregnancy, becoming apparent and necessitating further workup. Sometimes infarction may occur.

Breast infarct,[28, 29] which can affect any part of the breast tissue as well as sometimes a fibroadenoma,[30] is histologically characterized by a mass consisting of coagulation necrosis. The exact etiology of breast infarcts during pregnancy is not known.

Malignant. About 1–2% of breast cancers are considered concurrent with pregnancy or lactation. These include cancers that are detected during or within 1 year of pregnancy. Besides breast cancer, an association with pregnancy has been described for some rare lesions such as benign and malignant phyollodes tumor, Burkitt lymphoma, and angiosarcoma.

Risk of Breast Cancer

Breast cancer is an unusual disease in younger women. Even though malignancies have been described in the teenage group and women in their early twenties, a relevant increase of risk starts after about 25 years of age. At age 25, the incidence of breast cancer is about 1/10 000. After that it rises rapidly to about 1 : 1000 at age 40.[29, 31] Although malignant lesions are rare in these younger women, they do occur, and an attempt should be made to avoid unnecessary delay in diagnosis. In patients with genetic risk factors and in those with a family history of premenopausal breast cancer, the risk of breast cancer increases significantly even before 35–40 years of age.

The following paragraphs will summarize special issues in the diagnostic workup of young patients. Based on these considerations, recommendations of a diagnostic strategy will be suggested.

Clinical Findings

The great majority of young patients with breast problems present with a lump, lumpiness, localized pain, and occasionally with pathologic nipple discharge or other rare findings. Some young patients are referred because of an individual or strong family history of breast cancer or because of known genetic risk factors.

Benign causes of a palpable abnormality in the young patient include normal breast tissue, fibroadenoma, fibrocystic changes, papilloma, cyst, and, infrequently, juvenile papillomatosis. During pregnancy or lactation, benign causes include a galactocele, an abscess, puerperal mastitis, or a breast infarct.

Juvenile papillomatosis can present on palpation as an indeterminate mass or can be palpable like a fibroadenoma. Breast infarct becomes apparent as an indeterminate or suspicious mass of rubbery consistency.[29]

Unfortunately, in situ and invasive carcinoma, as well as other rare malignancies, have to be included in the differential diagnosis.

The differential diagnosis of very large masses should include the juvenile fibroadenoma, virginal hypertrophy, and rarely phyllodes tumor, lymphoma (e.g., Burkitt lymphoma during pregnancy), or sarcoma (periductal fibrosarcoma or angiosarcoma during pregnancy). The causes of pathologic discharge are similar to those in the older age-group and include papillomas, papillomatosis, duct ectasia, or fibrocystic changes, a lactating fibroadenoma (rarely), or, in about 10% of the cases, a carcinoma.

As in the older patients, sensitivity of the clinical examination for the detection of carcinoma varies with the lesion size and decreases strongly with smaller tumor size.[32, 33] As reported by Reintgen[33] on a large series of over 500 breast carcinomas, only about 50% of the carcinomas in the size range of 11–15 mm are palpable, and even experienced clinicians do not detect the majority of breast cancers until they are greater than 15 mm.

Overall, clinical evaluation of the young patient is more difficult because of the increased firmness and nodularity of the breast tissue. Because of even more pronounced nodularity and firmness of the breast tissue, evaluation frequently is significantly impaired during pregnancy and lactation.

Furthermore, the high prevalence of benign disease impairs assessment. During pregnancy and lactation, detection and diagnosis of malignancy and its differentiation from the physiological hypertrophic changes become even more difficult, as documented by the commonly encountered delays in diagnosis.[29, 34–36]

Mammography

Mammographic evaluation in the young patient is often impaired by dense glandular tissue that can obscure both benign and malignant masses. Therefore, the value of mammography is limited. However, because of the variability of parenchymal patterns—about 30% of the patients have sufficient amounts of interposed fat to be well-assessed mammographically—and because of its unique capability to image microcalcifications (which may be the only sign of malignancy in about 30% of the carcinomas), mammography can be useful (see Fig. 8.**10b**, **c**) below 35 years of age. It should therefore be utilized whenever indicated (see below).

When not obscured by dense tissue, **benign lesions** display large variations, as decribed in the respective chapters. Juvenile papillomatosis, an infrequent lesion seen predominantly in the young patient, usually cannot be distinguished from dense glandular tissue on mammography (Fig. 20.**51a**). This appearance together with the usual palpable encountered palpable abnormality does not allow exclusion of malignancy. Breast infarct, a rare finding associated with pregnancy or lactation, can be obscured by dense tissue or present as an ill-defined mass or asymmetry mammographically. It usually cannot be distinguished from malignancy. For lesions

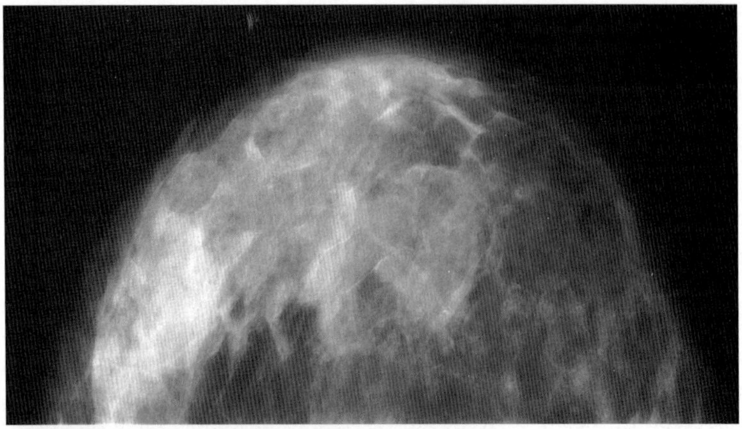

Fig. 20.**51** Fifteen-year-old patient with a family history of breast cancer. She presented with a palpable mass in the upper outer quadrant
a Mammogram cc-view. Dense breast tissue. No mass visible

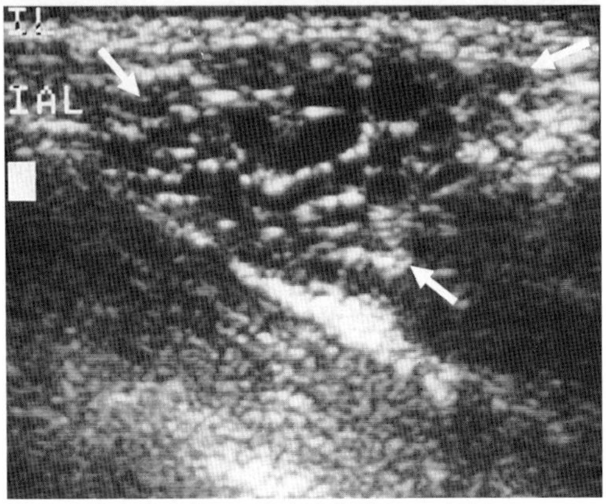

Fig. 20.**51 b** Sonogram displays a hypoechoic mass including small cystic spaces. *Histology:* juvenile papillomatosis

with typical benign features (fat-containing lymph node, hamartoma, etc.), no further assessment is needed. For those with a high probability of benignity (>98%), follow-up is justified. In the other cases, which unfortunately constitute the large majority in the young patients, biopsy remains necessary.

As to detection and diagnosis of **malignancy**, many authors have reported a decreased sensitivity of mammography and a lower positive predictive value for patients under 35 years of age.[21, 37–43]

The increased number of reported false positive calls is explained by the high prevalence of benign lesions (nodular breast tissue or fibroadenomas), where malignancy cannot be excluded because of uncharacteristic appearance or overall high radiodensity (Fig. 20.**52a**) (see also Figs. 11.**2c** and 11.**3a**).

Mammographic false negative interpretations have mainly been attributed to two facts:

- Owing to the higher amount of glandular or dense breast tissue, carcinomas without microcalcifications may be obscured (Fig. 20.**53a, b**)
- A relatively high percentage of carcinomas (15–20%) in young patients has been reported as having been misinterpreted as benign masses (like fibroadenomas) (Fig. 14.**12c, d**).[37, 39, 40, 44, 45]

In spite of these problems, mammography is able to detect nonpalpable carcinomas even in young patients[44] (Fig. 20.**54a–d**):

- In those younger patients (circa 30%) who have fatty or mixed dense/fatty breast patterns, accuracy is comparable to that achieved in older patients
- Detection of carcinomas presenting with suggestive microcalcifications is excellent in any breast type

During pregnancy and lactation, mammographic evaluation, which is only indicated in symptomatic patients, is even more difficult than in the nonpregnant young patient. This is caused by further increase in density due to glandular proliferation, increased water content, and hyperemia. Even though numerous lesions can be obscured mammographically and benign lesions can only rarely be unequivocally diagnosed by mammography, mammography should be applied in all indeterminate or suspicious lesions; mostly because of mammography's capability to image microcalcifications, a definite diagnosis of malignancy will be possible in at least some cases (Fig. 20.**55**, see also Figs. 19.**10b, c**). In these cases, mammography can accelerate the diagnosis of carcinoma. It is common for patients to be biopsied only after completion of pregnancy. Additionally, in the case of suspected malignancy, further foci may be detected, which can be important for adequate treatment planning.

When mammography is applied in the young patient, it must be remembered that the potential risk of radiation is higher for young patients than for older patients. Consideration of this potential increased risk of breast cancer is important when mammography is applied in asymptomatic patients. It is not important in those symptomatic patients whose symptoms cannot be explained by clinical or sonographic findings. Because of the low energy of the mammographically used X-rays, virtually no radiation will reach the fetus, particularly when the abdomen is shielded. Therefore, pregnancy is not a contraindication to mammography. To decrease mammographic density and thus improve mammographic evaluation during lactation, mammograms should be taken directly after breast feeding.

Based on the above considerations and the experiences reported in the literature, the following recommendations are given for the **use of mammography:**

- *Routine mammographic screening* is not advocated in the *asymptomatic patient younger than 40*.[40, 44, 46]
- In women with a first-degree relative with premenopausal breast cancer and in women with positive genetic testing, with a history of Hodgkin disease, with a prior breast cancer, or with a high-risk lesion of breast biopsy, routine screening before age 40 is indicated. In women with a first-degree relative with breast cancer, screening should begin at an age 10 years earlier than the cancer was diagnosed in that relative but not earlier than 25 years of age.[46, 47] In women treated for Hodgkin disease, screening should commence no later than 8 years after the completion of treatment.[48]

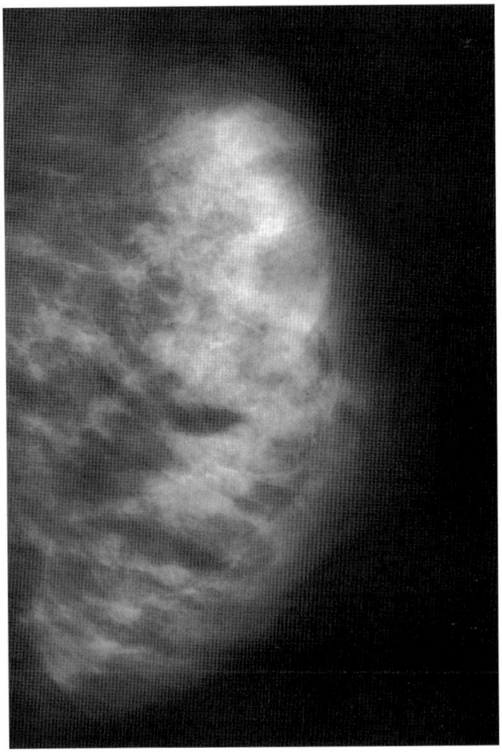

Fig. 20.**52** Eighteen-year-old patient with a palpable mass at 12 o'clock
a Mammographically the mass is obscured by dense tissue

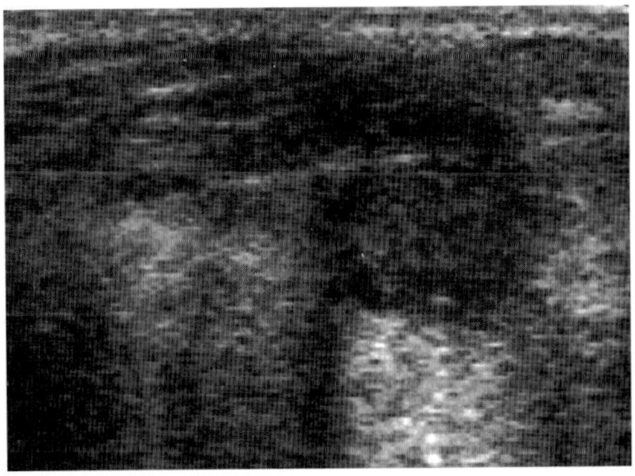

b Sonographically a hypoechoic round mass with posterior enhancement is seen, fairly mobile. Core biopsy revealed a fibroadenoma.

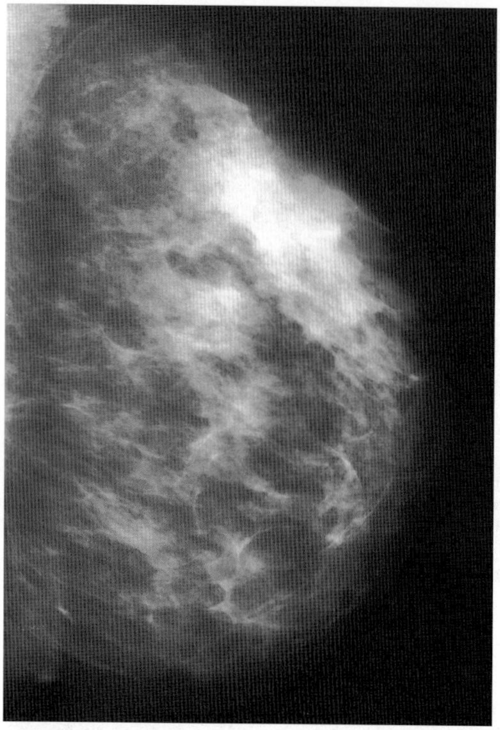

a

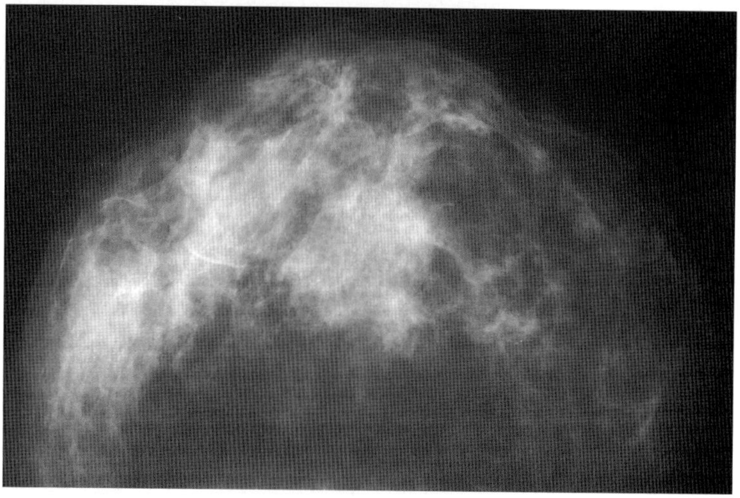

b

Fig. 20.**53** Two months after a normal screening mammogram and normal clinical examination, this 38-year-old patient with a family history of breast cancer noticed a palpable mass in the upper outer quadrant of her left breast

a, b Oblique and cc mammogram 2 months before showed dense breast tissue, no mass

- Considering the high prevalence of benign problems (e.g., cysts) that can at least partly be solved by ultrasound, *in symptomatic patients mammography should be used after sonography.*
- *In all symptomatic patients* without a definitely benign diagnosis established sonographically (cyst, galactocele, freely moveable typical benign solid mass as defined on p. 169), *mammography is strongly recommended* since it may be able to detect suggestive microcalcifications or masses.
- This also applies to symptomatic patients during pregnancy. Pregnancy is no contraindication to mammography.
- In the case of *absent mammographic findings in*

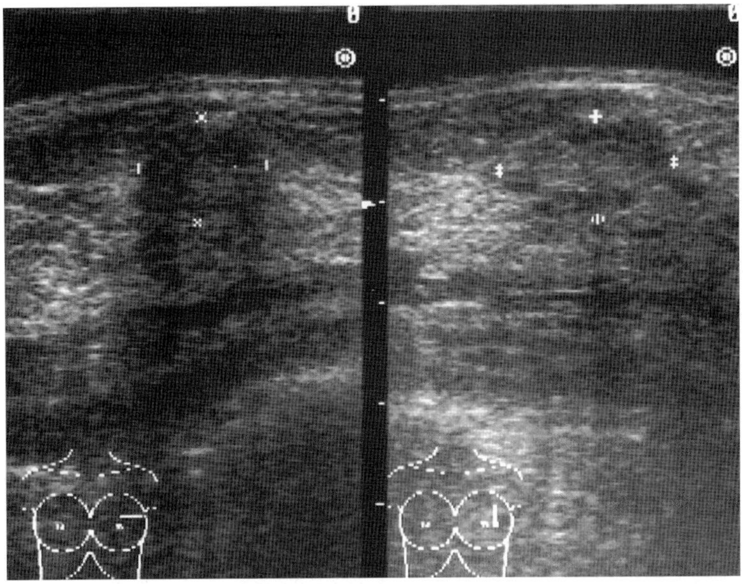

Fig. 20.**53c** Sonographically a 1.6 cm hypoechoic mass with heterogeneous internal echoes and distal shadowing is highly suscipious

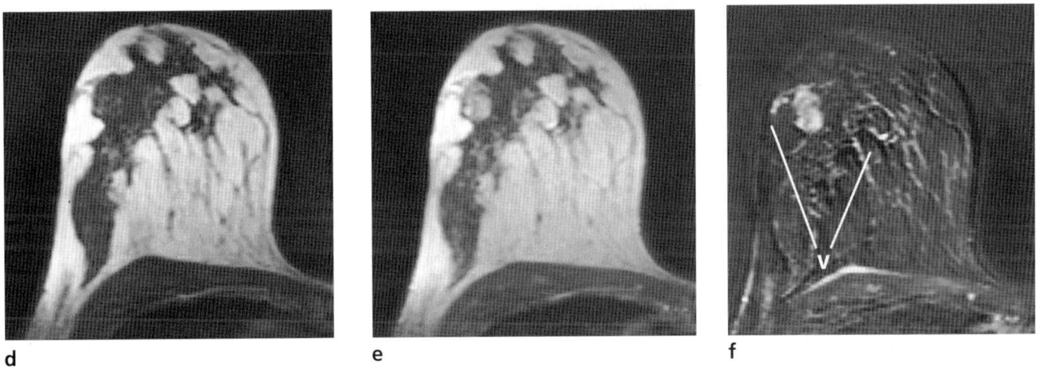

Fig. 20.**53d–f** Contrast-enhanced MRI, which was performed to exclude additional foci, confirmed the presence of an oval mass of about 1.8 cm with some irregularities. In spite of its delayed enhancement and fairly oval shape, the mass is suspicious. No further foci. (v = vessel)
d Precontrast image **e** Postcontrast image (3rd minute) **f** Subtraction of image (**e**) minus (**d**)
Histology: invasive ductal carcinoma NOS

dense tissue or potentially benign mammographic findings, a negative mammogram should not dissuade from *further workup* of suspicious or indeterminate clinical findings.

Sonography

In view of the difficulties surrounding mammographic detection and diagnosis of breast cancer in the young patient, sonography has been proposed as the method of choice in young patients.[49] Indeed, the use of sonography is recommended as the first method for the workup of symptomatic patients below the age of 35 years. The reasons are as follows:

- Since sonography is not associated with any radiation, it is completely harmless for the patient.
- In the case of a simple cyst, a definitive diagnosis is possible by sonography, and no further workup is necessary.
- In patients with mammographically dense tissue, a hypoechoic suggestive mass detected in an area of an indeterminate pal-

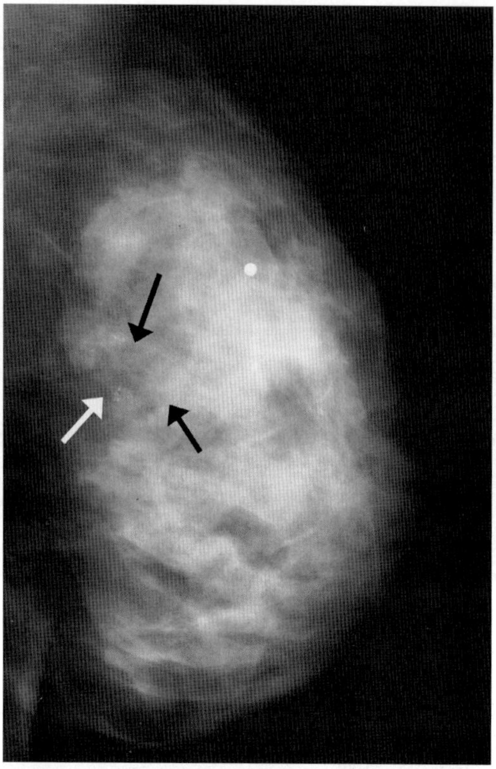

a

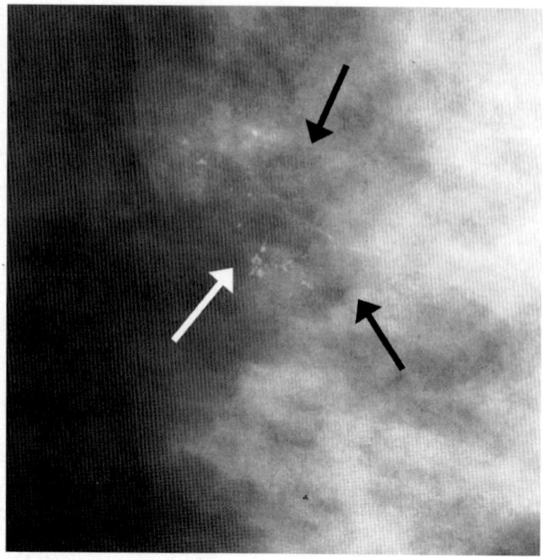

b

Fig. 20.**54** Breast cancer in young patients
a, b Twenty-two-year-old patient who presented with bone metastases. Search for primary tumor revealed mammographically suggestive microcalcifications, which are excellently seen in spite of the dense tissue
a Oblique view
b Magnification of the area of microcalcifications

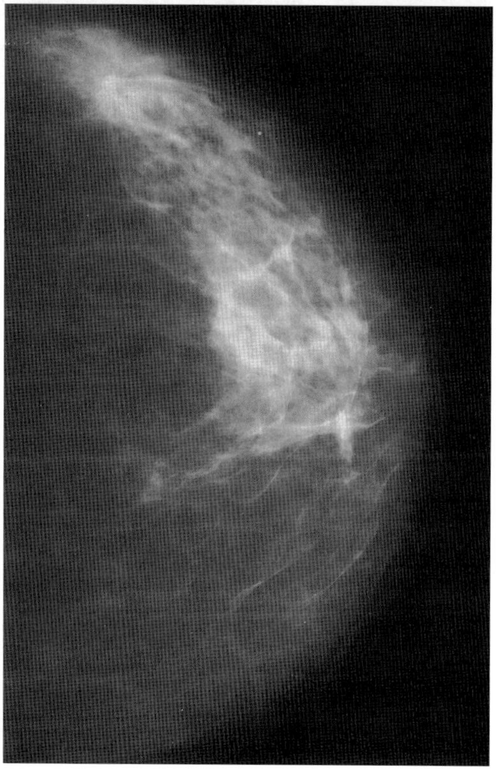

c

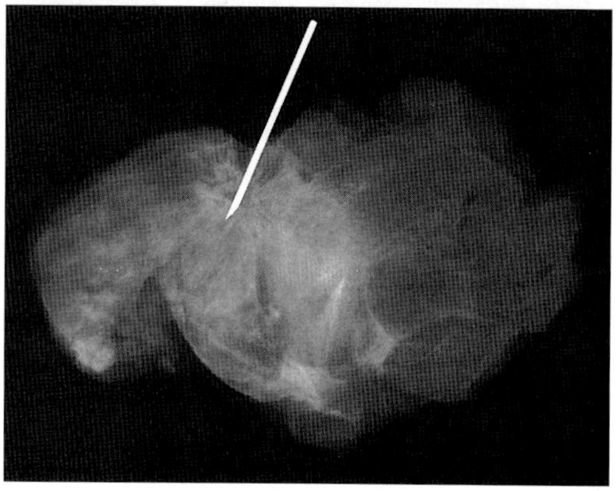

d

Fig. 20.**54 c–f** Thirty-two-year-old patient with carcinophobia
c Suggestive architectural distortion in the upper outer quadrant
d Specimen radiograph reveals a radiolucent center, which, however, does not prove benignity

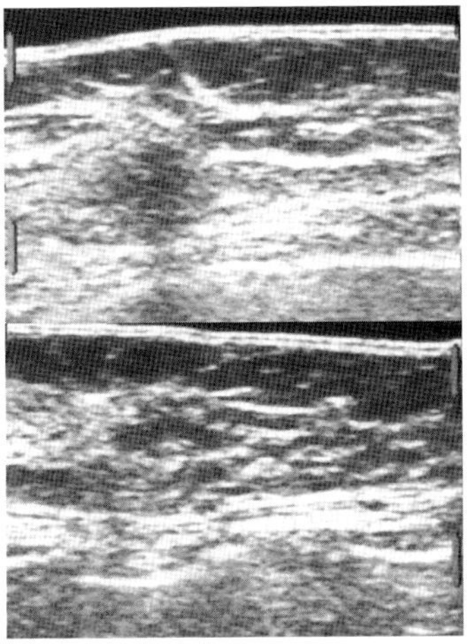
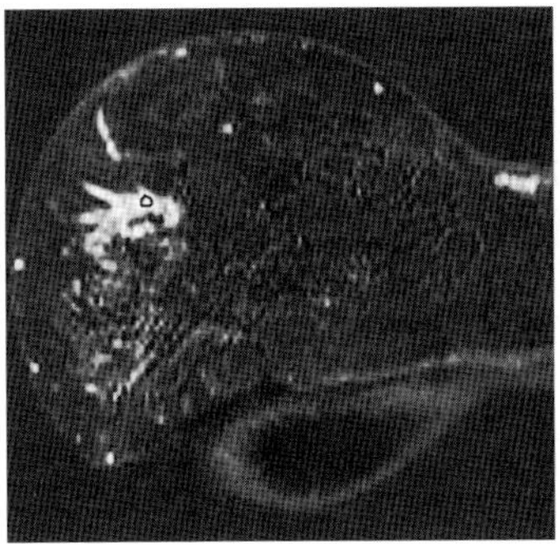
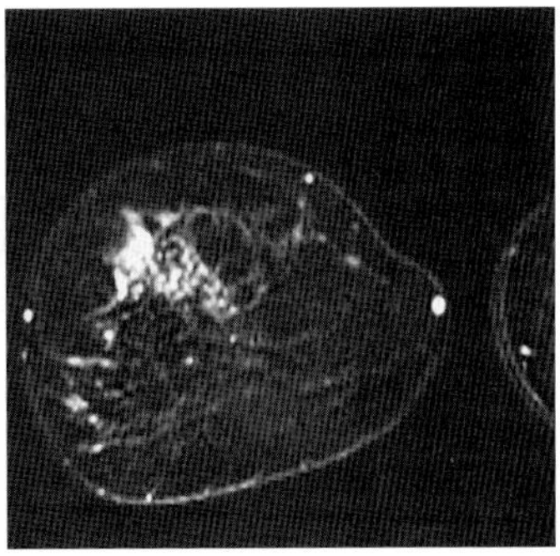

e f g

e Sonogram in two planes shows slight architectural distortion
f MR subtraction (post-CM minus pre-CM): a star-like enhancement is shown in the area of suspicion
g MR subtraction of another slice, 1 cm from slice (**e**). Further areas of enhancement are seen in other slices as well.
Histology: sclerosing adenosis, associated with noncomedo DCIS. The enhancement on the adjacent slices only corresponded to areas of adenosis

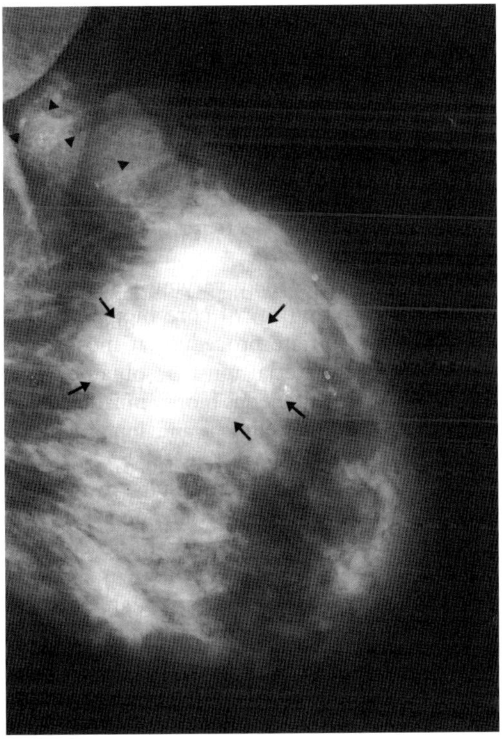

a

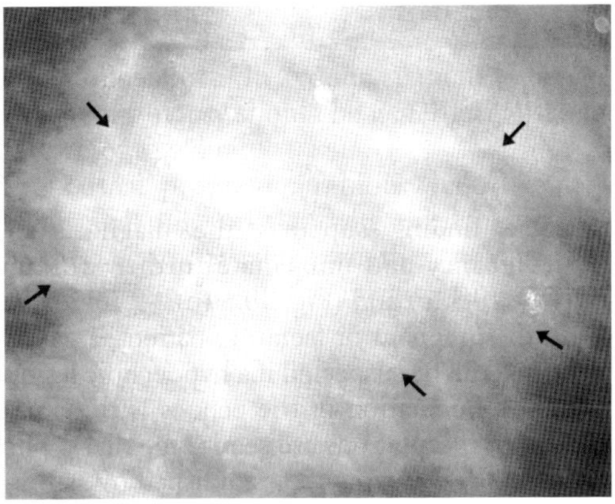

b

Fig. 20.**55** Forty-two-year-old lactating patient with left breast lump
55 a–c A large area with suspicious microcalcifications (arrows) is shown. Note microcalcifications within two suspicious lymph nodes in the axillary tail.
Histology: invasive ductal carcinoma

8. Fischer U, Vosshenrich R, Probst A et al. Preoperative MR mammography in patients with breast cancer – useful information or useless extravagance. Fortschr Rontgenstr. 1994;161:300
9. Harms SE, Flaming DP, Hesley KL et al. MR imaging of the breast with rotating delivery of excitation off resonance: clinical experience with pathology correlation. Radiology. 1993;187:493
10. Oellinger H, Heins S, Sander B et al. Gd-DTPA enhanced MR breast imaging: the most sensitive method for multicentric carcinomas of the female breast. Eur Radiol. 1993;3:223
11. Schulz-Wendtland R, Bauer M, Tontsch P, Döinghaus K. Validität der bildgebenden Diagnostik bei der Beurteilung des Mammakarzinoms und seiner Umgebung. Radiologe. 1995;(35):77
12. Tontsch P, Bauer M. Schulz-Wendtland R et al. Dynamische MR-Mammographie bei 160 Hochrisikopatientinnen. Radiologe. 1995;(35):83
13. Heywang-Köbrunner SH. Brustkrebsdiagnostik mit MR: Überblick nach 1250 Patientenuntersuchungen. Elektromedica. 1993;61/2: 43–52
14. Liberman L, Evans WP III, Dershaw DD, Hann LE, Deutch BM, Abramson AF, Rosen PP. Radiography of microcalcifications in stereotaxic mammary core biopsy specimens. Radiology. 1994;190:223–5
15. Lanyi M. Formanalyse von 5641 Mikroverkalkungen bei 100 Milchgangskarzinomen: die Polymorphie. Fortschr Rontgenstr. 1983;139:240
16. LeGal M, Chavanne D, Pellier D. Valeur diagnostique des microcalcifications groupées découvertes par mammographies. A propos de 227 cas avec vérification histologique et sans tumeur du sein palpable. Bull Cancer (Paris). 1984;71:57–64
17. Sickles EA. Breast calcifications: mammographic evaluation. Radiology. 1986;160:289
18. Bassett LW. Mammographic analysis of calcifications. Radiol Clin North Am. 1992;30:93–105
19. Boice JD Jr, Preston D, Davis FG, Monson RR. Radiat-Res. 1991, 125(2):214
20. Bassett L, Ysrael M. Gold R, Ysrael C. Usefulness of mammography and sonography in women less than 35 years of age. Radiology. 1991;180:831
21. Bennett JC, Freitas R Jr, Fentiman IS. Diagnosis of breast cancer in young women. Aust-NZ-J-Surg. 1991;61/4:284
22. Kerlikowske K, Grady D, Barclay I et al. Positive predictive value of screening mammography by age and family history of breast cancer. JAMA. 1993, Nov. 24;270(20):2444
23. Lamin DR, Harris RP, Swanson FH et al. Difficulties in diagnosis of carcinoma of the breast in patients less than 50 years of age. Surg Gynecol Obstet. 1993;177/5:457
24. Rosen PP, Holmes G, Lesser ML et al. Juvenile papillomatosis and breast carcinoma. Cancer. 1985;55:1345
25. Bazzocchi F, Santini D, Martinelli G et al. Juvenile papillomatosis (epitheliosis) of the breast: a clinical and pathological study of 13 cases. Am J Clin Pathol. 1986;86:745
26. Tokunaga M, Wakimoto J, Muramoto Y et al. Juvenile secretory carcinoma and juvenile papillomatosis. Japan J Clin Oncol. 1985;15:457
27. Ferguson TM, McCarty KS, Filston HC. Juvenile secretory carcinoma and juvenile papillomatosis: diagnosis and treatment. J Pediatr Surg. 1987;22:637
28. Hasson J, Pope CH. Mammary infarcts associated with pregnancy presenting as breast tumors. Surgery. 1961;49:313
29. Harris JR, Hellman S, Henderson C, Kinne DW. Breast Diseases. 2nd ed. Philadelphia: JB Lippincott; 1991
30. Wilkinson S, Green WO Jr. Infarction of breast lesions during pregnancy and lactation. Cancer. 1964;17:1567
31. Maass H. Mammakarzinom: Epidemiologie. Gynäkologe. 1994;27:3
32. Ciatto S, Roselli-del-Turco M, Cantarzi S et al. Causes of breast cancer misdiagnosis at physical examination. Neoplasma. 1991;38(5):523
33. Reintgen D, Berman C, Cox C et al. The anatomy of missed breast cancers. Surg Oncol. 1993;2(1):65
34. Appelwhite RR, Smith LR, De Vincenti F. Carcinoma of the breast associated with pregnancy and lactation. Am Surg. 1973;39:101
35. Fleming U, Sheridan B, Atkinson L et al. The effects of childbearing on carcinoma of the breast. Med J Aust. 1970;1:1252
36. Treves N, Holleb AI. A report of 549 cases of breast cancer in women 35 years of age or younger. Surg Gynecol Obstet. 1958;107:271
37. Meyer J, Kopans D, Oot R. Breast cancer visualized by mammography in patients under 35. Radiology. 1983;147:93
38. Ashley S, Royle G, Corder A et al. Clinical, radiological and cytological diagnosis of breast cancer in young women. Br J Surg. 1989;76:835
39. Harris V, Jackson V. Indications for breast imaging in women under age 35 years. Radiology. 1989;172:445
40. Jeffries D, Adler D. Mammographic detection of breast cancer in women under the age of 35. Invest Radiol. 1990;25:67
41. Bassett LW, Kimme-Smith C. Breast sonography. AJR. 1991;156:449
42. Joensuu H, Asola R, Holli K et al. Delayed diagnosis and large size of breast cancer after a false negative mammogram. Eur J Cancer. 1994;30A(9):1299
43. Yelland A, Graham MD, Trott PA et al. Diagnosing breast carcinoma in young women. BMJ. 1991, Mar 16;302(6777):618
44. de Paredes ES, Marsteller L, Eden B. Breast cancers in women 35 years of age and younger: mammographic findings. Radiology. 1990;177:117
45. Gilles R, Gallay X, Tardivon A et al. Breast cancer in women 35 years old or younger: clinical and mammographic features. Eur Radiol. 1995;5:630
46. Liberman L, Dershaw DD, Deutch BM et al. Screening mammography: value in women 35 – 39 years old. AJR. 1993;161(1):53
47. Moskowitz M. Breast cancer screening: all_s well that ends well, or much ado about nothing? AJR. 1988;151:659
48. Dershaw DD, Yahalom I, Petzek JA. Mammography of breast carcinoma developing in women treated for Hodgkin's disease. Radiology. 1992;184:421–3
49. Harper A, Kelly-Fry E, Noe J. Ultrasound breast imaging: the method of choice for examining the young patient. Ultrasound Med Biol. 1981;7:231
50. Kersschot EAJ, Hermans M, Pauwels C et al. Juvenile papillomatosis (Swiss cheese disease) of the breast: sonographic appearance. Radiology. 1988;169:631
51. Cantarzi S, Guiseppetti GM, Rizzato G et al. A multicenter study for the evaluation of the diagnostic efficiency of mammography and echography in nonpalpable breast neoplasms. Radio Med Torino. 1993;84(3):193
52. Balu-Maestro C. Bruneton JN, Melia P et al. High frequency ultrasound detection of breast calcifications. Eur J Ultrasound. 1994;3:247

53. Ciatto S, Roselli-del-Turco M, Catarzis M et al. The diagnostic role of breast echography. Radiol med. 1994;88:221
54. Pamilo M, Soiva M, Anttinen et al. Ultrasonography of breast lesions detected in mammography screening. Acta Radiol. 1991;32:220
55. Potterton AJ, Peakman DJ, Young IR. Ultrasound demonstration of small breast cancers detected by mammographic screening. Clin Radiol. 1994;49:808
56. Jackson V. The role of US in breast imaging. Radiology. 1990;177:305
57. Adler DD, Heyde DL, Ikeda DM. Quantitative sonographic parameters as means of distinguishing breast cancers from benign solid masses. J Ultrasound Med. 1991;10:505
58. Fornage BD, Lorigan JG, Andry E. Fibroadenoma of the breast: sonographic appearance. Radiology. 1989;172:671
59. Harris J, Lippmann M, Veronesi U, Willett W. Breast cancer. N Engl J Med. 1992;327:319
60. Azavedo E, Svane G, Auer G. Stereotactic fine-needle biopsy in 2594 mammographically detected non-palpable lesions. Lancet. 1989:1033
61. Dent DM, Kirkpatrick AE, McGoogan E, Chetty U, Anderson TJ. Stereotaxic localization and aspiration cytology of impalpable breast lesions. Clin Radiol. 1989;40:380
62. Dowlatshahi K, Yaremko ML, Kluskens LF, Jokich PM. Nonpalpable breast lesions: findings of stereotaxic needle-core biopsy and fine-needle aspiration cytology. Radiology. 1991;185:639
63. Dempsey P, Rubin E. The roles of needle biopsy and periodic follow-up in the evaluation and diagnosis of breast lesions. Semin Roentgenol. 1993;28:252
64. Kuhl CK, Seibert C, Kneft BP et al. Focal and diffuse contrast enhancement in dynamic MR mammography of healthy volunteers. Radiology. 1995b;193(P):121

■ Suggested Reading

Heywang-Köbrunner SH, Beck R. Contrast-enhanced MRI of the Breast. 2nd ed. Heidelberg, New York: Springer; 1995

Lafontan DB, Daures JP, Salicru B et al. Isolated clustered microcalcifications: diagnostic value of mammography – series of 400 cases with surgical verification. Radiology. 1994;190:479

Lanyi M, Neufang KFR. Möglichkeiten und Grenzen der Differentialdiagnostik gruppierter intramammärer Mikroverkalkungen. Fortschr Rontgenstr. 1984;141:430

Morrone D, Ambrogetti D, Bravetti P et al. Diagnostic errors in mammography. I. False negative results. Radiol Med Torino. 1991;82/3:212

Index

Page numbers in **bold type** refer to illustrations.

A

abnormalities
  and normal breast, 131
  summary, 135
abscesses, and mastitis, 199–201, **202**
  summary, 202
accessory breast tissue, 134
accuracy
  biopsy, 101–2, 105, 107, 261
  cyst diagnosis, 160
  fibroadenoma diagnosis, 173
  and legal aspects, 223
  mammography, 11–12
    ductal carcinoma in situ, 215
  MRI, 92–3
    cysts, 162
    ductal carcinoma in situ, 218
    fibroadenoma, 179
  percutaneous biopsy, invasive carcinoma, 261–2
  sonography
    fibroadenoma, 173–4, 176
    invasive carcinoma, 256
adenofibrolipoma, 166–7
adenofibroma, 167
adenolipoma, 166
adenoma, 168
  papillary, of nipple, 180
adenosis, 142
  microcystic, and calcification, 385
  sclerosing, **399**
adolescent breast, 122–3, **124**
  see also young patient
air, after pneumocystography, **78**
air gap, in magnification mammography, **52,** 53
anatomy, normal breast, 122
angiolipoma, 188
angioma, 188
angiosarcoma, 269
anisomastia, 132
appearance, 121–324
application of diagnostic imaging of the breast, 329–403
architectural distortion, **398**
  with calcification, **381**
  diagnostic algorithm, **347**
  differential diagnosis, 346–8, **348–53**
  and invasive carcinoma, 248, 250, 253
arteriosclerosis, **379**
artifacts, 377–8, **378**
  nipple, contralateral, 339, **343**
aspiration, cysts, 160–1
asymmetry, 131, 132, **132–3,** 135
  and calcifications, 376
  diagnostic algorithm, **357–8**
asymptomatic patient, 67
attenuation
  compensation, 86
  and invasive carcinoma, 250
atypia, 142
  ductal, 110
atypical hyperplasia, 142
augmentation of breast
  changes after, 311–12
  summary, 313
autoimmune disease, and granuloma, 203, 204
automatic exposure control, 31
  assessment, 60–1
axillary view, 43, 46

B

BCDDP, 333, 334
B-cell lymphoma, 272
beam quality, assessment, 60
benefits of screening
  and cost, 335–6
  and risk, 334–5
benign disorders, 141–55
  clinical findings, 143
  cysts, 148–9
  definition, 141
  focal changes, 149
  histopathology, 141–3
  mammographic appearance, 144, **145**
  MRI, 151–4, **152, 153**
  summary, 154–5
  sonography, 149, **150**
benign tumors, 166–94
  angioma, 188
  diabetic mastopathy, 189–10
  fibroadenoma, 167–80
  fibrosis mammae, 190
  focal fibrous disease, 190
  granular cell, 188
  hamartoma, 166–7
  lipoma, 186–7
  lymph nodes, intramammary, 190–2
  myoblastoma, 188
  papilloma, 180–6
  rare, 187–8
  young patient, 393–4
biopsy
  excisional, 144, 199
  guns, **104**
  percutaneous, *see* percutaneous biopsy
  punch, and skin thickening, 322
  see also fine-needle aspiration cytology
BI-RADS
  category, 66
  lexicon, 64–5
  scale, 66
bleeding
  percutaneous biopsy, 103
  and preoperative localization, 112, 113
blunt duct adenosis, 142
blurring, 23–4
breast
  accessory tissue, 134
  adolescent, 122–3, **124**
  benign disorders, 141–55
    summary, 154–5
  clinical examination, 7–10
  compression, *see* compression of breast
  contour, 7
  cyst examination, 157
  dense, *see* dense breast
  and hormone replacement therapy, 138–9
    summary, 139
  implants, *see* implants
  mature, 125–30
  MRI, 128–30, **129**
  normal, 122–40
    anatomy, 122
  size, 7
  thickness, and radiation dose, 36
  sonography, 126, **126–8,** 128
  young patient, changes, 392

Breast Cancer Detection Demonstration Project (BCDDP), 333, 334
breast cancer in men, 326–28, **327**, **328**
breast-conserving therapy
with irradiation
changes after, 292–306
mammography, 293–301
MRI, 303, **304**, 305, **305**
percutaneous biopsy, 305–6
summary, 306
sonography, 301–3, **302**, **304**
without irradiation, changes after, 292
breast feeding, and image interpretation, 6
Burkitt lymphoma, 272
butterfly arrangement, calcifications, 376

C

calcifications, 65–6
after breast-conserving therapy, **285**
and angiomas, 188
associated changes, 66
benign, 65, 377–86
distribution, 383, 385–6
extramammary, 377, **377**, **378**
morphology, 379, **380**, 381, **381**, **382**
and benign disorders, 146–8
bizarre, 379, 381
branching, 373, **373**, **375**
clustered, 383, **383**, 385
and cysts, 161
differential diagnosis, 259
diffuse, 383
distribution, segmental, 376, **376**
ductal arrangement, 376
ductal carcinoma in situ, 212, 213–14
dystrophic, 281, 283, **381**
eggshell-like, **382**
fibroadenoma, 169, **170**, **171**, **172**, 381
fine-granular, 374, **376**
granular, 373–4
indeterminate, 65
linear, 373, **373**, **379**
magnification mammography, 371
malignant, 373–7
summary, 377
and mammographic detection, 370–2
necrotic, **380**, 381
needle-like, 373, **373**, 381
periductal, and plasma-cell mastitis, 198, **198**
pleomorphic, 373–4, **375**, **383**, **388**
popcorn-like, 379, 381
post-therapeutic, 297
psammomatous, **387**
punctate, **377**, **383**
ring-like, **377**, **380**
rounded, 379, **379**
semicircular, 379
shell-like, 379, **382**
solitary, 383
suture material, **286**
symmetric, 383
track-like, 385
see also macrocalcifications; microcalcifications
Cameco handle, **104**
Canadian screening study, 332
cancer risk
radiation dose, 34–5
screening, 334–5
young patient, 392–3, 395
capsular fibrosis, MRI findings, 98
carbon solution, for lesion marking, 118
carcinoma
adenoid cystic, 227
carcinosarcoma, 227
cribriform, 211, 213, 227
cyst wall, 164
diffusely growing, 241–3, **242–3**
ductal, *see* ductal carcinoma
inflammatory, 227, 243, **243**
intraductal, **244**
invasive, *see* invasive carcinoma
lobular, *see* lobular carcinoma
medullary, 226–7
micropapillary, 213
mucinous, 227
mucoepidermoid, 227
noncalcifying, 241
Paget, 227
papillary, 211, 227
in situ, 209–20
definition, 209
spindle cell, 227
squamous cell, 227
tubular, 227, **245**
types, 225–7
sonographic diagnosis, 81–2
young patient, **398–9**
see also breast cancer in men; lesions; malignancy; tumors; *specific types*
carcinosarcoma, 227
case control studies, screening, 332–3
summary, 333–4
casting microcalcifications, 373, **375**
CC, *see* craniocaudal view
CCD sensors, 67
checklist, visual, 61
chloroma, 272
chondroma, 187–8
chondrosarcoma, 269
cicatricial changes, *see* scars
circumscribed nodule, 169
classifications
ductal carcinoma in situ, 211–12
epithelial hyperplasia, 143
Holland, 212
papilloma, 180–1
Van Nuys, 211–12
cleavage view, 43, 46, **48**
clinical examination
asymmetry, 132
breast, 7–10
adolescent, 122
mature, 125
inverted nipple, 134
involution, 130
lactation, 136
macromastia, 133
papilloma, 181
polymastia, 134
pregnancy, 136
clinical findings, 7–10, 62
abscess, in mastitis, 200
benign breast disorders, 143
breast cancer in men, 326–7
changes after trauma and surgery, 280
cysts, 156
diabetic mastopathy, 189
ductal carcinoma in situ, 212
fibroadenoma, 168
fistulae, in mastitis, 200
granuloma, 203
gynecomastia, 326
hamartoma, 166
hematologic malignancies, 273
invasive carcinoma, 227–8
lipoma, 186
male breast, 324, 326–7
mastitis, 195
metastases, 276
nodular changes in skin, 317
papilloma, 181
phyllodes tumor, 265
post-therapeutic, 292–3
sarcomas, 269
skin thickening, 320–1
summary, 10
young patient, 393
clock face description, 62
club arrangement, calcifications, 376
cluster shapes, 65
documentation, **63**
microcalcifications, 148
coffee-bean shape, lymph nodes, **191**
collimation assessment, 60
comedo ductal carcinoma in situ, 211, **237**
calcifications, 213, **214**, **215**, 373
MRI, 218
compressibility
and solid masses, 91
sonographic assessment, 88, **89**
compression of breast, 37–9, **38**, 61
and contrast, 29

and fibroadenoma, 173, **175**
and patient information, 39
for scatter reduction, 18–19
spot, 49, **49, 50**
compression paddle/cone, 41
in spot compression, 49
compression plate, 113, **114**
computer-aided image analysis, 372
contour of breast, 7
and solid masses, 90
contraindications
galactography, 69
percutaneous biopsy, 101
pneumocystography, 76
contrast, 26–33
definitions, 26, 27
film, 20–1
and film selection, **32,** 32–3
MRI, 92–3, 97–8
optimizing, 27
radiation spectrum, 15–16
resolution, in sonography, 83
Cooper's ligaments, 125, **125,** 128
core biopsy, *see* percutaneous biopsy
costs and benefits, screening, 66–7, 335–6
craniocaudal (CC) view, 41–2, **42**
exaggerated lateral, 44–6, **45**
exaggerated medial, 43, 46
cribriform carcinoma, 211, 213, **216,** 227
curve, characteristic, density and radiation dose, 20, **22,**23
cutaneous changes, post-therapeutic, 295, **297**
cut sausage pattern, 166
cystosarcoma phyllodes, 265–8, **266–7,** 268, **268**
cysts, **77,** 142, 156–65
air-fluid level, **78**
aspiration, 160–1
in benign disorders, 148–9
breast examination, 157
and calcifications, 161
complicated, 156
differential diagnosis, **163**
mammography, 161, **162, 163**
milk of calcium, **382**
pathognomonic findings, 338
oil, *see* oil cysts
pathognomonic findings, 338
pneumocystography, 161, **162, 163**
simple, 156
summary, 164
sonography, **163**
diagnosis, 81
findings, 90
typical appearance, 157, **158–60,** 160
see also pneumocystography
cytology
nipple discharge, 181
smear, invasive carcinoma, 228
see also fine-needle aspiration cytology

D

darkroom
cleanliness, 61
fog, 61
DCIS, *see* ductal carcinoma in situ
definitions
abnormalities, 131
breast-conserving treatment, 292
circumscribed nodule, 169
contrast, 26, 27
cysts, 156
galactoceles, 164
galactography, 69
gynecomastia, 324
inflammatory changes, 391
magnification technique, mammography, 49
microcalcifications, indeterminate, 386
multicentricity, 224
nipple discharge, 389
pathognomonic findings, 338
percutaneous biopsy, 101
pneumocystography, 76
preoperative localization, 112
reconstruction, 306
screening, 331
in situ carcinoma, 209
skin thickening, 317–18
spot compression, 49
demarcation, sonography, invasive carcinoma, 250
dense breast
asymptomatic patients
high risk, 359–61, **361–2, 362–3**
low risk, 357–9
differential diagnosis and work-up, 357–70
and nipple retraction, diagnostic algorithm, **371**
with palpable finding, 364–7, **365**
diagnostic algorithm, **366**
search for primary tumor, diagnostic algorithm, **367**
special considerations, 367, **368, 369,** 370, **370**
density
film, 20, **22,** 23
and masses, 64
not smoothly outlined, 344, 346
diagnostic algorithm, **345**
radiographic, invasive carcinoma, 229
smoothly outlined, 339, 341, **342–4**
diagnostic algorithm, **340**
soft, and microcalcifications, **388,** 388–9, **389**
depth localization, in percutaneous biopsy, **106**
description of masses, 64–5
desmoid, extra-abdominal, 278
detectability, invasive carcinoma, 221–2
deviation of nipple, 6, 8
diabetic mastopathy, summary, 190
diagnosis
abscesses, in mastitis, 200
benign disorders, 143–4
changes
after augmentation, 311–12
after reconstruction, 307
after reduction, 313
cysts, 157, 160
diabetic mastopathy, 189
ductal carcinoma in situ, 212
fibroadenoma, 179–80
findings at screening, 338–403
fistulae, in mastitis, 200
granuloma, 203–4
gynecomastia, 326–7
hamartoma, 166
hematologic malignancies, 273
imaging, 329–403
invasive carcinoma, 222–5
lipoma, 186
lymph nodes
intramammary, 191
in invasive carcinoma, 225
mastitis, 195
metastases, 276
nodular changes in skin, 317
papilloma, 181–2
phyllodes tumor, 265–6
post-therapeutic, 293
sarcomas, 269
skin thickening, 320
young patient, 401
see also diagnostic algorithms; differential diagnosis
diagnostic algorithms
architectural distortion, **347**
asymmetry, **357–8**
dense breast
and nipple retraction, **371**
with palpable finding, **366**
search for primary tumor, **367**
inflammatory changes, **390**
lesions not smoothly outlined, **345**
microcalcifications, **385–5**
nipple retraction, **371**
smoothly outlined density, **340–1**
see also differential diagnosis
differential diagnosis, 339–91
asymmetry, 353, **354,** 355, **355, 356**
calcifications, 259
cysts, **163**
dense breast, 357–70
fibroadenoma *vs.* tumor, 168
invasive carcinoma, 248, 256
lesions not smoothly outlined, 344–6

microcalcifications, 370–89
indeterminate, 387–8
differential nipple discharge, 389–90
papilloma *vs.* papillary carcinoma, 181
recurrence, 297, 300
smoothly outlined density, 339–44
diagnostic algorithm, **340–1**
soft density and microcalcifications, **388,** 388–9
see also diagnosis; diagnostic algorithms
diffuse changes, and malignancy, 248
diffusely growing carcinoma, 241–3, **242–3**
digital mammography, 67–8
and microcalcifications, 371–2
summary, 68
discharge, *see* nipple discharge
distance, source to image-receptor, 15, **15**
distortion, *see* architectural distortion
documentation, 62
cluster shapes, **63**
focal lesions, **63**
microcalcifications, **63**
MRI, 96–7
previous findings, 62–3
screening findings, 66–7
dose, *see* radiation dose
drill biopsy, 101
ductal atypia, 110
ductal carcinoma, 226, **233, 238, 252, 259**
diffusely growing, **242**
follow-up mammography, **244**
galactography, **247**
histology, 246
hypercellular, **253**
invasive, 226, **399–400**
after false negative findings, **396–7**
multifocal, **257**
nodular, **234**
scirrhous, **232**
sonography and histology, 254
see also comedo ductal carcinoma; ductal carcinoma in situ; noncomedo carcinoma
ductal carcinoma in situ (DCIS), **74,** 210–20
classification, 211–12
clinical findings, 212
cribriform, **216**
definition, 210
diagnosis, 212
histology, 211–12
mammography, 212–16, **214, 215,** 215–16, **216–17**
accuracy, 215
follow-up, **245**
and microcalcifications, 212, 213–14, **214, 215**
MRI, 218
papillary, **216, 217**
percutaneous biopsy, 110, 218
specimen radiography, 216, **216**
staging, 224
sonography, 218
summary, 219
ductal hyperplasia, 142
atypical, 142–3
duct ectasia, 71, **72**
dye marking, 118
dystrophic calcification, **381**

E

echoes, 86–7
echogenicity, invasive carcinoma, 250
ectasia, lactiferous ducts, 71
Edinburgh screening study, 331–2
Eklund's method, breast implant imaging, 55, **55,** 56
elasticity, invasive carcinoma, 253
epithelial hyperplasia, 142–3
classification, 143
epitheliosis, 142
equipment, visual inspection, 61
erythema, 248
examination
clinical, *see* clinical examination
technique
MRI, 95–6
sonography, 86–8
exposure, 21
and contrast, 30–1
control, 58
automatic, 31
manual, 31–2
and sensitive film, 33, **33**
technique, dose-related optimization, 35
extension of tumor, 224
MRI, 256–7
extra-abdominal desmoid, 278

F

fat necrosis, 280, 281, **286,** 289, **380**
fibroadenoma, 156, 167–80
accuracy of diagnosis
mammography, 173
sonography, 173–4, 176
adult, 168
age and incidence, 167–8
appearance, **170**
and calcifications, **382,** 385
pleomorphic, **388**
calcified, 381
pathognomonic findings, 338
clinical findings, 168
diagnosis, 179–80
edematous, **175,** 177, **178**
fibrosis, sonographic features, 173, **176**
giant, 392
histology, 168
incidence, 167
intracanalicular, 169
juvenile, 167, 168, **172,** 392
mammography, 169, **170–2,** 173
MRI, 176–9, **177, 178**
myxoid, **171**
old, 169, **177**
percutaneous biopsy, 176
pericanalicular, 169, **172**
sclerosed, 176, **177**
summary, 180
therapeutic recommendations, **170**
sonography, **84, 172,** 173–4, **175,** 176, **176**
characteristic features, 173
young, **178**
in young patient, **395**
fibroepithelial mixed tumors, 167–80
fibromatosis, 278
fibrosarcoma, 269
fibrosis
benign, 189
diabetic, **189,** 189–90
in fibroadenoma, 173, **176**
focal, 142
strands, imaging, 13
fibrosis mammae, 190
filling defects, galactography, 71, **72, 73, 74**
filling in, cyst echoes, **159**
film, **19,** 19–21, **20**
density, 36
exposure, 21
fixture retention, 61
labelling, 44
noise, 34
processing, 21, 33, 37
and image quality, 59
reading, 23
selection, and contrast, **32,** 32–3
sensitive, and exposure time, 33, **33**
filtering, radiation spectrum, 16
findings
clinical, *see* clinical findings
documentation, 62
evaluation, 338–403
galactography, 70–1
MRI, interpreting, 96–9
normal, *see* normal findings
palpable, 67
pathognomonic, 338
pneumocystography, 77
previous, and documentation, 62–3
screening, examples, 67
sonography
interpreting, 88–91
normal, 88, 90
fine-needle aspiration cytology, 101

accuracy, 101–2
and cyst fluids, 161
materials, 103
stereotaxic biopsy, 105
fingerprint artifact, 377, **378**
fistulae, and mastitis, 199–201
summary, 202
fixture retention, film, 61
FLASH 3D imaging, 94, 128, **129**
benign disorder, **152**
fibroadenoma, **177**
Florence screening study, 332–3
focal changes
in benign disorders, 149
post-therapeutic, **298**
focal enhancement, 97
focal fibrosis, 142
focal fibrous disease, 190
focal lesions, documentation, **63**
focal spot performance, 60
focal spot size, 15
focusing
sonography, 83
in ultrasound examination, 87–8
fog, darkroom, 61
follow-up mammography, 62
ductal carcinoma, **244**
invasive carcinoma, 243, **244–5**
foreign body granuloma, 203
fungal infection, 203

G

gadolinium diethylenetriaminepentaacetic acid (Gd-DTPA), 94, 129
gain, in ultrasound examination, 86
for cyst diagnosis, 157
galactoceles, 164, **165**
pathognomonic findings, 338
galactography, 69–75
contraindications, 69
definition, 69
ductal carcinoma, **247**
guided localization, 118
indications, 69
invasive carcinoma, 223
normal, **71**
papilloma, 183, **183**
preoperative marking, 71
procedure, 69–70
side effects, 69
summary, 71
galactophoritis, 285
galactorrhea, 69
Gd-DTPA, 94, 129
gel, in sonographic examination, 85, 86
gelplate, 85
generator, 57
geometric blurring, 24
giant fibroadenoma, 167, 392
glandular tissue, normal, 126
granular cell tumor, 188, **188**
granularity, 49
granuloma, 203–8, **284**
clinical findings, 203
histology, 203
Kveim test, 203
lipophagic, 297, **299**
mammography, 203
percutaneous biopsy, 207
and scarring, 204, **205**, 207
silicone, 204, 205, **205**, **206**, 207
summary, 207–8
sonography, 203–4
grid mammography, 18, 36
and contrast, 29
in magnification mammography, 53
for scatter reduction, 18
gynecomastia, 324–5, **325**, **326**
summary, 328

H

hamartoma, 166–7, **167**
pathognomonic findings, 338
hardware, and image quality, 57–8
Health Insurance Plan of Greater New York study, 331
heel effect, 17–18, **18**
hemangioma, 188
hematologic malignancies, 272–4, **274**, **275**
summary, 274
hematoma
after trauma and surgery, 280, 281
mammography, **288**
MRI, 291
sonographic appearance, 288, **288**
hemorrhage
MRI, 291
sonographic appearance, 287–8
histiocytoma, malignant fibrous, 269
histology
abscess, in mastitis, 199–200
adolescent breast, 122
breast cancer in men, 326
changes after trauma and surgery, 280
cysts, 156
diabetic mastopathy, 189
ductal carcinoma in situ, 211–12
fibroadenoma, 168
fistulae, in mastitis, 200
granuloma, 203
gynecomastia, 326
hamartoma, 166
invasive carcinoma, 225–7
and mammographic presentation, 246, **247**, 248
and sonographic findings, 254, 256
lactation, 136
lobular carcinoma in situ, 209–10
mature breast, normal, 125
metastases, 275–6
phyllodes tumor, 265
pregnancy, 136
sarcomas, 269
histopathology
benign disorders, 141–3
papilloma, 180–1
history, *see* patient history
Hodgkin lymphoma, 272
screening after, 395
Holland classification, 212
hormone replacement therapy, 6
breast response, 138–9
summary, 139
hypercellular carcinoma, **255**
hyperplasia, epithelial, 142–3
hyperthermia, 248

I

ill-defined mass, 344, **345**, 346
illumination, 22, 23
image analysis
computer-aided, 67, 372
and medical history data, 6
image intensifier, selenium, 67
image quality
evaluation, 61
and hardware, 57–8
and screen–film system, 58–9
sonography, 83, **84**, 85–6
near field, 85
phantoms, 85
summary, 86
imaging
comparison with earlier findings, 6
diagnostic, 329–403
digital, and microcalcifications, 371–1
receptor system, **19**, 19–21, **20**
repeated, and radiation dose, 37
sharpness, 23–6
sonography, 86
subtraction, 94
technique, components, **14**, 14–22
viewing, 22–3
implants, 306
failure, and unenhanced MRI, 93
and mammography, 53, **55**, 55–6
normal MRI findings, 98
parenchymal areas obscured, **309**
rupture, 98–9, **99**, **307–8**
see also prosthesis
incidence
ductal carcinoma in situ, 210–11
fibroadenoma, 167
lobular carcinoma in situ, 209
microcalcifications, indeterminate, 386
skin thickening, 318, 320
indications
galactography, 69
mammography, 11

magnification, 53
indications
MRI, 93
cysts, 162
invasive carcinoma, 260
percutaneous biopsy, 101, 102
invasive carcinoma, 262
pneumocystography, 76
preoperative localization, 112
spot compression, 49
sonography, invasive carcinoma, 249
inflammatory carcinoma, 227, 243, **243**
histology, 246, 256
sonography, 256
inflammatory conditions, 194–208, 391
diagnostic algorithm, **390**
in-phase condition, in MRI, 94
inspection of equipment, 61
interference, sonography, 85
interpretation
of imaging
computer-assisted, 67
and medical history data, 6
of screening findings, 66–7
intracanalicular fibroadenoma, 169
intracapsular rupture, 98, **308**
intraductal carcinoma, **244, 258**
intraductal papilloma, 180
intramammary lymph nodes, 190–2, **191, 192**
summary, 192
invasive carcinoma, 221–64
clinical findings, 227–8
cytology, 228
definition, 221
detectability, 221–2
diagnosis, 222–5
elasticity, 253
histology, 225–7
and mammographic presentation, 246, **247,** 248
imaging methods, 223
indirect signs, 238, **239–41**
mammography, 228–48, **232–6**
sensitivity and specificity, 11–12, 248
signs, 229, **230**
and microcalcifications, 236–7, **237–8**
mobility, 254
MRI, 256–60, **257–9**
mucinous, **235**
percutaneous biopsy, 260–2
screening, 222
spectrum, 221–2
staging, 224–5
summary, 262–3
types, 225–7
sonography, 249–56
accuracy, 256
appearance, **251, 252–3**
inverted nipple, 6, 8, 131, 134, 135, **135**
involution, 130–1
summary, 131

J

Jackson sign, 8
juvenile fibroadenoma, 167, **172,** 392
juvenile papillomatosis, **394,** 400
Swiss-cheese appearance, 400

K

keyhole sign, 98
Kveim test, and granuloma, 203

L

lactation, 136, **137,** 138
lactiferous ducts, 69–75, 122, **123**
ectasia, 71, **72**
normal mature breast, 126
sonographic imaging, 73, **74, 75**
Lanyi distribution, 66
lateral view, 90°, **43,** 43–4
lateromedial view, **43**
latissimus dorsi flap, 307
LCIS, *see* lobular carcinoma
legal aspects, 223
leiomyoma, 187, **187**
leiomyosarcoma, 269
lesions
benign, *see* benign tumors
depth calculation, 106
differentiation, ultrasound, 81
excised, radiography, 56
orientation, and malignancy, 250
palpable, percutaneous biopsy, 110
structure, and malignancy, 250
see also carcinoma; density; localization; malignancy; tumors
leukemia, 272
linear calcifications, **379**
line pairs per millimeter (LP/mm), 25
linguini sign, 99, **99**
lipoma, 186, **187**
pathognomonic findings, 338
liponecrosis, calcifying, 283, 285, **285, 286,** 385
lipophagic granuloma, 297, **299**
liposarcoma, 269
litigation, and accuracy of detection, 223
lobular carcinoma, **255**
diffusely growing, **242**
histology, 246
invasive, 226
in situ (LCIS), 209–10
sonography and histology, 254
lobular hyperplasia, 142
atypical, 143
lobulated mass, 248
localization
calcifications, 65
carbon solution marking, 118
with compression plate, 113, **114**
galactographically guided, 118
manual, 113, **114,** 115, **116–17**
marker wires, 119, **119**
materials, 118–19, **119**
MRI-guided, 118
preoperative, 112–20
stereotaxic, 113–14
needle biopsy, **108**
summary, 120
techniques, 113–15, **114, 116–17,** 119
ultrasound-guided, **117,** 117–18
see also preoperative localization
location, describing, 62
LP/mm, *see* line pairs per millimeter
lumps, clinical findings, 8, 10
lymphangioma, 188
lymph nodes
axillary, and staging, 225
intramammary, 190–2, **191, 192**
summary, 192
pathognomonic findings, 338
lymphoma, 272

M

macrocalcifications, **382**
macromastia, 131, 133
magnetic resonance imaging (MRI), 92–100
abscesses, in mastitis, 201, **202**
accuracy, ductal carcinoma in situ, 218
benign disorders, 151–4, **152, 153**
changes after trauma or surgery, 291
cysts, 162–4
diabetic mastopathy, 190
documentation, 96–7
ductal carcinoma in situ, 218
and extension of tumor, 256–7
fibroadenoma, 176–9
diagnosis, 179
fistulae, in mastitis, 201
granuloma, 205–7, **206**
hematologic malignancies, 273, **274**
hemorrhage, 291
and hormone replacement therapy, 139
indications, 93, 260
interpreting findings, 96–9
invasive carcinoma, 223, 256–60, **257–9**
involution, 131
lactation, 138

localization, guided, 118
lymph nodes, intramammary, 192, **193**
mastitis, **197,** 199
and menstrual cycle, scheduling, 2, 130
metastases, 277
and microcalcifications, 372
needle biopsy, guided, 110
nipple, inverted, 135
normal mature breast, 128–30, **129**
papilloma, **185,** 185–6
patient acceptance, 2–3
phyllodes tumor, 267, **267**
pitfalls, 258–9
polymastia, 134
post-therapeutic, 303, **304,** 305, **305**
pregnancy, 138
and reconstruction, 310–11, **310–11**
sarcoma, 270, 272
silicone-only sequence, 95, 98
skin thickening, 322
technical requirements, 93–5
unenhanced, 93
young patient, 401
magnification mammography, 49, 51–3, **52**
and calcification, 371
definition, 49
and digital technology, 67
ductal carcinoma in situ, **216**
focal fibrous breast disease, **147**
indications, 53
oil cyst, **286**
technique, 57
male breast, 324–28
leiomyoma, **187**
malignancy
hematologic, 272–4, **274, 275**
indirect signs, 238, **239–41**
and microcalcifications, 373–7
and MRI contrast enhancement, 97
young patient, 394
see also carcinoma; density; malignancy; tumors; *specific types*
mammographic unit, assembly evaluation, 60
mammography, 11–80
abscesses, in mastitis, 201, **202**
accuracy, 11–12
adolescent breast, 122, **124**
asymmetry, 132, **132–3**
and benign disorders, 144, **145**
breast cancer in men, 327, **327, 328**
calcifications, detection, 370–2
changes
after augmentation, 312
after reconstruction, 307–10
after trauma and surgery, 281–5, **281–7**
cysts, 161, **162, 163**
dense breast, 357
diabetic mastopathy, 189, **189**
diffusely growing carcinoma, **242**
digital, 67–8
summary, 68
ductal carcinoma in situ, 212–16, **214–17**
accuracy, 215
false negative findings, 394, **396–7**
fistulae, in mastitis, 201
follow-up, 243, **244–5**
galactoceles, 164, **165**
granuloma, 203
grid, 18, 36
and contrast, 29
and magnification, 53
scatter reduction, 18
guided localization techniques, 113–15, **114, 116–17,** 119
gynecomastia, 327, **327**
hamartoma, 166, **167**
hematologic malignancies, 273, **274, 275**
hematoma, **288**
and histology, in invasive carcinoma, 246, **247,** 248
and hormone replacement therapy, 138, **139**
indications, 11
intramammary lymph nodes, 191, **191**
invasive carcinoma, 223, 228–48, **232–6**
sensitivity and specificity, 11–12, 248
inverted nipple, 134, **135**
involution, 130
lactation, 136, **136, 137**
lipoma, 186, **187**
magnification, *see* magnification mammography
male breast, 326
mastitis, 195–8, **196, 197–8**
metastases, 276, **277, 278**
and microcalcifications, summary, 372
microfocus, 67
nodular changes in skin, 317, **318–19**
normal mature breast, **125,** 125–6
oil cysts, **289**
and palpation, 10
papilloma, **182,** 182–3
patient information, 2
phyllodes tumor, 266, **266, 268**
polymastia, 134
post-therapeutic, 293–301
pregnancy, 136, **137**
problem solving, 13
quality factors, 57–61
questionnaire, 4–5
radiation dose, 34
recurrence, **300–2**
report, 62–7
sarcoma, 269–70, **270–1**
scars, 282, **282–3, 284**
screening, 12
sensitivity, 13
skin thickening, 321
slot, 67
standard views, 39–43
technique, 12–14
components, **14,** 14–22
technological improvement, 67
viewing areas, 23
young patient, 393–7
Mammography Quality Assurance Act, 59
mammoplasty, *see* augmentation of breast; reduction of breast
manual exposure, 31–2
manual localization, 113, **114,** 115, **116–17**
margins, sonography, invasive carcinoma, 250
marker wires, for lesion localization, 119, **119**
masses
associated changes, 66
and densities, 64
description, 64–5
granulomatous, 203
ill-defined, 344, **345,** 346
intraductal, **72, 73, 74**
ultrasound findings, 90
see also density; lesions; tumors
mastectomy, reconstruction after, 306
mastitis, 194–9
abscesses, 199–201, **202**
acute, 195, **196**
chronic, 195, **197**
clinical findings, 195
diagnosis, 195
etiology, 194–5
fistulae, 199–201
mammography, 195–8, **196, 197–8**
MRI, **197,** 199
plasma cell, 198, **198,** 285, 373, **375,** 381, **383**
tuberculous, 203
sonography, 198–9
mastodynia, 143
mastopathy
diabetic, **189,** 189–90
proliferative, **241**
medical physicist, responsibilities, 59–61
mediolateral oblique (MLO) view, 39–41, **40**
mediolateral view, **43**
medullary carcinoma, 226–7, **247, 252**

histology, 246
sonography and histology, 254
menstrual cycle, and MRI scheduling, 2, 130, 151
metastases, 275–8
summary, 278
methods, 1–120
microbiology, granuloma, 203
microcalcifications, 53, **54**, 236–7
analysis, 372
benign, 377–86
summary, 385
and benign disorders, 146–8
clusters, 148
diagnostic algorithm, **384–5**
differential diagnosis, 370–89
documentation, **63**
in ductal carcinoma, invasive, **399–400**
in ductal carcinoma in situ, 212, 213–14, **214, 215**
extramammary, 386
and fibroadenoma, **382**
imaging, 12, 13
indeterminate, 386–8
differential diagnosis, 387–8
intramammary
distribution pattern, 386
morphology, 385
and invasive carcinoma, **231**, 236–7, **237–8**, 248
linear, **387**
malignant, 373–7
and mastitis, 195–6
monomorphic, **387**
parallel, 381
pleomorphic, **387, 389**
post-therapeutic, **286–7**
punctate, **387**
and recurrence, 300–1
in specimen radiography, 56
summary, 372
microcystic adenosis, and calcification, 385
microcysts, 142
microfocus mammography, 67, 372
microglandular adenosis, 142
micropapillary carcinoma, 213
milk, witch's, 164
milk of calcium cysts, **145**, 147, **382**
pathognomonic findings, 338
MLO, *see* mediolateral oblique view
mobility
invasive carcinoma, 254
and solid masses, 91
ultrasound assessment, 88, **89**
modulation transfer function (MTF), 26, **26**
molybdenum, target/filter combinations, 16, **17**
Mondor disease, 8
motion blur, 23–4
MRI, *see* magnetic resonance imaging
mucinous carcinoma, 227, **235**
histology, 246, 254
ultrasound, 254
multicentricity, definition, 224
multifocus, ultrasonography, 83
myoblastoma, 188, **188**
myocutaneous flap, 308, **309**, 310

N

near field, 85
necrosis, 280
needle biopsy, *see* percutaneous biopsy
needle-like calcifications, **373, 375**, 381
needle positioning, percutaneous biopsy, **107**
neurofibroma, 187
Nijmegen screening study, 332–3
90° lateral view, **43**, 43–4
nipple
contralateral, as artifact, 339, **343**
inverted, 6, 8, 131, 134, 135, **135**
papillary adenoma, 180
retraction, in dense breast, 370
diagnostic algorithm, **371**
shadow, **127**, 128
and signs of malignancy, 6, 8
see also nipple discharge
nipple discharge
benign disorders, 143
cytology, 181
definition, 389
in dense breast, 370
differential diagnosis and workup, 389–90
and galactography, 69
and invasive carcinoma, 246, 248
and signs of malignancy, 6
nodular changes, skin, 317, **318–19**
nodule, circumscribed, 169
noise, 33–4, 49
quantum, 33
non-comedo carcinoma, 211, **399**
calcifications, 213
MRI, 218
non-Hodgkin lymphoma, 272
diffuse, **275**
nodular, **274**
normal findings, 122–40
anatomy, 122
galactography, **71**
glandular tissue, 126
histology, 125
implants, MRI, 98
lactiferous ducts, 126
male breast, **325**
mammography, **125**, 125–6
MRI, 98, 128–30, **129**
parenchyma, 126
sonography, 88, 90, 126, **126–8**, 128

O

oblique view, 46
offset pad, 85, **85**, 87
oil cysts, 283, 285, **286**, 297
calcifying, **382**
mammography, **289**
pathognomonic findings, 338
sonographic appearance, **289**
ointment artifact, 377, **378**
optical density, 20, **22**, 23
osteochondrosarcoma, 269
osteoma, 187–8

P

Paget disease, 8, 227
histology, 246
pain
in dense breast, 367
percutaneous biopsy, 103
and preoperative localization, 112
see also mastodynia
palpation, 8–10, 62
and invasive carcinoma, 228
and mammography, 10
papillary carcinoma, 211, **216, 217**, 227, **259**
sonography and histology, 254, 256
vs. papilloma, 181
papilloma, 180–6
and calcification, 385
classification, 180–1
clinical findings, 181
cyst wall, 164
diagnosis, 181–2
galactography, 183, **183**
mammography, **182**, 182–3
percutaneous biopsy, 186
summary, 186
sonography, 183, **184**
papillomatosis, **72, 73**
juvenile, 180–1, **394**, 400
parasitosis, 203
parenchyma
changes, post-therapeutic, 294, 295, **296, 297**
normal mature breast, 126
pattern, 64
pathognomonic findings, 338
patient history, 3–6
cysts, 156
fibroadenoma, 168
invasive carcinoma, 228
in MRI, 96–7
patients
asymptomatic, 67
informing, 2–3
breast compression, 39
mammography, 2
percutaneous biopsy, 103
puncture, 3
questionnaire, 4–5

symptomatic, evaluation, 338–403
young, 391–401
peak kilovoltage (kVp), 16
accuracy, 60
and contrast, 28
in magnification mammography, 52–3
optimizing for contrast, 29
and radiation quality, 35
setting, 16
peau d'orange, 248
penetration
heel effect, 17–18, **18**
radiation spectrum, 15–16
percutaneous biopsy
accuracy, 101–2, 105, 107
invasive carcinoma, 261–2
and benign disorders, 144, 154
changes after augmentation, 312
contraindications, 101
core
accuracy, 261
and microcalcifications, 372
definitions, 101
depth localization, **106**
diabetic mastopathy, 190
drill, 101
ductal carcinoma in situ, 218
and fibroadenoma, 176
granulomas, 207
hamartoma, 167
and hormone replacement therapy, 139
indications, 101, 102
invasive carcinoma, 262
intramammary lymph nodes, 192
invasive carcinoma, 223, 260–2
lymphoma, 274
materials, 103
metastases, 277
methods, 101–11
needle, 101, 102
materials, 103
MRI-guided, 110
positioning, **107**
ultrasound-guided, 108–10, **109, 110**
palpable lesions, 110
papilloma, 186
patient information, 103
phyllodes tumor, 267
post-therapeutic, 305–6
scar tissue, 291
side effects, 101, 103
stereotaxic, 101, 104–8
summary, 111
young patient, 400–1
pericanalicular fibroadenoma, 169, **172**
phantom images
mammography, 61
sonography, 85
photocell, 21
and automatic exposure control, 31
positioning, **23,** 31, 42
phyllodes tumor, 265–8, **266–7, 268**
summary, 268
physician's work sheet, 9
physicist, medical, 59–61
plasma cell mastitis, 285, 373, **375,** 381, **383**
plasmacytoma, 272
pneumocystography, 76–8, **77,** 157, 161, **162, 163**
definition, 76
papilloma, 183, 185
summary, 78
polymastia, 131, 134, 135
popcorn-like calcifications, 379, 381
positioning, 37
abbreviations, 44
additional views, 43–4
optimum, 43
of photocell, **23**
standard views, 39–43
for stereotaxic needle biopsy, **108**
sonographic examination, 86, **87**
post-surgical changes, 280–91
post-traumatic changes, 280–91
Prechtel grades, epithelial hyperplasia, 143
pregnancy, 136, **137,** 138
and image interpretation, 6
young patient, 392
preoperative localization, 112–20
definition, 112
indications, 112
side effects, 112–13
primary tumor, search, 367, **367**
problem solving, in mammography, 13
processing, film, 21
processor, quality control, 61
proliferative mastopathy, **241**
prosthesis, silicone, 307–8
evaluating defects, 311
and recurrence, **309**
types, 306
pseudogynecomastia, **326**
puerperal mastitis, 194
pulse sequence
in MRI, selection, 94
unenhanced MRI, 95
punch biopsy, for skin thickening, 322
punctate calcifications, **377**
puncture, patient information, 3

Q

quadrant, 62
quality assurance, mammography, 57–61, 59–61
quantum noise, 33–4
questionnaire
patient information, 4–5
physician's work sheet, 9

R

radial scar, 110, 142
radiation
protection, 58
quality, 35–6, 57
and contrast, 27
risk
in screening, 334–5
young patient, 395
scattered, 18–19
spectrum, 15–16, **17**
see also scatter reduction; X-ray
radiation dose, 13, 34–6
and film processing time, 37
in magnification mammography, 53
minimizing, 36
and repeat images, 37
radiography
specimen, 56, **56,** 216, **216**
see also mammography
radiologic technologist, responsibilities, 61
radiotherapy
changes after, **295**
and image interpretation, 6
randomized screening studies, 331–2
summary, 333–4
reconstruction of breast
changes after, 306–10
definition, 306
and MRI, 310–11, **310–11**
summary, 313
and sonography, 310
recurrence
detection, 297, 300
focally growing, 300
mammography, **300–2**
and microcalcifications, 300–1
with prosthesis, **309**
reduction of breast
changes after, 312–13, **313–15**
summary, 313
repeat analysis, 61
repeat images, 37
reporting, 62–7
resolution, 57
in magnification mammography, 51
and modulation transfer function, 26, **26**
and screen-film system, 24–6, **25**
total, in magnification mammography, 51
sonography, 83
reverberation echoes, 85, **85**
cyst wall, **158**
reverse C sign, 98, **99**
rhabdomyosarcoma, 269

rhodium, target/filter combinations, 16, **17**
ring-like calcifications, **377, 380**
risk, 3
  and benefit, in screening, 334–5
  radiation dose, 34–5
rolled views, 43, 48, **48**
round calcifications, 379, **379**
round changes, and malignancy, 248
rupture, implants, 98–9, **99**

S

salad oil sign, 99
sarcoidosis, 203
  and granuloma, 203, 204
sarcomas, 269–72, **270–1**
  summary, 272
sausage pattern, 166
scar granulomas, 204, **205**, 207
scars, 281
  after reduction mammoplasty, **313–15**
  after trauma or surgery, 289, **290**, 291
  and calcifications, 381, 385
  mammography, 282, **282–3, 284**
  post-therapeutic, 295
  radial, 110, 142
scatter echoes, 87
scatter reduction, 18–19, **30**
  and contrast, 29
  grid, and radiation dose, 36
  in magnification mammography, 53
scheduling of examinations, 2, 130, 151
scirrhous ductal carcinoma, **232**
sclerosing adenosis, 142
screen
  cleanliness, 61
  noise, 33–4
  speed, 61
screen-film system, **19**, 19–21, **20**
  blurring, 24
  contact, 24–5, 61
  and contrast, 33
  and image quality, 58–9
  and radiation dose, 36–7
  and resolution, 24–6, **25**
screening, 331–7
  after Hodgkin disease, 395
  benefit-cost, 335–6
  benefit-risk, 334–5
  case control studies, 332–3
    summary, 333–4
  definition, 331
  findings
    documenting, 66–7
    evaluating, 338–403
    example, 67
    interpreting, 66–7
  invasive carcinoma, 222
  mammography, 12
  and mediolateral oblique view, 39
  randomized studies, 331–2
    summary, 333–4
  recommendations, 336
segmentectomy, changes after, **294–4**
sensitivity of mammography, 11–12, 248
seroma
  after trauma and surgery, 280, 281
  MRI, 291
  sonographic appearance, 288
setting, peak kilovoltage, 16
sharpness
  image, 23–6
    sonography, 86
  imaging technique, 15, **15**
  screen-film system, 20
shell-like calcifications, 379
side effects
  galactography, 69
  percutaneous biopsy, 101, 103
  pneumocystography, 76
  preoperative localization, 112–13
silicone granulomas, 204, 205, **205, 206**, 207
silicone prosthesis, 307–8
  rupture, 98
size of breast, 7
skin changes, 7–8, 317–23
  and invasive carcinoma, 228
skin thickening, 317–18, 320–2, **320–2**
  clinical findings, 320–1
  definition, 317–18
  diagnosis, 320
  incidence, 318, 320
  and malignancy, 248
  mammography, 321
  MRI, 322
  punch biopsy, 322
  summary, 322
slice thickness
  contrast MRI, 93–4
  sonography, 85
  unenhanced MRI, 95
slot mammography, 67
smoothly outlined density
  differential diagnosis and work-up, 339–41, **342–4**
  and malignancy, 248
soft density, and microcalcifications, **388**, 388–9, **389**
sonography, 81–91
source to image-receptor distance (SID), 15, **15**
specificity of mammography, 12
specimen radiography, 56, **56**
  ductal carcinoma in situ, 216, **216**
specular echoes, 86–7
spiculated masses, 248
spiculation, 282, **284**
spindle cell tumor, benign, 187
spot compression, 49, **49, 50**
spotlight, 22
staging, invasive carcinoma, 224–5
stereotaxic biopsy, 104–8
stereotaxic localization, 113–14
subtraction images, 94
surgery, and image interpretation, 6
suture material, calcified, **286**
Swedish screening studies, 331–2
Swiss-cheese appearance, in juvenile papillomatosis, 400

T

tangential view, 46, **47**
target/filter combinations, 16, **17**
  and contrast, 28, **28**
  optimizing, 29
  and radiation quality, 35
TDLU, *see* terminal ductulobular unit
teacup sign, **145**, 148, 381, **382**
technologist, radiologic, responsibilities, 61
terminal ductulobular unit (TDLU), 122, **122**
terminology, lactiferous duct system, **123**
three-dimensional (3D) sequences, contrast MRI, 94
thyroid hormone, 6
time-gain compensation, 86–7, **87**
tissue necrosis, 280
transducer, selecting, 83
transverse rectus abdominis flap, 307
trigger point, papilloma diagnosis, 181
Tru-Cut needle, **104**
true lateral view, **43**, 43–4
tube power, 57
tuberculosis, 203
tubular carcinoma, 227, **245**
  histology, 246
tumors
  benign, *see* benign tumors
  localizing, **64**
  phyllodes, 265–8, **266–7**, 268, **268**
  primary, search, 367, **367**
  see also carcinoma; lesions; malignancy; *specific types*
tungsten, target/filter combinations, 16, **17**

U

ultrasonography, *see* sonography
  abscesses, in mastitis, 200–1, **202**
  adolescent breast, 122–3, **124**
  beam, **84**
  benign disorders, 144, 149, **150**
  changes
    after augmentation, 312

after trauma and surgery, 287–91
cysts, 157, **158–60,** 160, **163**
diabetic mastopathy, **189,** 190
ductal carcinoma in situ, 218
equipment, 83
examination technique, 86–8
fibroadenoma, **172,** 173–4, **175,** 176, **176**
characteristic features, 173, **174**
filling in, cyst echoes, **159**
findings, interpreting, 88–91
fistulae, in mastitis, 200–1
granuloma, 203–4
guided localization, **117,** 117–18
hamartoma, 166–7
hematologic malignancies, 273, **274, 275**
hematoma, 288, **288**
hemorrhage, 287–8
and histology, invasive carcinoma, 254, 256
and hormone replacement therapy, 138
intramammary lymph nodes, 191–2, **192**
invasive carcinoma, 223, 249–56
advantages, **255**
appearance, **251, 252–3**
indications, 249
limitations, **255**
inverted nipple, 134, **135**
involution, 130–1
lactation, 138
macromastia, 133
male breast, 327
mastitis, 198–9
metastases, 276, **277**
and microcalcifications, 372
needle biopsy, guided, 108–10, **109, 110**
normal mature breast, 126, **126–8,** 128
oil cysts, **289**
papilloma, 183, **184**
patient acceptance, 2
phyllodes tumor, 266–7, **267, 268**
polymastia, 134
post-therapeutic, 301–3, **302, 304**
pregnancy, 138
and reconstruction, 310
sarcomas, 270, **270**
scar formation, 289, **290,** 291
seroma, 288
skin thickening, 321
summary, 82
young patient, 397, 400
ultrasound, *see* sonography
Utrecht screening study, 332–3

V

Van Nuys classification, 211–12
vasovagal attacks
and percutaneous biopsy, 103
and preoperative localization, 112, 113
verruca, pathognomonic findings, 338
viewbox, 23
viewing conditions, 61
views
abbreviations, 44
additional, positioning, 43–4
axillary, 43, 46
cleavage, 43, 46, **48**
craniocaudal, 41–2, **42**
lateral, exaggerated, 44–6, **45**
medial, exaggerated, 46
lateromedial, **43**
mediolateral, **43**
mediolateral oblique, 39–41, **40**
90° lateral, **43,** 43–4
oblique, 46
rolled, 43, 48, **48**
standard, positioning, 39–43
tangential, 46, **47**
visual inspection, 7–8
V-shapes, microcalcifications, 373, 381

W

wax granulomas, 204, 205
Wegener granulomatosis, 203, **207**
witch's milk, 164

X

xeromammography, 67
X-ray tubes, 14
heel effect, 17–18, **18**
with microfocus, 372
see also radiation

Y

young patient
breast cancer, **398–9**
cancer risk, 392–3
diagnostic strategy, 401
differential diagnosis and work-up, 391–401
fibroadenoma, **395**
mammography, 395
MRI, 401
papillomatosis, juvenile, **394**
percutaneous biopsy, 400–1
sonography, 397, 400
Y-shapes, microcalcifications, 373, 381